MW. 2A 80

GW00697074

HANDBOOK OF PSYCHIATRY

HANDBOOK OF PSYCHIATRY

for social workers and health visitors

Charles Bagg,

M.A.(Cantab.), M.R.C.S., L.R.C.P., M.R.C. Psych., D.P.M.

Constable London

First published in Great Britain 1977
by Constable and Company Limited
10 Orange Street London WC2H 7EG
Copyright © 1977 Charles Bagg

Hardback ISBN 0 09 460180 1
Paperback SBN 0 09 461520 9

Set in Monotype Joanna
Printed in Great Britain by The Anchor Press Ltd
and bound by Wm Brendon & Son Ltd
both of Tiptree, Essex

To Cathy

The quality of the imagination is to flow and not to freeze

R. W. Emerson

Contents

Preface

After I had completed the manuscript of this book I gave it to a social worker colleague whose opinions I hold in high regard, with a request for any comments that might seem useful. The suggestion received was 'There are so many men in the profession these days that you can't keep referring to social workers as "she". You should use the term "they".'

I started to read through it again in an attempt to comply with her suggestion but it proved impracticable. Members of all professional groups, including social workers, psychologists, educational welfare officers, art therapists etc., therefore remain referred to as 'she', although most of these professions contain a large number—in some fields a preponderance—of male members. In leaving the manuscript unchanged I adopted the broad, if facetious, principle that 'she embraces he'. I myself doubt whether much male objection will be raised to this simplification of sexual references. Also for simplicity, I have in the main adopted the convention of referring to the client, patient or relative, whether adult or child, as 'he', except in particular circumstances such as in the chapters on childhood disturbances where the maternal role has been given the main emphasis in description.

The other criticism made by my colleague was that in some places the text tended to state the obvious or imply a vulnerability to the stresses of work that might seem almost denigratory to some readers. Again, while I valued the comment, it would have been impracticable to re-write the manuscript with this aspect in mind. Indeed, I am not convinced that it would have been wholly desirable to do so.

Like the members of all professions, social workers vary widely in their experience. On the whole those who are still

students will have had little background in dealing directly
with families with psychological problems. Similarly they will
have had comparatively little opportunity of accumulating
much psychiatric knowledge from theoretical studies in a
heavily loaded curriculum. Even quite elementary information
on the subject may therefore sometimes have its importance.

On the other hand, many workers with years of professional
practice behind them will have acquired a considerable
understanding of the psychiatric side of their work. This
understanding will have included not only a grasp of the
problems of their clients, but also an insight into the reactions
which this branch of work may produce in themselves and
how they may best cope with any such reactions. Some of the
material dealing with these aspects may therefore be found
unnecessary. But, here again, for the less experienced worker
it may provide some pointers that are much needed on occasions.

Social work presents a wide spectrum of interests. Psychological material in its deeper aspects is only one. Psychiatry
and its related casework do not appeal equally to everybody.
Not unnaturally, different areas of social work make differing
appeals to its various practitioners. Some workers rate most
highly their function of remedying their clients' social
circumstances—clients poorly housed, undernourished, or
intensely worried about finances tend to find cold comfort
from exclusively psychological help. Often these requirements
must claim, at least initially, a predominance of attention and
action. Other workers regard their casework function as being
of high importance—remedying material inadequacies will be
of little value to a client suffering, for example, from an
endogenous depression that causes him to believe himself
unworthy of anything better. To concentrate predominantly
on the machinery for giving help to a client to claim social
benefits may be to mishandle a situation in which an unrecognized but disabling preoccupation with less obvious
emotional problems has prevented him from taking the
necessary measures for attending to his own practical welfare.

It is this lack of uniformity in readers' outlook, experience
and knowledge that presents the difficulty to an author. I hope

that students still struggling to amass a general knowledge of the social sciences will not find that the study of these psychological aspects imposes too much additional strain, though for a time they may need to be selective in the areas on which they concentrate. I hope also that beginners in their earlier years of professional practice, who are as yet tentatively feeling their way into burdensome and perplexing situations, will not find the more extreme problems described here too daunting. It should be remembered that no single situation at any one time involves more than a small proportion of the many types of difficulty encountered over the course of a working lifetime.

To those seasoned workers who have already met many of these problems, who have acquired a knowledge of clients' difficulties and who have also long ago passed through the somewhat disturbing reactions that assail everyone to some extent during the earlier phases of working in the field, I apologize for the inclusion of the material that may be platitudinous in relation to their individual levels of experience. However, I hope there will be something that is of interest to most readers, and much that is of interest to some. The needs of both students and practitioners have received consideration.

Finally, the object is not to produce irrelevant involvement in 'amateur psychology' nor to encourage social workers to engage in unwarrantable interest in a client's psychological problems. With the great majority of clients requiring social work, no such problems exist and they should not be assumed. Nevertheless, in those situations in which they do exist, the social worker's role—if undertaken with professional enlightenment as well as human sympathy—can often supply a service whose beneficial influence will extend far beyond the needs of the particular clients or families for whom she is currently working.

C.B.

Acknowledgements

I would like to express my warm thanks to a number of colleagues for their very helpful suggestions and for having read through those parts of the manuscript which relate to their particular fields: Mr John Ayres, Headteacher, E.S.N.(M) School; Mr Graham Bowe, Hospital Administrator; Miss Jeannie Burlingham, Art Therapist; Mrs Hazel Creaser, Social Worker; Mr Tom Crookes, Clinical Psychologist; Miss Gillian Dobson, Child Psychotherapist; Sister Beryl Dugdale, Community Sister; Sister Brenda Enticknap, Day Hospital Sister; Miss Josephine Freeman, Educational Psychologist; Mrs Ann Gillings, Dietician; Mr David Haddock, Headteacher, E.S.N.(S) School; Mrs Jean Jukes, Social Worker; Mrs Anne Lambley, Occupational Therapist; Mrs Muriel Lloyd, Nursery School Headteacher; Mrs Margaret Oakley, Psychiatric Social Worker; Sister Audrey Pearce, Community Sister; Mrs Renata Whurr, Speech Therapist.

Although the responsibility for the book is my own, their discussions and comments have been invaluable. I would also like to thank Miss Elfreda Powell, Senior Editor, Constable & Company Limited, for her tolerance and encouragement when the manuscript failed to materialize on the date for which it was commissioned and for a considerable time thereafter.

In the home sphere I am extremely grateful to Cathy, my elder daughter, without whose assistance the task would have been impossible, for receiving the dictation and typing the manuscript with an invariably good grace; and last but not least to Diana, my wife, who repeatedly sheltered me from distractions and kept me fed, watered and comfortable.

Introduction

This book has been written in an attempt to meet the need of social workers and health visitors for a digest of the psychological and psychiatric aspects of their work—a need that is particularly urgent during the current era of rapid expansion of the functions of social service departments and the increasing involvement of health visitors in the psychological needs of their clients. It is intended to supplement, not in any way to replace, standard works already available on social work as a whole. However, it provides a particular slant—that of presenting the psychological aspects as observed through the eyes of a practising psychiatrist. It is concerned only with some of the aspects of psychiatry. Large areas of this field that are considered to be of only marginal relevance to the social worker receive no mention or are accorded merely passing reference.

For convenience of presentation, the term 'social worker' rather than 'social worker and health visitor' is used throughout. The latter phrase would be too cumbersome for constant repetition. However, it should be constantly remembered that all remarks are addressed equally to health visitors.

The book enters little into rarefied atmosphere. The domains of the sociologist, the biochemist, the neurophysiologist, are scarcely touched on. Specific research findings are not discussed. In its scope and its content it is essentially psychological and clinical. Nor is it conceived as a platform from which to campaign for or against current trends. It does not undertake to dissect administrative concepts or to unravel organizational tangles. It is assumed that the social worker already has the necessary knowledge of the administrative procedures by which help is obtained through standard social agencies, or at least that when required this knowledge will be obtained by reference to the relevant departments of the local authority or voluntary organizations. The institutions and systems which will be encountered by the social worker will naturally differ in detail from the composite descriptions necessarily presented in this book.

The material it presents, however, is based on the experience of continuous practice of psychiatry with adults and children and the teaching of its principles and methods in relation to the needs of the supportive workers in these fields. It aims to provide a distillation of the sort of psychological material about which such workers frequently express ignorance, and about which they ask frequent questions. They themselves are constantly on the receiving end of questions put to them by patients and clients. A patient may ask, for instance, exactly what lies before him when faced with a prospective stay in a mental hospital. A parent may feel uncertain as to how to handle the problems arising from an emotionally disturbed child's timidity or school failures. A mother may need guidance on how to handle her rejecting child after her return home from hospital.

Innumerable situations, infinitely variable, can pose problems to the social worker which she will find perplexing and disturbing unless guiding principles are readily to hand. In their absence the opportunity for giving certain types of service of crucial importance to clients and their families can be lost irretrievably. An attempt has been made to provide information that will nourish the social worker's efforts to meet this need.

This then is the *raison d'être* of the book. In so far as it may have succeeded in its aims the credit is due to those social workers and health visitors who over the years have taught me of their difficulties and needs. I am grateful for having learnt about them and for the thoughts they have stimulated. It is to be hoped that these thoughts and observations will now be passed on with advantage to other members of these and allied professions. If they obtain from these pages any of the interest and pleasure I have derived in writing them, the task will have been well worth while.

Part One

Emotional disturbances of childhood

Some common manifestations

The social worker has, and will always have, a fascinating job. In the past, the accent has been on specialization; in the present era, the role of the general social worker receives much of the emphasis; the future is a picture which nobody can see with much clarity. But however far the specialist services may be retained in, for instance, the mental hospitals and the child guidance clinics, the era of the generalist is here; and to a greater or lesser extent it seems here to stay.

The general practitioner of social work, like her counterpart in the general practice of medicine, must now cover a wide range of fields. Because of the great number of areas to be covered, none can be pursued at student stage at great length or in much depth. It is therefore sometimes said by the antagonists of this system that the psychological content must inevitably be so superficial as to make it impssioble for the social worker to bring enough understanding to any but the simplest type of situations involving psychological knowledge.

That this danger exists there can be no doubt. But on a more constructive level one may usefully accept this criticism of superficiality as reflecting a need for students and practising social workers to grasp as much specialized knowledge as possible through discussion with the specialists they encounter —psychiatrists, psychologists, educational welfare officers, remedial teachers and so on.

The crucial point for the social worker to remember is that discussions with these specialists are liable to prove relatively fruitless, uneconomical of the precious commodity of time, and even on occasions misleading, unless they are buttressed by enough prior knowledge to make them sufficiently meaningful. Asking questions may be of little value when the content of the enquiries has not first been thought out with care and formulated with lucidity. The questions may well be asked in a floundering unstructured nebulous form, evoking responses that will therefore have far less value than they might.

Precise formulations for the questions most usefully asked are not given in this book. Social workers must obviously use their own initiative when they set about this. The intention will in general be to enable social workers to pursue their own enquiries with a maximum of benefit to their knowledge and thinking and within a reasonable space of time, rather than awaiting a lifetime of experience during which understanding may dawn all too slowly. Nothing of course can replace experience; but it can be catalysed, or it can pass by with much of its significance making little impact, and even then only at the margins of awareness. The material discussed in this chapter, and indeed throughout the book, is designed to help towards the former of these two processes.

It is impossible to assign to any one field of work an importance supreme over the others, or to arrange a hierarchy of priorities for attention. The choice of relative values must necessarily be to some extent an arbitrary decision. However, amongst all the experience to which individuals are exposed, those occurring in childhood are often the most fundamental. For the social worker to become as familiar as possible with the work and nature of child guidance clinics is therefore one of the basic needs.

THE CONCEPT OF THE CHILD GUIDANCE CLINIC

That the child is father to the man is a paradox whose essential truth can be recognized on the instant. That by the same token the child is also grandfather and even great grandfather is, however, an extension to this adage that is seen less spontaneously.

Yet anyone perusing a moderate-sized batch of well-recorded casenotes in a busy child guidance clinic, which for reasons of confidentiality would in practice be available only to the professional workers in the clinic itself, would soon discover that this extension of the child's personal influence into more distant generations is more than a mere abstract conception. It is tangible reality.

Moreover, anyone who has worked in a clinic for long enough to have known the members of three generations of any family attending there—which in these days of early marriage and pregnancies need involve only a comparatively short span of years—will almost certainly have seen instances of the process in his personal experience. And this passage of emotional disturbance from one generation to the next can often be convincingly explained without any need for references to genetic factors—which may or may not coexist.

Genetic aspects of transmission are of little concern to the social worker. In spite of their obvious importance, in the majority of conditions relevant to child psychiatry they are as yet ill-defined and ill-understood. And sometimes the thoughts in this essentially scientific field are presented with a perplexing diversity of opinion, and with an obscurity that leaves the non-geneticist unclear. So far as present knowledge takes us, the main area of genetic application is in the field of mental subnormality. Some of the mechanisms that may be involved in the environmental forms of transmission, however, will be discussed later.

In the meanwhile a few words should be said about the child guidance clinics themselves. The child guidance movement was born in Chicago in the 1920s. In the intervening years its scope has increased enormously. Yet though changes have occurred, basic principles have remained. Variations on the basic theme there have been; but the theme itself, which consists of the provision of a comprehensive and expert understanding of traumatic factors, psychological reactions and methods of management, has remained based on the time-honoured principle of specialized teamwork that comprises a continuity of therapeutic relationship for both the family and the child himself.

This principle of teamwork and specialization will continue to be irreplaceable. Nevertheless, within this framework the passage of time has brought, and will rightly continue to bring, additional orientations of the clinic's work towards providing advisory functions for children's homes, hospital wards, schools for maladjusted children, ordinary schools and indeed any of the other establishments outside its own walls to which the continuing focus on the welfare of children will no doubt give birth in the future. Indeed, the extension of the work carried out within the clinics themselves has in some cases led to their adopting a more clearly expressive designation such as 'Family and Child Guidance Clinic'.

The personnel working in the child guidance clinic consists basically of the psychiatrist, the educational psychologist and the clinic social worker. Their individual functions will be discussed in chapter 3. In addition workers in other disciplines, such as child psychotherapists—who receive an intensive training which includes a personal psychoanalysis—and highly trained speech therapists and remedial teachers, can, when available, provide services of very great value for selected children.

In addition to the work carried out within the clinic itself, steps may also be undertaken there to initiate measures that operate outside its own immediate ambit—and these actions often comprise a fundamental part of its function. For instance, measures to obtain placements in special classes for educationally backward or emotionally disturbed children (chapter 5) on a daily basis while living at home, transfer to a boarding school for maladjusted children (chapter 5)—in which case the child may be seen during the school holidays—help over rehousing, or assistance for children or parents to acquire diversionary activities and supportive relationships outside the home, may all dovetail to form a therapeutic service which supports any value conferred specifically by the team members and may even provide a basis for progress when their own direct efforts with the child and family are proving ineffective. A 'pull here and a push there', mediated by the clinic and implemented in many external as well as internal directions, will often diminish isolation, produce realignments of relationships, and restore the capacity for normal feelings and functioning.

SOME MANIFESTATIONS OF EMOTIONAL INSECURITY
AND THEIR CAUSES

It is obvious that the manifestations of childhood insecurity often embody features that are also found in normal children. The question is therefore sometimes asked as to how states of normality and morbidity can be distinguished one from the other. Such a question is understandable; but in practice this problem is often less perplexing than might be thought. Intermittently all children present in minor degree some of those disturbances which when occurring in more florid form characterize the symptoms encountered in child guidance work. But differentiation between the normal and abnormal, by reference to the degree or persistence of features, is not usually difficult.

For example, crying on occasions is obviously normal; frequently recurring, excessive and bitter tears, perhaps associated with insatiable demands for consolation, are clearly pathological. Similarly, patches of difficulty over certain subjects at school are so common as to be of little significance. On the other hand, continuous failure to concentrate and severe mental underfunctioning in spite of indications of average intelligence call for a search for underlying areas of insecurity. Often they may be found lying buried beneath an outward show of academic indifference or even an attitude of calculated recalcitrance.

This same diagnostic principle of differentiation by the degree of severity ranges over most of the childhood attributes. And it relates to the social virtues as well as the vices. Quietness and compliant behaviour when they are relevant are not only socially desirable but also psychologically healthy. In excess, however, they may reveal to the discerning eye a state whose pathological quality is at least as significant as that which is betokened by an undue inclination to aggression. Indeed, morbid compliance may at times conceal this very attribute. A child can be too good to be healthy. It is the excessive degree of an attribute, or its exceptionally long duration, that may furnish pointers to the existence of psychopathology.

There are many other features which, if evoked with undue readiness, are unduly intense or persistent, or occur at an inappropriate age, may comprise pointers to insecurity. They need not be enumerated exhaustively. But severe backwardness at school, delinquency in any of its forms, bedwetting and soiling, inordinate general timidity or specific phobic anxieties, severe sleep disturbances, outstandingly intense sibling jealousies, excessive dreaminess, attention-craving, thumb-sucking, nail-biting, and many other major or minor deviations from the norm of any age group may all validly suggest states of insecurity whose origins require elucidation.

On the whole, symptoms in child psychiatry do not occur as narrowly specific responses to correspondingly specific causes. The same causes of insecurity may produce a variety of symptoms by which they are manifested. Likewise, the same symptoms may arise from a variety of causes—aggressiveness, for example, may derive from sources as various as disturbing changes of environment or an intrinsic lack of intelligence—though it is obvious that all causal factors will have as their common denominator the property of making for emotional insecurity.

FORMS OF EDUCATIONAL BACKWARDNESS

A few symptoms nevertheless arise more directly from situations connected with themselves. Backwardness in a particular school subject is a common example of a specific difficulty that can sometimes arise from particular types of circumstances, in the presence of normal or even superior general intelligence. Reading and spelling problems may fall into this category, and it will be worth our giving some passing consideration to the possible origins of these two particular learning problems.

Firstly, neurophysiological defects may lie at the root of these educational difficulties. In chapter 13 'word blindness', or as it has sometimes been termed 'dyslexia', is discussed in connection with the condition termed sensory aphasia. The essence of extreme word blindness is that written words have no meaning. Just as in extreme word deafness words sound like a foreign language, so in extreme word blindness written words may convey little more meaning than undifferentiated squiggles. It is thought that the difficulty may occur in children as a congenital condition. Unfortunately minor degrees of the anomaly are liable to be overlooked, their presence remaining obscured beneath the superstructure of emotional reactions and other symptoms to which they have given rise. Only psychometric testing will then reveal them.

Naturally the child suffering from congenital word blindness, while able to see without any visual impairment—he does not need glasses—has great difficulty in learning the symbols of the alphabet. Thus he will inevitably develop problems over learning to read, write and spell in spite of normal intelligence. Unless this condition is suspected and, when confirmed by psychometric tests for perceptual anomalies, is then dealt with by means of special educational techniques and a skilled management of its attendant psychological difficulties, the child will be destined for a life that is crippled and unfulfilled.

Primary difficulties in the emotional sphere, however, in contrast to those of a primarily neurophysiological nature, may constitute the sole factors leading to the learning blocks that include reading, writing and spelling backwardness. Indeed in severe cases ineptitudes in the various scholastic subjects that arise on an emotional basis may eventually prove as disastrous to educational progress, as great a challenge to techniques of remedy, and as much in need of patient skill and management, as those which arise from physically based anomalies of perception.

Purely emotional blocks to the learning of particular subjects —whether due to aversion to a particular teacher at an early point, loss of schooling at a stage vital to the further understanding of the subject-matter, or failure of concentration as a result of emotional problems of any sort—may, when once started, soon prove very difficult to reverse. They are best dealt with by the application of skilled understanding early in the 'blocking' process. The part played by emotional factors in the impairment of language development and verbal facility is looked at in chapter 5.

DELINQUENCY

We have now taken a look at a particular problem, namely some of the areas of educational backwardness that may arise from either physical or emotional causes. Before proceeding to consider further causes of insecurity, a few other symptoms commonly found particularly distressing may be usefully looked at. And amongst all the situations that may point to the fact that a child is emotionally disturbed, there is one about which the social worker is usually approached with the greatest pleas of urgency, and often with the most frantic requests for advice and help.

This sympton, as any reader already engaged in the practice of social work may have guessed, is delinquent behaviour. Not unnaturally, the anxieties generated in parents by this discovery are usually greatest when the delinquent acts have taken place outside the home. But there are also circumstances in which their occurrence within the family may act as the fuse to serious distress and turbulence there, or may intensify any such emotions that already exist within the home setting.

Every social worker, therefore, whether or not her work is carried out in a child guidance clinic, needs clear-cut thoughts on some of the possible origins of delinquency.

Delinquency, or at any rate indictable and officially recorded delinquency, has been rising fluctuatingly over the years and much thought has been given to its possible causes. For convenience they may be viewed under two headings. There are the sociological factors, and there are those disturbances of interpersonal relationships within the family that are comparatively unrelated to the more general climate of society as a whole. Clearly, however, these two groups overlap.

The sociological factors blamed for rising delinquency are diverse and often frankly speculative. The suggested possibilities range through the greater amount of money available to young people, the influence of the mass media, the absence of compulsory military service, the increased accent on academic values amongst the population as a whole, the widening of the gap between adolescents and their parents, unemployment, boredom, the younger age of marriage, problems of housing, increased employment of women outside the home and shifts of population. This list is of course by no means comprehensive.

Each sociological factor will have its relevance to some situations; no single factor will apply to all; and during the course of their careers social workers will often observe circumstances of delinquency in which one of these factors is clearly operative but where its particular influence, having in ignorance been regarded as basic, is in fact very far from being the basic cause in spite of the obtrusive quality of its presence.

Money, proverbially described as the root of all evil, may certainly lie at the roots, or at least within the soil, of some delinquent behaviour. For example, with increased money in the possession of the age group at greatest risk of delinquent development it is obvious that not only pop records but also drugs and motor scooters for gang activities will become more freely available.

Obviously too the presentation of violence and crime by the mass media of entertainment must sometimes imply to the simple-minded, if only tacitly, that these activities render their participants worthy of special interest and capable of obtaining a welcome exhilaration from their criminal exploits—and may even lead to a crude copying of the exploits enacted. In addition, the deification of personal possessions, again implicit in the constant mass media advertisements, is likely to generate in those people unduly influenced in this direction the philosophy that material possessions are of such paramount importance that the means of their acquisition become relatively unimportant. Naturally these considerations do not argue against the overall importance of material standards and security. But they highlight some potential side-effects. An over-acquisitive society may clearly bring itself its own problems.

Whether or not the loss of the opportunity for vicarious release of aggression (sometimes assumed to have been associated with peace-time military service) can be regarded as playing a part in the rise of violence is more speculative, though it is sometimes advanced as an explanation of the increase of violence amongst the age group concerned. A more cogent factor in this age group would appear to be the jealousy felt by those of the older generation who are sometimes inclined to resent the fact that their children's generation appears more fortunately placed than they were in their own youth.

On balance such feelings of jealousy are not usually justified. The loss of the former clear-cut boundaries can bring traumatic uncertainties as well as advantages. Nevertheless when adult resentment exists, it will clearly widen the natural psychological gap between the generations and tend to push the younger person into a limbo of indeterminate identity and a disconcerting sense of isolation. To weld themselves together into groups, sometimes set on delinquent retaliation, is an understandable response.

The emphasis on academic achievement may also produce its side-effects. Nobody could reasonably dispute the value of education and the psychological need of the individual to receive it to the full extent of his capacity. There is no doubt, however, that this good general principle throws up its casualties. Every child guidance clinic sees cases in which a young adolescent of essentially non-academic turn of mind remains at school denigrated, resentful, bored, incarcerated in a situation redolent with potentialities for delinquent development and totally unrelieved by any compensating advantages. And even before this age is reached, the scholastic race takes an undoubted toll on those less academically able but intrinsically worthy and admirable children who become the victims of miserable and unjustified self-contempt and on occasions franky antisocial reactions.

Sometimes, then it is social factors that appear to have exerted the most influential weight in producing delinquent reactions. But not uncommonly these sociological aspects are subsidiary to, or heavily supplemented by, disturbing effects in the more intimate and fundamental area of relationships within the family or the substitute family.

The constitutional make up of the child may also play its part. There are reasons for suspecting that in some cases genetic factors, and at other times non-genetic factors within the womb, may have rendered the person prone to delinquency.

Genetic factors have been regarded by some research workers as sometimes relevant in those rare cases of abnormality in which a combination of XYY sex chromosomes is found in the genetic makeup. The normal female sex chromosomes are XX and those of normal males are XY, these letters being used because the shapes of the chromosomes bear a vague resemblance to them. Some research workers believe that in maximum security prisons there is an unusually high number of individuals with XYY makeup, this chromosomal abnormality being due to genetic changes termed mutations.

Much of this, however, is a relatively vague and uncharted area, though it can be predicted that further evidence for chromosomal abnormalities associated with criminal tendencies may come to light with more research into the genetic aspects of psychiatry. And, with the passage of time, brain damage may also become indictable, with a greater degree of clarity than exists at present, as a basic cause of the perverted conduct in certain individuals with delinquent propensities. Again, however, at the moment such physical explanations are often so indeterminate that they are sometimes embraced or rejected almost according to taste. Even poor intelligence, which is a state widely believed to be often genetically or antenatally determined, and whose contribution to antisocial conduct is well recognized and common, is far from clearly understood in its hereditary aspects.

Notwithstanding our ignorance of hereditary transmission of attitudes of mind, low intelligence is frequently, though not of course invariably, found unequivocally amongst perpetrators of antisocial behaviour. In these people the ability to understand abstract concepts may be largely absent, or seriously curtailed. Only tangible and concrete facts can be clearly grasped. Abstractions such as honesty and virtue, which of necessity are presented by verbal communication and grasped through verbal understanding, are likely to be beyond precise and easy understanding by some dullards. And the need for compensatory self-aggrandisement, the feelings of resentment against the world for its frequently shown contempt for their innate deprivations, and the inability to communicate their emotions by the more subtle and delicate means open to the

H.O.P.—B

person of normal intelligence, may palpably lead to reactions of defence by delinquency. Relatively crude and primitive instincts may be the only real weapons they possess. At the same time the power of imagination which enables those of normal intelligence to identify in detail with their victims, and which is therefore necessary for sympathetic involvement with other people, may be poorly developed.

Nevertheless, we do well to remember here that the large majority of dull people are of course kindly and entirely law-abiding.

Even in delinquent children of normal or above-average intelligence, however, the nature of the morbidly-engendered insecurity and aggression that rank so highly in their various motivations is not usually clear to themselves. This is not surprising, since the full motivations are often not perceived even by onlookers, whose reactions, although partly dictated by their own emotional involvement, should at least be less distorted than those of the perpetrators of the offences. If supposedly objective adults cannot see the reasons clearly, either because of their own emotions or as a result of an un-tutored ignorance of the mechanisms involved, then the emotionally-disturbed child himself is hardly likely to do so. The child at a clinic or with a probation officer who answers 'don't know' when asked the reason for his stealing is often telling the truth.

Some of the possible causes of insecurity have already been stated and others will be dealt with later. At the present point, however, it is axiomatic that an abnormal degree of aggression will often exist within many states of insecurity. Even when its presence is not found in other directions, it is still often exercised in restricted forms towards the people to whom it primarily relates. A simple example is seen in the child who in his manner reveals little conventional evidence of hostility towards his parents, but who steals money directly from the home. On the other hand these hostile emotions may become projected on to inappropriate people and situations. Hence by 'projection of affect' (chapter 2) the antisocial behaviour may express itself elsewhere—at school, for example, or in the community in general, and vice versa.

Motivations to delinquency other than aggression also abound amongst insecure children. Of these, attention-craving is one of the commonest; and even though children have received a heavy surfeit of attention they may still experience this craving if it has not been of the sort required to fulfil their psychological needs. Thus subtle factors like resentment against the stifling effects of a morbidly over-possessive parent may introduce a reaction more complex than that which is associated with the more easily recognized 'spoiling' in the ordinary sense. In these cases of morbid over-protectiveness, delinquent behaviour compounded both of attention-craving and aggressive response is a common finding.

A concept widely held amongst child psychiatrists is that of 'testing out'. Some cases of 'naughty behaviour', and indeed of frank delinquency, appear to contain this element of 'testing out'. In this concept it is postulated that if a child is unsure about the depth of the love on which he can rely, he may engage in unattractive behaviour in order to prove to himself that, contrary to his fear, he is acceptable in all circumstances. The child himself, and unfortunately often the adult also, is unaware of this motivation. In these circumstances, while it may be recognized by the adults that he is clearly 'trying it on', the fact that he is prompted by this particular emotional need, and not by pure love of battle of wills, may well have escaped notice.

While the contents of the child's acts must be conveyed to him as deserving of disapproval in themselves, the importance of convincing him at the same time that he is loved and accepted as a person, however bad his behaviour, is the logical and necessary corollary to this concept. If he fails to receive the comfort of this reassurance, the internal provocation to persist in the exploratory antisocial behaviour will naturally remain. And experience shows that if uneradicated by means related to its origins it is all too likely to become reinforced by habituation. In this group of cases, if the child's anxiety about his basic acceptability can be relieved, then the undesirable stimulus and its antisocial response will sometimes subside quite rapidly. Nevertheless, more often the insecurity is too ingrained for rapid or complete abolition, and an immediate improvement may not occur, or a relapse may take place. The parents will need to anticipate this likelihood and persist, possibly for a prolonged period, without discouragement.

A child guidance clinic is often able to help parents directly in these efforts, by removing their discouragement through disclosing to them the child's own feelings found at the clinic. It is surprising how often a child at home seems to have made it repeatedly clear to his family beyond all doubt that he does not care what they feel about him, while at the clinic he provides glaring evidence, quite often by direct statement, that in point of fact he cares very much. Great comfort can be given on this basis to discouraged parents; and secondary benefits can thus be conferred on the child, with recession of his symptoms of insecurity as a result of the parents' reorientation of outlook and management. By presenting parents with this slightly deeper psychological perception, not previously available, the mutually-reinforcing misunderstandings may dissolve.

Certain other subtleties that play their part in motivations to delinquency may repay mention. Material possessions symbolize security. They may therefore be sought as substitutes for the values of secure relationships when these cannot be obtained naturally. A previously law-abiding but immature young man stole a car, probably in the main on this basis, after his wife had left him. The acquisition of money, or indeed of any other form of status symbol for which the individual so motivated has pushed himself perhaps to the outer limits of endurance or beyond, may in some cases spring from an attempt, foredoomed to failure, to achieve compensatory comfort for love that is unobtainable or which is thought, sometimes erroneously, to be sparse or absent.

It occasionally happens that a child by direct statement puts forward as the motivation for his delinquent conduct that he has been impelled by his wish to be removed from home, knowing that detection may lead to transfer to a foster home, a local authority children's home, a boarding school for maladjusted children, or even to an approved school (nowadays termed a Community Home). This motivation is unusual but it appears to exist rather more frequently than is often supposed, though like the others it commonly lies outside the child's clear understanding. It is likely to occur most often amongst children of problem families who have become aware of the possibility through a history of removal of their own siblings, or as a result of witnessing this destiny amongst other children of their acquaintance. It should always be suspected when the child has made little effort to obscure his offence, though of course the wish to be caught may well carry other implications, such as the craving of attention or the seeking of help along lines apart from removal.

In concluding this brief sketch of a few of the causes of delinquency there is a final aspect that must be given its due emphasis. The processes leading to diversion into delinquent behaviour do not always consist of adverse factors within the family, or even problems related to sociological evils. There is the child, for example, who is sensitive by constitutional makeup rather than insecure through environmental background. It is natural that the introverted child whose temperament precludes smooth and spontaneous relationships may sometimes find that the only, or at least the easiest, portal of entry to his peer groups is through ingratiating himself by joining their gang activities.

This child may, but not necessarily, possess an intelligence of above average level, which has itself imposed a barrier against group acceptance. He may then crave for a social life other than that arising from intellectual pursuits, which indeed he may have vaguely come to regard as the weakness of eccentrics. In these circumstances he may offer his ability for use by the gang. And such a child may, though again not necessarily, show an exemplary record of scholastic achievement and general cooperation, both at school and at home.

An inept management of this situation may then direct him along a road of antisocial progression from which he might well have been deflected by timely understanding of his problems. The child who steals to buy popularity through distributing his bounty often falls into the same general category of craving for admission to the group which he cannot enter unaided. And of course any of the various causes of emotional insecurity discussed in later chapters sometimes become transmuted into delinquency in this and other ways. Both immediate and root causes always need thought and sometimes action.

Sometimes a particular form of delinquency, once started, sets the tone for different examples of delinquent behaviour in other directions. Thus a child who has deceitfully truanted from a particular lesson which he believes he cannot cope with may start to lie about matters with no direct relation to this particular circumstance, probably unconsciously influenced not so much by the views of others as by the low regard in which he has now come to hold himself. At the most basic level he feels that morally he has nothing to lose.

Punishment may deter or assuage his guilt-feelings by engendering a comfortable sense of redressed balance and thus a beneficial feeling of restoration to the ranks of group normality; but it may also simply reinforce his sense of belonging to an antisocial subculture, to which he may then come to regard himself as being still more deservedly affiliated. In consequence he can develop feelings of resentment that foster further delinquency, with a resulting sense of delinquent camaraderie which offers him its own perverted comfort.

Dogmatic statements cannot be made. Nevertheless the principle of attempting to restore self-regard and avoiding punitive reactions frequently intended to deter, but which are often destined more to belittle, clearly merits high priority when evaluating the pros and cons of the various alternatives contemplated for attempts at correction. Cool logic, rather than responses based on anxiety, status consciousness or vindictiveness, is the paramount need. The social worker may be well placed to provide some tactful and insightful guidance along these lines when the accent would otherwise fall on the irrational and retaliatory emotions of exasperation that too often aggravate an already difficult situation.

Serious lying and stealing are particularly apt to arise as reactions to feelings of insecurity that are deeply based. Constant marital discord, for instance, with its disorderly emotions, wounding disregard of the other partner's feelings, and its chaotic reactions of ill-considered reprisals may sometimes instil into a child such a lack of belief in the existence of fundamental order and individual rights that a failure to assimilate a basic and solid sense of moral order is hardly surprising, even when formal moral training and specific exhortation to honesty have been conscientiously given. Lying and stealing are sometimes grounded in fundamental emotional insecurity stronger than the value of moral training.

Most people with commonsense and without any special taste for psychological interpretations would accept all these concepts as basically applicable on occasions. And it is only a short cry, and not an essentially irrational one, from recognizing their existence to relating them to some of the torrential force which a child's need to receive and observe reliable love, and his disturbing reactions against its apparent absence, will generate. Given that these ideas of the origins of delinquency are worthy of belief and relevant at times, which to most people would seem a reasonable assumption, then the logic of a comparably basic approach on apt occasions to the ensuing offences in terms of these causal factors involves no essential discrepancy. Applied early enough—even if the causal factors have been prolonged but are still not too heavily weighted— it is a matter of experience in child guidance practice that an approach based on these perceptions often proves effective when other approaches, such as punitive methods, have been persistently tried and found persistently ineffective or even deleterious.

SCHOOL REFUSAL

Only two other manifestations of insecurity will be mentioned. Each merits particular consideration since, like delinquency, it is very apt to form a source of distress that is exceptionally disturbing, leading to urgent demands for the social worker's help or advice. The first is school aversion that overwhelms the child; the second is wetting and soiling.

Severe school aversion can be potentially very serious, for in child guidance practice a child's incapacity to face school without intense anxiety has all too often led to a total inability, and consequently a blatant refusal, to do so. This seemingly stubborn refusal to cooperate often masks to a greater or lesser extent the extreme anxiety lying beneath it. Such a degree of aversion, when it appears to have affinities with the phobic features described in connection with psychoneurosis in chapter 9, is sometimes termed school phobia. It is a situation that not only plagues the child and the family, but also presents to various fields of officialdom—the school, the education department of the local authority, and even potentially the courts—problems that perplex, frustrate, sadden and on occasions anger.

School aversion severe enough to constitute a pathological state has become a moderately common problem at every child guidance clinic, and it has been the subject of much detailed study and published material. Its origins have been explored; successes and failures in its management have been recorded; concepts about its nature have been propounded. But one aspect stands out sharply as an important factor common to a large number of these cases. It is that if once the child ceases to attend school totally for an uninterrupted period of a few weeks, the prospect of achieving success declines very sharply, and a level is soon reached at which the aversion is so entrenched that his refusal to return has become an irreversible state. Threats, bribes, imploring, may all be greeted with the same negative response. The child's anxieties mount, his determination to resist continues to harden, and its particular manifestations—perhaps psychosomatic symptoms such as vomiting or abdominal pain, withdrawal, a defensive air of nonchalance—become correspondingly pronounced.

At any point along this course the social worker may be approached by parents desperately requesting practical help for arrangements over special transport facilities, for intercession with the school, for the further weight of her authority to be brought to bear against the child in support of their own unsuccessful attempts and those of the educational welfare officer, or simply for a sympathetic and understanding person on to whom they can pour out these problems.

A period of erratic attendances commonly precedes the complete breakdown. Prevention of the symptom itself at this point is likely to be better than cure; but it must be remembered that the general family setting within which the problem has arisen will also require immediate psychological review in its own right. And, if the child guidance clinic considers that the child should be kept at school, the social worker may usefully exert her influence to ensure that he does not succeed in remaining away as a continuous pattern of reaction to his anxieties, while at the same time supporting the family in their doubts and uncertainties.

To adopt this function towards a manifestly anxious child may demand a robustness of attitude not always within the easy reach of a social worker witnessing the child's distress and sometimes mixed motives in the family. The pull of her own sympathy together perhaps with some fear of recrimination from parents, who while asking for her assistance may nevertheless be clearly ambivalent and even hostile in their ideas about how it should be exercised, may combine to discourage her from throwing her weight on to the right side of the scales at the crucial point.

She may be helped to stiffen her resolve by recognizing that distressing situations are to be anticipated in any eventuality, and that their development need not cause her automatic self-accusation. Moreover it is open to her to discuss the progress with the child guidance clinic if she so wishes—and if she is wise she will do so without hesitation. When the child guidance clinic has entered the picture, its techniques of management will usually not differ basically from those adopted in relation to many of the other features of insecurity that give grounds for clinic involvement. But frequently in these particular cases evidence will emerge of a child having undue emotional dependence on his mother, and sometimes of having severe and irrational anxieties concerning her welfare combined with complex feelings which include a clinging dominance over her that may be more clearly apparent when they are seen together.

The general methods of psychological management and advice adopted by the child guidance clinic will vary according to the nature and causes of the situation; and no doubt they will undergo refinement as further observations accumulate. As always, the child's condition cannot be considered in isolation from the emotional problem of the family as a whole. Sometimes a group of one sort of another will form the central

therapeutic pivot. At other times any psychotherapeutic success
may revolve around individual interviews. Some of the relevant principles that apply both to individual and group
approaches to therapy will be looked at in chapters 2, 3 and 5.

Certain measures more specific to this condition will also
be required. The immediate processes of attempting to persuade the child to return to school are on the whole best
undertaken by an educational welfare officer, since the air of
firmness so often required is likely to be more easily available
within the ambit of the functions of an educational welfare
officer than those of a social worker. Nevertheless on occasions,
perhaps because of the personal predilections of an individual
child or his potentially more compliant responsiveness to someone without formal associations with the school, the services
of a social worker may be preferable.

Failures are common. If the child remains continuously
within the home, the situation will become redolent with
adverse emotions. Unless steps are taken at least to dilute these
problems he will often be left continuously imbibing anxieties
from within the family, battening on the sometimes morbid
sympathies of the other members while at the same time
generating reactions of resentment amongst them, reciprocat-
ing and intensifying their feelings of resentment by reacting
with his own counter-hostility, and progressively committing
himself to an attitude of refusal to cooperate with anyone in
the home which he will find more and more difficult to
relinquish, partly through fear of loss of face. Inevitably he
will develop a growing sense of unworthiness mingled with a
morbid taste for power which nevertheless frightens him. And
he sometimes gradually withdraws from contact with the
children of his own age group in his area.

It is clear therefore that any suitable diversionary activities
available outside the home are urgently needed. The social
worker may be of great help in seeking them and persuading
him to attend. For those children whose psychological difficulties stand to gain from the sort of class for emotionally
disturbed children described in chapter 5, a system of attendance there for one or more sesssions each week is sometimes
practicable if recommended by the psychiatrist and agreed by

the teacher of the class. The object there is to provide psychological rather than educational help. And it will be realized that, in suitable cases, some at least of the circumstances needed for children with these problems will be obtainable in a special class of this nature. Those children with difficulties in relating to peer groups, and those in need of management in an atmosphere that is free from adverse anxiety and which they cannot manipulate—two of the factors most commonly required—form obvious examples of types of school refusers likely to benefit in this sort of setting.

FAULTY ELIMINATION

The final symptom that will be discussed in this chapter is faulty elimination of excreta.

In this group of problems are to be found bedwetting, daytime wetting, constipation and soiling. Wetting is termed enuresis, and the technical term for soiling is encopresis. Each is apt to evoke emotions of revulsion and shame within the child and the parents, resulting in defensive reactions in both generations which unfortunately often contribute more harm than relief to an already unhappy situation.

Sometimes these features merely represent a delay in physiological development frequently on a familial basis—a parent having had similar difficulty in childhood. Occasionally, however, they are manifestations of physical abnormality. If they persist, therefore, they should be drawn to medical attention. When on the other hand they occur as psychosomatic phenomena—whether as direct physiological responses to sheer anxiety or as physical features of regression to earlier levels of development, or include a large element of purposively-motivated symptoms such as aggression or attention-seeking whose purpose is not within the child's awareness—they are amongst the most troublesome of the childhood features that can arise on a psychosomatic basis. And if prolonged and mismanaged they can be highly destructive of the healthy self-image that is so necessary for a child's sound emotional development.

Sometimes they occur together, but the soiling may be concealed from the social worker by the parent, or indeed by the child, for fear that the family will be regarded as slummy or sluttish. Tactful introduction of the fact that weakness of control in one system is sometimes linked with weakness of control in the other, unrelated to the presence or absence of ordinary social cleanliness, may reassure the parents and open the way to comforting disclosure and then to maintaining a therapeutic support over the symptom as well as providing the benefit of the relationship for unburdening anxieties in general. If necessary the social worker should ask directly whether both symptoms are present.

Whether the wetting occurs by day or by night, whether the urinary symptom is frequency of micturition or incontinence of urine, and whether the abnormality of bowel function consists of constipation or soiling or alternations of both, once again the management is basically directed towards evaluation and resolution of the causal problems.

In addition to her work within this general context of psychological management, the social worker should be aware of certain special measures that may also be required in individual cases. Some of these measures can only be instituted on medical recommendation. Nevertheless when the recommendations have been made she can be of considerable help in encouraging parents and children to persevere with them. And if she is prepared to familiarize herself with the necessary details she may also give practical supervision and assistance. Discussion between the social worker, the health visitor and the medical staff may be necessary to pave the way for a well informed and well organized regime of management.

These special measures will vary. Sometimes the only recommendation is for restriction of fluid intake; at other times medicines or tablets may be prescribed as a temporary measure, including laxatives or drugs designed to lighten sleep; in some instances a system of bowel or bladder training will be advised; and for enuresis the use of an 'alarm system' in selected cases may be felt appropriate.

The decision as to whether the alarm system should be prescribed or withheld includes considerations based on broad principles that are used throughout the whole of medicine. The social worker will already have realized that in psychiatry, as in medicine as a whole, those responsible for the treatment of any sufferer, from whatever condition he may be suffering, are liable to face the problem of whether the case predominantly calls for treatment of the symptom, or attempts to remove the basic causes. And if the former of these approaches is indicated, then the problem is for how long and on what criteria should the symptomatic treatment alone be continued before the regime should be extended or altered fundamentally.

In general medicine, if the warning discomfort caused by a gastric ulcer is merely suppressed by medicines there is the possibility that a continuing and increasing process of ulceration may bring serious consequences. In psychiatry, the elimination of hysterical symptoms that are serving a protective purpose, without complementary action to deal with the causal factors that exist within the individual or to remove the environmental stresses provoking his reaction, will often prove ineffective at best. The isolated removal of the 'prop' by which the patient is unknowingly seeking some form of gain is liable to be followed by substitute symptoms designed for the same purpose. Similarly, even if a symptom is a direct outcome of anxiety, and does not contain any element of protective motivation, still any attempts at removing it without reference to the underlying factors provoking the anxiety —though perhaps destined for success within the symptom's own restricted area of operation—often prove of only limited assistance to the totality of the maladjustment.

Yet though consideration of basic needs must be given to every case when the best type of management is being assessed, the fact remains that not every symptom necessarily falls into the category in which the eradication of fundamental causes is the paramount need. Vulnerability that is innate, for example, cannot be eradicated. External stresses may likewise defy all efforts at removal or even modification. But the symptom itself adds its own distress, often without conferring satisfactory advantage and goes on to produce its own secondary problems.

In spite of the intractability of underlying factors, therefore, any facility that exists for removing such a symptom may well need to be utilized. The fact that the treatment is merely on a symptomatic level does not detract from its need in these cases. Evaluation is thus a broadly based clinical matter that will not rest with the social worker in the first instance. It must be based on medical advice. When the clinical decision has been made, however, she will often have a great deal to offer towards success in implementing it.

These concepts can now be applied to the problem of enuresis. On their basis, a decision may sometimes be made that a particular case of enuresis is one that falls into the category in which the treatment should be most heavily directed towards the symptom itself—only accompanied by as little or as much attention to other aspects as is merited by the individual circumstances.

There is a particular form of inborn vulnerability that often comprises a possible indication for the use of the technique of treatment, already referred to, termed the 'alarm system', also known as the 'buzzer'. This form of vulnerability consists not of proneness to psychological weakness but a constitutional tendency towards delay in the acquisition of bladder control. It is the type of enuresis in which this liability to occur as a constitutional physiological tendency may be revealed by parents' admissions that they themselves were afflicted by this particular problem in childhood. Enuresis of different origins too may sometimes be judged as open to benefit by this treatment, after its advantages and disadvantages have been carefully weighed. And such cases are of fairly frequent occurrence.

The broad principles of the buzzer and the details of its use should therefore be known to the social worker. The former are founded on the concept of Pavlovian conditioning which is described in chapter 8 and will not be repeated at this point. The essence of the aim is to establish habituation—or conditioning—into the successful achievement of dry nights, and to consolidate any success as a conditioned pattern. Very briefly, the apparatus consists of a bell or rattle which is powered by an electric circuit run off a battery. Two metal foils are placed in the bed and connected to the circuit. When urine, which is a conductor of electricity, is passed into the bed it closes the electric circuit and the buzzer becomes activated, awakening the child, who gets up and after emptying his bladder returns to a comfortably dry bed, the mother having in the meanwhile reassured the child that a useful means of help has been started, and having also changed the wet sheet. Eventually, if the treatment is successful, the child starts to wake up by his bladder signal alone without requiring any stimulus by means of apparatus.

The suggestion has been put forward, with fair likelihood of validity in relation to their poor capacity for control of their bedwetting tendencies, that some of these children have a less than average capacity for conditioning. The treatment rests in part on this basis of theory, as well as on the practical successes that it often, though by no means invariably, obtains in practice. And if the reader now turns to the Pavlovian experiment described in chapter 8, in which the experimental subjects ultimately respond in the absence of the unconditioned stimulus—a reflex action that has become a conditioned response—it will be appreciated that the end-point at which the child eventually wakes up in response to the bladder signal alone points to a fundamental physiological relationship between the two situations. The treatment is fundamentally based on the acquisition of conditioned reflex response.

Parents will not always be capable of carrying out the practical steps without guidance and encouragement. They may need the social worker's help. A mother may be unable to summon up the necessary hope, too discouraged by the repeated failures that have greeted all previous attempts by discipline, exhortation or bribery. She may have reached a stage at which suppressed anger and resentment about all the labours of sheet-changing and washing have undermined even her wish to help the child. Her concentration may be impaired by depression, or she may basically lack the intelligence to grasp and carry out the practical details.

The social worker should therefore take full care to read the instructions supplied with the apparatus and if necessary discuss its operation with those more experienced in its use. She should if possible become familiar with the details for setting up the apparatus in the bed, the need for a second dry set of foils and sheets during the night, the testing of the battery, the reasons for occasional failure of the rattle, the care of the foils, the need for the parent to encourage the child during the night at least initially, and so on. And, as with all the techniques with which she is concerned, it will always be her practical experience which, in the final analysis, will prove the most valuable and indeed an indispensable element in her work.

AUTISM
Finally, a condition which although very uncommon has nevertheless more and more come to be recognized as an individual entity and has received increasing and intensive study, is the state referred to as autism. Its essential nature, management and outcome remain so speculative that all that can be usefully said in the present context is that the main characteristic is in general a striking state of withdrawal from relationships, from ordinary activities and from interest in the environment. The child develops an impenetrably abstracted manner and a gross inaccessibility to conversational and other forms of approach, all of these features being different both in quality and degree from those seen in children whose withdrawal is a psychoneurotic defence mechanism against emotional insecurity. Experience is needed for recognition of this distinction in practice.

Within the withdrawn condition other phenomena may sometimes be seen. An obsessive type of preoccupation with objects or parts of the body, the intermittent emergence of areas of intelligence within the matrix of the child's apparently gross incomprehension of the environment, and even behaviour suggestive of hallucinatory experiences are amongst the features recorded. Its causes are ill-understood, and it is variously and nebulously ascribed to physical factors, influences in the environment, or a mixture of each.

Recognition can be particularly difficult when there is a history of severe psychological trauma or of hearing impairment. Any contributory influences from the environment can be hard to evaluate, while the assessment of hearing loss in a child showing withdrawal severe enough to raise the suspicion of autism may well prove insuperable. An incorrect diagnosis of mental subnormality may be made by those who were unfamiliar with his condition before the onset of the illness, or there may be a frankly conjectural assumption, based on unclear and retrospective data, that a brain-damaging occurrence such as a virus infection or degeneration of brain nerve fibres from other causes may have brought on the clinical picture.

It will be clear, therefore, that any advice given to the family by the social worker about the management of the child can only be undertaken in the closest cooperation with those involved in the diagnosis and treatment. And a similarly close cooperation will be needed to ensure that any general support also accords with the views and recommendations of the specialists involved in the particular case.

2

Causes of emotional insecurity in childhood

We shall now consider some of the most important of the general causes of emotional insecurity in a child; namely, friction in the home, emotional immaturity in the parents, various forms of disciplinary mismanagement, intense sibling jealousies, excessive ambition in parents, and changes to substitute families. For convenience the emphasis will be placed on the role of the mother. But naturally these factors apply similarly to the father.

FRICTION IN THE HOME

Friction between the adults is amongst the most significant causes of emotional insecurity in a child. Of course this phrase does not refer to the ordinary ups and downs of married life or the sparks that fly off the normal clashes in human relationships. Most children are organisms of sufficient resilience to withstand these ordinary circumstances of life. The sort of friction amongst adults that may lead to psychological damage in the children tends, as will be seen, to spring from sources that are more pathological and to relate to their own immaturity.

It is axiomatic that a state of pathological friction—or its equivalent expression in the form of emotionally-charged coldness—cannot supply the sense of security needed by a child, at whatever age in his development it may occur. Its effects can be as adverse during the earlier stages of life as during later years. Indeed for two broad reasons these earlier developmental phases are those that carry the greatest vulnerability. First, the child is less open to reassurance, because he has not yet acquired the necessary understanding of language to render him accessible to it. Secondly, it is thought that during these earlier stages his normal inner emotional turmoil arising from frustration of instincts tends to be at its highest peak of intensity, and therefore in greatest need to be counter-balanced by evidence of stability in the outside world.

The hypothesis is that if in the eyes of the child the quarrel-ling parents' emotions are as potentially destructive as those which, with his love-hate feelings, are within himself at this stage, then he experiences a sense of insecurity both from within and from without. Security thus seems non-existent; and where prolonged and severe marital discord surrounds the child's early life, the curtain may rise on a lifelong tragedy of ineradicable anxiety and maladjustment.

If in addition he is used by his parents as ammunition in their attempts to hurt one another, either before marital separation or in subsequent situations such as those of custody and access, then factors within the child—such as divided loyalties, guilt, uncertainties through the inconsistencies of handling received, and fears of his own capacity for the manipulation of those on whose strength both his emotional and material security depend—may all add their own momen-tum to the process of deterioration caused by the marital friction itself. The nebulous nature of these feelings within the child does not diminish their significance.

EMOTIONAL IMMATURITY IN MARRIAGE

Such pathological discord between marital partners is fairly common due to a degree of immaturity of emotional makeup in one or both partners. An impression often gained in clinical practice is that immature personalities marry one another very frequently. This marital correlation occurs with a frequency that implies very strongly that it takes place in excess of that which could be explained in terms of chance relationships. The social worker will find innumerable examples of marriages between immature partners amongst problem families.

Commonly it will be found that these immature personalities themselves have a history of emotional deprivation in their own childhoods. Moreover, the social worker with eyes to see, and an open mind with which to receive, will soon realize that such people, having been deprived of the healthy love in their own childhoods necessary to ensure their continued emotional development, have quite obviously failed to pass the developmental milestones successfully, and have remained stuck at a stage of emotional immaturity—either as a permanent state or as one into which they regress all too readily under the impact of stress. The forty-year-old woman with a personality-immaturity shown by attacks of screaming tantrums will often be found to have been subjected to experiences in her own childhood which prevented her developing or maintaining emotional development beyond the emotional age of three. Although she is the perpetrator of the three-year-old tantrums at the present time, nevertheless she was not responsible for the emotionally retarding circumstances of her childhood. Social workers may be rendered better able to tolerate and cope with these irritating and at first even alarming episodes or chronic states if they remember this causal principle that is frequently so relevant.

These immature personalities continue in adult life in the anxieties of their childhoods. Commonly they marry on a pathologically brittle basis of conditional love; and the formula 'I can only love you if you always completely love me' is the rock towards which sooner or later the marriage often hurtles, and on which in the more severe cases it too easily becomes shattered. The basis of this unhappy course is that since each partner has become conditioned through childhood deprivation into the belief that he or she is unworthy, neither can sustain reassurance by the other of being worth loving. They lack the capacity for self-acceptance.

True and mature self-acceptance is the basis of the capacity to accept others, and vice versa. The person who perpetually denigrates other people is often unwittingly proclaiming an insecurity in himself. The defence mechanism involved—ascribing to other people the inadequacies we feel ourselves to possess—is termed 'projection'. Sometimes, as in the case of a person constantly expressing contempt for the intelligence of others, it may point to a sense of inferiority of a comparatively specific nature. But frequently it is more generalized. And it is understandable that the marital situation provides an area of life where this sense of insecurity is often at its most sensitive, and where the associated defence mechanisms are therefore most readily evoked and productive of the most fundamental type of havoc.

It is a matter of frequent observation that unrequited love can lead to emotions of severe hostility. These situations are often made all the more poignant by the fact that in the first instance they were based on a mistaken assumption. At that stage the love was not in fact unrequited. But for antecedent reasons it was automatically assumed to be so; and the attitudes arising from the resulting defence mechanisms then themselves stimulated a true rejection by the partner on a secondary basis.

Defence mechanisms in neurotic marriages, however, do not always consist of those that give rise to the open 'thunder-and-lightning' atmospherics of this sort. They may also operate in terms that are more tacit and less overt. The partners may shut down on their feelings, and find themselves unable to express them openly or even to experience them directly in consciousness. The surface atmosphere may then be compara-tively unruffled; but it will consist of a cold and stilted in-capacity for basic communication which at best comprises only a psychoneurotic adjustment and is certainly not a marital fulfilment. Its effects on the child can be quite as deleterious as those produced by scenes of florid hostility.

However, in spite of its high incidence found in casework problems, union between immature personalities is only a tendency. Obviously it is far from being an invariable fact, and should not be overassumed. Relationships are too complex to permit of rigid generalization on this point. In the first place, instances are often seen of an immature personality receiving a great deal of therapeutic support from the understanding and acceptance supplied by a stable partner, though the latter often experiences considerable distress and finds burdensome diffi-culties in maintaining these accepting attitudes at a continu-ous level. Secondly, it would obviously be fallacious to assume that all marital discord reaching excessive proportions is necessarily the outcome of emotional immaturity in either partner. Incompatibility of basic temperament may be the essential factor, unassociated with any signs of deficiency in personality or psychoneurotic attributes of primary origin.

DISCIPLINARY MISMANAGEMENT

Disciplinary mismanagement is a significant cause of childhood insecurity, and is to be rated as equal in its significance to friction in the home. In practice the two often coexist. The child treated with excessive harshness, unhealthy indulgence, or serious inconsistency of handling is as much at risk of developing emotional insecurity as is the child subjected to the impact of discord between the parents.

In the complexities of child psychiatry, the causes of the causes themselves often need inspection. When one looks at each of these three forms of disciplinary mismanagement, for instance, one may find more distant circumstances that can account for the current situation. And in many cases it will therefore prove impossible to produce the necessary improvement without reference to these earlier levels of causation.

EXCESSIVE HARSHNESS: SOME CAUSES

Sometimes the sequence of reactions that have already been described as leading to discord between two immature personalities may not erupt during the first stage of marriage. In the less severe cases a relatively healthy and happy adjustment may have been achieved throughout this phase. But with the arrival of the first child storm clouds may rapidly gather.

In the seriously insecure parent, the triangular relationship that follows the birth of the child is often found to bring about a situation in which predetermined though latent jealousies then burst into fruition. Either parent may be the one to react initially. Often it is the mother, tired in her puerperal state and suffering from the various effects of the pregnancy, the labour and the postnatal hormonal changes, who first displays disturbance. If the father directs attention to the baby, more particularly if it is a girl, she feels unfavoured;

if on the other hand he pays less attention to the child, she feels unsupported.

Resentments then multiply, tensions between the couple increase, her handling of the baby becomes correspondingly abrupt and uncomfortably jerky with arms that are unconsolingly stiff. The baby reacts with reciprocal tension, perhaps crying incessantly and refusing her offering of feeding. This latter situation not only lights up further the sense of rejection residual from her own childhood but it does so in a way which, because it occurs in the context of the feeding situation, violates the most fundamental of the maternal biological instincts. Commensurate hostility towards the baby as well as the father then follows.

Other causes of excessive harshness are so protean and wide-ranging that in general they defy clear classification. Sometimes one finds them associated with relatively recognizable conditions, such as psychopathic personalities (chapter 9) or occasionally the emotional coldness and loss of former capacity for sympathy that has resulted from schizophrenic illness (chapter 11). In psychotic situations a child may even become directly implicated in a parent's delusional system. In a different sphere of illness, the irritability and aggressive outbursts that sometimes form part of known epileptic tendencies may lie behind unduly punitive and heavy-handed reactions adopted towards a child.

At the other end of the diagnostic scale are the more subtle states, whose recognition must often be inferential and based to a greater extent on deductions that are made from a combination of casework experience, an intuitive facility for perception, and a readiness to recognize the tentative nature of any diagnosis made on this basis. With sensible use of these three factors, however, the essence of the situations may often be seen.

This group of situations in which the origins may be somewhat subtler will be our main concern for the next few pages. Not infrequently, inordinate harshness in parents is a direct reflection and outcome of their own patterning. During their formative years they have had no better experience, and basically and predominantly it is therefore the only model and

mode of understanding within them. At other times the opposite obtains, and they react against too lax an early model, feeling that they themselves received too little guidance and therefore deciding, with grimly overcompensatory determination
and perhaps a sense of personal expiation against their own
'spoilt' behaviour, that their own child shall be spared this
deficiency of handling.

When parents appear to have too serious a fear of the chaos
that is part of their own aggressive feelings, in whatever way
these feelings arose, they may also experience quite unrealistic
anxiety as to where the child's behaviour will lead, at the
extremes of doubt being even intermittently haunted by the
spectre of the child growing up into almost a murderer if he
stamps and expresses hatred. They have the feeling, obviously
valid as a fact, that the child is an extension of themselves.
Accordingly any loss of self-control by the child may become
vaguely but significantly equated with their own fear of loss
of self-control. So, in so far as they find it necessary to keep
themselves under strict control, it follows that they cannot
easily face this piece of themselves which is represented by the
child, and which contains the self-willed and unruly element
from which they suffer in their own makeup. The child is unwittingly revealing their own Achilles' heel. Thus, in summary,
they clamp down on him with heavy self-protectiveness, only
to find that this action merely proves counter-productive in
the child, accentuating the existing problems of management.

In other words, since anxiety and dislike about what is
within oneself sometimes forms material which is dealt with
by the mechanism of projection—a defence mechanism in
which there is a tendency to be particularly intolerant of those
faults in others from which the individual himself suffers—it
follows that if a child shows features possessed by parents that
are too disturbing to themselves, this excessive reaction against
him is apt to happen. Furthermore, if he displays an attribute
that is identified with that of another person also towards
whom the parent is antipathetic, possibly even the marital
partner or an in-law, then here again projected hostility may
be directed towards the child. If these origins are present in the
parent's consciousness, the responses may be controlled; but

if there is no real awareness, then a situation where a detrimental sense of rejection becomes fostered in the child can operate without any beneficial modifications through insight.

Sexual rivalry may constitute another source of dissension within a family, and it too may lead to undeserved hostility towards a child. One of the most contentious areas arising from Freudian concepts is to be found in relation to the Oedipus situation (chapter 8). Early-life sexuality, and the sequels arising from it, is a concept that to many people does not come naturally or easily. But without entering into details of this often misunderstood area it can be said that the occurrence of a degree of sexual jealousy within many families is recognized by even the most prosaic of observers. The coy little 'daddy's girl' who arouses conflicting feelings in the mother, and the 'mother's boy' whose maternal mollycoddling evokes in the father emotions of jealousy that go beyond those of cool reasoning, and may exacerbate in the boy the already disturbing effects of the overpossessiveness to which he has been subjected, are common and easily recognized examples.

The final form of harshness that will be mentioned here is perhaps the most subtle. This is the overindulgence that has affinities with destructiveness. Chaos is the obverse of security. For a parent to abandon the task of producing secure orderliness of behaviour may itself be a subtle expression of harshness. Sometimes it is reflected quite frankly in the phrase 'Let him get on with it then'; but on occasions it may be a motivating factor operating less obviously.

EXCESSIVE HARSHNESS: SOME EFFECTS

Turning now from our consideration of some of the causes of harshness in parents to a brief survey of a few of its effects, a number are seen with particular frequency in child and family guidance practice. Not unnaturally the simplest and most straightforward reaction is for the child to become overtly cowed and timid. Sometimes this state is confined to his behaviour in the presence of his parents, while it is associated with outlet reactions of aggression elsewhere, often in school. But ultimately the initial cowed timidity may give place to an attitude in which the child himself becomes rigid, controlling and authoritarian as a generalized characteristic.

Alternatively these children may react by open rebellion at home from the outset. They become aggressive and, feeling themselves unloved, develop attention-seeking devices, including delinquency, that partly seem designed to incur the wrath of others and thus gain their attention. And in the service of aggression and attention-seeking, even very young children often have an uncanny knack of sensing the form of behaviour that will prove the most distressing and successful in violating whichever area of good conduct constitutes the cardinal virtue in the eyes of the parent. If graciousness is highly valued, the child becomes uncouth and boorish; if strict honesty is the idol of the parents, the child steals—often from within the family, where the secret will be let out to the grandparents; and so on.

A common result of harshness is seen in its paralysing effect not only on emotional but also on intellectual growth. Then the spirit becomes stunted, and confidence fails to develop. At school such a child is often unable to venture intellectually. He makes little effort, functioning below his potential; and of course his confidence will be still further reduced if an unwise type of opprobrium at school or at home follows in the wake of his academic ineptitude. At the same time he may be driven to a very active fantasy life in compensation, becoming dreamy and preoccupied with matters that are of little practical value and fail to commend themselves either to teachers or parents.

Not only does the child have difficulty with adults. Relationship problems with other children frequently complicate the situation. The child himself becomes reciprocally hypercritical and thereby antagonizes children as well as adults. He then finds himself unable to make friends and develops a feeling of desperation that nobody likes him. Eventually he may either abandon his efforts in this sphere also or in a desperate bid for popularity become clinging and overcompliant, hovering around other children and adults and again finding himself repelled in consequence.

OVERINDULGENCE: SOME CAUSES

We should now look at the other side of the coin of disciplinary mismanagement, namely overindulgence. A very high degree of parental attention and tolerance are of course essential in the management of infancy. With a complete absence of parental attention future trouble is inevitable—and in other pathological situations there is a sliding scale commensurate with its lack. But as time passes the form and the focal intensity with which parental attention is expressed must change to allow the child to develop. If a good relationship exists between the parents, the marital balance which was altered by the inevitable insertion of the child's needs should gradually return to its original state, though richer in content. The intensity of the cocooning of the child should progressively diminish as he passes the milestones of development. Failure on the part of the parents to do this constitutes morbid indulgence.

Morbid overindulgence may have roots that are broadly comparable with those relating to harshness. For example if the mother has had a harsh upbringing she may swing to the opposite extreme and overindulge, feeling that her own creativity was extinguished as a child. In severe instances she may become obsessed with the feeling that her own child has an almost divine spark that should not be put at risk of stultification by any form of direction whatsoever.

If, on the other hand, she herself was overindulged, there may again be a direct tendency to build on the same model; but here there is often a modification in that an overindulgent background may have left her with a streak of egocentricity that acts against her sacrificing her own comfort in the service of indulging her child.

In some instances, in giving the child an excess of material goods an overindulgent parent may be vicariously acting as a self-donor, presenting the child with things that she herself wanted in childhood but was unable to obtain. This concept does not, of course, deny the validity and value of the true and healthy love that finds its expression in giving generously to the child a chance better than the parents themselves received;

it merely points out that sometimes motivations may contain a pathological element nullifying the value of the act. In other cases an excess of material goods may be showered on to the child because the parents, having had too little emotional involvement of real depth in their own childhoods, are left without the ability to give it easily except in terms of what they 'know'. They will therefore wear themselves out in providing material comforts; but to the extent that they express love in predominantly material forms, the child is deprived of an ingredient essential for his psychological welfare. And any fear in the parents that he will fail to respond is apt to add further stimulus to their efforts in the same restricted and fruitless direction.

There is also the form of morbid overindulgence that is morbid overpossessiveness. This is a controlling form of overindulgence—one engaged in predominantly to maintain power. Like all the causal influences we are considering, it may exist either in severe or in quite mild degrees. In addition to its effect in preventing the development of independence it tends to contain a disguised quality of moral blackmail, since while it may be resented by the child it is nevertheless exercised in the name of love. But it is only one component in an emotional amalgam, being accompanied by genuine and unselfish feelings in the same parent. Hence, while resented, it is difficult for the child to rebel against it without arousing within himself the trauma of painful ambivalence in the most fundamental sphere of his emotional life.

OVERINDULGENCE: SOME EFFECTS

The broad result of overindulgence is that the child remains immature. Maturity consists of the ability to look not only at one's own needs but also at the needs of others. The overindulged child remains immature and therefore self-centred, retaining, or too easily regressing into, the attributes of egocentricity that characterize normal early life.

Associated with this egocentricity there is often a manifest lack of confidence. It operates on two levels. First, since the child has had too little opportunity to discover what he can do, he lacks confidence about matters of ordinary achievement, perhaps being scarcely competent to lace his shoes or go shopping. Secondly, and more fundamentally, there is the lack of confidence which relates to a failure of emotional emancipation from his parents and is associated with a close and stifling neurotic attachment that sometimes has a paralysing effect on even those achievements that he has successfully acquired. For instance he may not wish to go to the school camp simply because it involves being away from his mother. He can only operate effectively within the orbit of her presence, showing severe delay in developing the capacity to perform within the world as a whole those same tasks in which he can succeed at home. He goes to pieces because he is insufficiently emancipated emotionally; and this insecurity may be heavily coloured with a resentment about the low status in which he is held both inside and outside the home, though he is only vaguely aware of the nature of this resentment. A whole range of symptoms due to insecurity and hostility are often present.

In circumstances of this sort, social workers should not come to consider their role as that of an immediate diagnostician. Faced with the enigma of a timid child, especially when decision-making requires a hypothesis to explain the timidity, erroneous explanations which are not of the essence of the problem can spring to mind too readily. Ill-conceived steps to remedy the situation may follow on premature, subjective judgement; and as the situation unfolds itself these unfortunate errors may become belatedly apparent. With experience, however, workers will come to look correctly at the second levels of meaning, recognizing, shrewdly and sympathetically, the emotionally over-assiduous mother who doles out love like a stifling feather blanket, subtly dominating rather than basically encouraging, and sadly paying the price of seeing her child becoming progressively insecure when her real wish is that he should be happy and normal.

INCONSISTENCY

Although the origins and modes of action of these two excessive types of management are sometimes perplexing, the bald fact that they are liable to be attended by psychological damage is one that is obvious to anybody who is not unintelligent, ignorant, or rendered imperceptive by emotional factors. However, the significance and nature of the third major form of mishandling, namely inconsistency, does not always receive the same degree of recognition. But it too can sometimes be the source of serious damage.

It must be constantly remembered that we are only considering those cases at the morbid end of the scale of ordinary variation amongst the population as a whole. The term 'inconsistency' in this context contains two components in its meaning. First, a mother's morbid inconsistency of attitude commonly involves rapid changes of mood. Secondly, it may embody morbidly unrealistic reactions by the parent to the demands of reality. In other words, the child is forced to fit in rapidly with changing reactions, which are also ones for which he is given no reason and which in his eyes make no sense. Hence he becomes conditioned into the automatic assumption that irrational emotional reactions are the norm—and his expectations from other people and his own habitual reactions become moulded by this process.

Naturally, when these two components of inconsistency exist together the situation is maximally traumatic. But the frequent changes of mood can in themselves force on to the child the need for rapid adaptations which produce in him a pattern of slick and highly reactive changeability that soon outlives its usefulness and becomes an automatic and unhealthy mode of response.

We may take a simplified example. A child is behaving in a way that reasonably could be rewarded, such as drawing well or building lego, at the same time trying to catch his mother's eye for approval. If she ignores him he may then make a demand, for a biscuit for instance, which he does not really need.

We can see that in these circumstances not only has the child switched his behaviour in a way that runs counter to the maintenance of his stability of mood, but he has also himself become an active practitioner of inconsistency in the second sense we mentioned, the content of his reaction, as well as the changeability itself, embodying a quality of inconsistency. He demands something that he does not need in itself; and he is becoming conditioned into processes of falsity which may well become almost spontaneous and in relation to whose unrealistic content he will soon start to feel quite frank within himself. Insight into his own inconsistency becomes blurred and lost. His responses will thus become irrational and neurotic.

Next perhaps this mother may shout at him for her own relief when she is under stress that is not realistically to be related to the child. She may have heard bad news from a neighbour, for instance. At that time he may have been merely innocently bored or even playing quite constructively. However, in order to deal with her inconsistent emotion, disturbing in the rapidity of its change and threatening in its quality, he too engages in a reaction of inconsistency, pretending for expediency to feel affectionate towards her at the time.

She may then exploit him by grabbing him for comfort. He too rapidly exploits the situation by pestering her for a reward. Eventually he receives it. But he did not receive it when behaving in a way that might reasonably have been rewarded. The child has been giving no thought to his mother's need for comfort—nor she for his. They have each operated quite selfishly, functioning in a way that is not only inconsistent in being changeable but is also inconsistent with each other's needs and demands. In all these ways, therefore, while still only in his childhood his outlook and reactions can start to become twisted in their nature and automatic in their occurrence.

These few illustrations of the effects of severe inconsistency of parental management are simple and direct. But more complex and subtle reactions, less easily detected, sometimes may be found to require help either at a child guidance clinic or through casework in the community if the child's emotional development is to be safeguarded.

UNFAVOURITISM

Favouritism towards a child is a common cause of over-indulgence. Some of the effects of the latter have already been discussed. In the discussion that follows we shall concern ourselves with 'unfavouritism'.

A severely unfavoured child is always at risk of developing

a greater or lesser degree of emotional disturbance. A few of the possible reasons why parents may hold one of their children in disfavour by comparison with the others are therefore worth considering. Some were dealt with when looking at causes of excessive harshness. I shall only repeat here that by the process of projection we tend to be particularly intolerant in others of those features which we dislike in ourselves.

Vis-à-vis an unfavoured child, this tendency to hostility through projection may also apply in the context of unacceptable features possessed by, or thought to be possessed by, others such as a marital partner, a sibling or a parent. In other words, family members of either the present or the past may provide material in relation to which this mechanism leads to an unjustified aversion towards a child who is psychologically identified with them. For instance, symbolically-based jealousy may be present in a mother if her brother was favoured in her own childhood; a kind of sibling rivalry situation may have ensued in later life, a mother who is exceptionally insecure then assuming that people prefer her male child to herself—and she may feel an unrecognized element of resentment towards him in consequence.

Some children are clearly unfavoured because of their sex. 'She's a girl and sly', or 'I can't stand rough and untidy boys' are the sort of phrases that can point to an unfavouritism on this basis, which may not have been recognized or admitted by direct statement. Again, parents whose own siblings have all been of one sex may find a child of the opposite sex more difficult to cope with and prone to arouse their unease and hostility through fear of the unknown. Patterns then laid down may become progressively ingrained. An unwanted child is frequently unfavoured by comparison with his wanted siblings. In extreme cases it can happen that the child has proved to be one too many, and the father has left home; at other times the child has forced a disastrous marriage on a reluctant girl or man.

In the abstract these and many other causes are obvious; but in real-life situations they often need to be specifically sought. And many severely unfavoured children, all too readily regarded as unattractive and troublesome, thereupon proceed to give grounds in reality for the unfavoured role into which they have been so unhappily and undeservedly cast.

SIBLING JEALOUSIES

A degree of sibling rivalry between children forms part of the natural family scene. Intense and intractable sibling jealousy, however, may indicate significant insecurity, and even sow the seeds of later maladjustment.

Like so many other features in child psychiatry, sibling jealousy is one which while stemming from its own sources of insecurity can in itself, because of the guilt and hostility it evokes, also bring the sufferer a severe increase of the insecurity already present. It can be both an effect and a cause of insecurity. The bulk of our discussion of this topic will be reserved for chapter 3, where its more complex aspects will be dealt with. The only reference to sibling jealousies here will be to point out one or two of the more obvious facts that relate to the problem when it exists in severe form.

Firstly, many of the causes of 'unfavouritism' already touched on may themselves result in severe sibling jealousies. Another factor, which is common and will be dealt with later under separation anxiety, is the loss of the undivided attention of the parent when another child is born. The sibling jealousy resulting from this situation tends to be less severe when a large age-gap exists, because by the time of the birth of the second child the first child may have to a corresponding extent developed his own world. Quite often, therefore, the larger the gap the less the competition—unless the second child has been long-awaited, for example after a period of sterility, in which case the baby may be valued by the parents in such a floridly colourful manner that a reaction of jealousy in the older child is almost inevitably incited.

Sibling rivalry may result from quite ordinary and everyday circumstances whose significance may have passed unrecognized —a father taking only one of his boys fishing for example. Indeed the very fact that the parents wanted another child may have been construed by a young and already insecure child as an indication that he himself has failed to fufil his parents' needs. Any pre-existing tendency to think of himself as un-wanted may become reinforced by the next birth, and symptoms may be aggravated. As an antidote it is important for parents to emphasize to the child the pleasant and attractive attributes of himself and his own age group, as well as revealing their reac-tions to the charm of babyhood. This principle of course applies through the whole range of the years.

EXCESSIVE AMBITION IN PARENTS

Parents' over-ambitiousness for a child's success at school stands high amongst the sources of insecurity in childhood. Indeed, for them to over-identify themselves with a child's academic activities is one of the commonest methods of obtaining the sort of vicarious satisfaction sometimes found amongst parents in child guidance practice.

Manipulating a child into delinquent situations which bring release of parents' own aggression seems to occur at times; but it is unusual. Creating easy sexual opportunities between teenagers while experiencing sexually-charged anxiety about their effects is another paradoxical ploy for vicarious satisfac-tion that appears to be seen in parents from time to time; but this too is relatively rare. However, the impression that parents are redressing their own lack of scholastic success by attempt-ing to set the stage for the fulfilment by the child of their own frustrated academic hopes seems one that is valid all too frequently. But sometimes, also, it is the over-anxious obses-sional type of person, whose anxiety leads to a more general need to control the environment, who may fasten on to the child's academic welfare, and thereby produce the opposite result to that which is intended.

It is, of course, healthy and desirable for loving parents to entertain high hopes for their children's success. It is obviously also natural for them to hope that the child will do them credit. If, however, the child is pressed for this purpose beyond the powers of his ability or temperament, a serious danger point may be easily reached. In the abstract this principle is so clear as to render its statement almost platitudinous; in the living situation its presence is often overlooked. It is sometimes to be found in social circles in which competition is rampant, perhaps in smart executive set-ups, in which an additionally disturbing factor may lie in the father's frequent absences from home. If the seeking of status symbols is carried out too ruthlessly through the child it is liable to prove patently unsuccessful, often with the child in fact becoming humiliatingly unattractive and incapable.

When discussing causes of delinquency we noted a few of the psychological defence mechanisms through which dullness of intellect may give rise to delinquency of behaviour. Many features of insecurity other than delinquency may also arise in these circumstances. Sometimes, however, they occur in children whose intelligence level is average or even well above average, but who are the victims of a disparity between this level and the level of expectation which, rightly or wrongly, they believe their parents to hold of them. When the parents do in fact cherish unduly high expectations they may express them either by direct statement to the child or indirectly by generating a climate of feeling that tacitly leaves him in little doubt of their disappointment.

Sometimes, on the contrary, a child may for various reasons interpret the situation as one in which he is falling below the level his parents would wish, when such is not the case. For example, a child who can recognize that his parents are of far higher intellectual calibre than himself, but who is unable to perceive that they are not expecting him to become their equal, may develop an unjustified sense of inability to satisfy them that acts as a threat to his feelings of security. And in the sphere of moral worth also, as well as in other forms of personal quality, the very worthiness of admirable parents may in itself automatically eclipse the child's sense of his own capacity. The right balance of good parental example and a tolerant and visible acceptance of the child's potential as lower than their own may need to be suitably achieved and clearly conveyed.

The child who, within a situation either real or derived from his own fantasy, fails to reach a sense of being fundamentally at one with his parents is liable to undergo various other reactions. Love on merit, at least when it dominates the child's self-image, can, as we have seen, be a destructive formula. In addition to his doubts and insecurities vis-à-vis his own parents, the child on reaching adult life is at risk of developing the general belief that he is only acceptable if he succeeds in supplying, in its extreme and its entirety, whatever form of virtue he conceives as appealing to those to whom he wishes to relate. He grows up frequently seeing authority figures— first in the earlier stages at school and subsequently in life as a whole—as people who are to be feared as critical adversaries or abandoned as objects of unattainable relationship, rather than sought as benevolent helpers; to be shunned as threats rather than embraced as allies.

Moreover, since these are the criteria on which their outlook has fundamentally been built, such children are themselves apt to become capable only of accepting others primarily on merit. Although as they grow older they may lean over backwards to counteract this tendency, in the end by the strength of their conditioning and their in-built philosophy they tend to be attracted basically if ambivalently to those of 'superior' calibre and achievement—only to be disillusioned if they find that in other and more fundamental respects such idols have feet of clay. Their ultimate capacities for human relationships may become directed to limited ends, resting on a foundation laid down by the morbid expectations demanded in their child-hoods, with the resulting restrictions on their adult value systems. These and other long-term effects are of course only tendencies rather than inevitabilities; but they have their significance on occasions.

CHANGES TO SUBSTITUTE PARENTS

A particularly potent cause of emotional insecurity in early childhood may lie in the separation of a child from his parents. Some of the most appallingly disturbed of all the children seen in child guidance practice have a history of repeated changes of substitute parents and family figures. Readers are recommended to turn to chapter 5 and familiarize themselves with the theoretical concepts dealt with in relation to separation at an early age.

At any age, and even in the best of circumstances, changes of environment in childhood are liable to produce some degree of emotional difficulty. When this risk arises it will of course be minimized by a sense of continuing security in personal relationships within the family. The moves of domicile imposed merely by working requirements, as in many military families where the traumatic effects of changes of locality can be largely nullified by the integrity of the family itself, is a case in point. Nevertheless problems arising from dislocation of school progress may sometimes be difficult to mitigate, and disruption of the continuity of relationships will always comprise a hazard to be overcome. Occasionally the insecurities involved will defeat the most well thought out of efforts to forestall or eradicate them.

Changes to substitute parents, however, can generate emotional disturbances that are far more fundamental. Every social worker meets these situations. Frequently her involvement will be in relation to the management of difficulties attendant on separations due to eviction, death, divorce or desertion. Separation through admission to hospital of the mother or the child (chapter 5) is also very common, and the social worker's help may be sought with this problem too.

All gradations exist, from the child who is simply separated during a single hospital admission, traumatic though even this separation may be, to the unfortunate young victim foredoomed to the shattering sequence of events that arises for example when a promiscuous mother embarks on a series of abortive partnerships that takes the child into ever-changing accommodation and imposes on him inconstant, multiple and often hostile contacts that leave him emotionally insecure and socially inept beyond much hope of redemption. Within this pattern there are often interspersed periods of care in local authority homes or foster homes while his inadequately supported mother takes residential jobs. The highly responsible task of arranging for the care of the child with relatives, with foster parents, or in a local authority home will fall on the shoulders of social workers. It is therefore important for them to have acquired as much understanding as possible of the psychological responses which the separated child may undergo.

Conditioned on a foundation of confusion, jealousy, superficiality of feeling and expectations of broken relationships, there inevitably lies before such a child the risk of a future of insecurity governed by a combination of the laws of Pavlovian physiology and the distorting pressures laid down within his unconscious mind (chapter 8). Much will depend on the stage at which the separation occurs, the frequency with which it takes place, and the circumstances that precede and follow it. If the mother has been loving, which of course is the usual history in cases of hospital separation, the child may become more manifestly disturbed than if his only concept of life has been one based on an absence of concentrated love. The fully loved child with more to lose may well react against the loss more acutely, though when the intensity of the child's relationship with his mother has been diluted by the frequent presence of other members of the family, such as grandparents, he may react to her loss less acutely.

This last fact does not imply that a very young child stands to benefit by a general multiplicity of parent figures. On the contrary, it seems important for him to receive the stabilizing sense of security that derives from a basic one-to-one relationship with a mother on whose predominance and consistency he can depend without confusion. It is likely to be important that whenever possible the mother should be the central figure in his awareness as the reliable and key person. But if this healthy relationship has been present, the separated child who has had the advantage of an experience of multiple relationships may find that this situation has stood him in good stead —even though the separation, particularly in the pre-verbal stage before he has become accessible to adequate explanation, will inevitably bring its trauma. In any circumstances, however, the effect of a series of separations may be highly destructive, fragmenting the child's development and rendering him unable to put trust in any human relationship or invest emotionally in any human being for fear of abandonment or betrayal.

The child may then look to material things for security. He may even cling to a bar of chocolate which he thinks cannot disappear. Yet the child who has revealed himself as in need of clinging to material objects for symbolic support may, with the ambivalence found in psychological sufferers in all age groups, then proceed to destroy the very possessions from which he is drawing his comfort, tearing them up and finishing with nothing. Even the substitutes for human beings may become hated because they too let the child down in their intrinsic insufficiency.

It also seems possible that repeated separations may impede the development of the ordinary processes of guilt and reparation. On this hypothesis, with the disappearance of each person against whom the abandoned child assumes himself to have transgressed he is deprived of the opportunity to make amends or to maintain any state of reparation already achieved. A very young child, unable to formulate abstractions, needs for these purposes the physical presence of the same individual during this unsophisticated and formative stage. He cannot sustain guilt towards anyone who is not available to receive the feelings. So the feelings of guilt can neither be repaired nor maintained. Eventually, if the process of repeated separations from ever-changing adult figures continues, there has existed no constant person on to whom the child's guilt and reparation processes can be focused. The process is abandoned, and guilt development grinds to a halt. The development of healthy guilt is clearly bound up with the development of healthy conscience and is likely to depend on having a relationship to maintain. Degrees exist, but total lack of conscience characterizes the complete psychopath.

The social worker should keep these findings and hypotheses in mind when planning the arrangements for separated children. These are situations in which the exercise of preventive insight is likely to be far more effective than any later attempts through child guidance and casework to achieve impracticable cures. As was mentioned earlier, some of the most grossly disturbed of all the children attending child guidance clinics have a history of repeated separations.

3

The management of emotional disturbances of childhood

Probably the most useful means of presenting to the community social worker the salient concepts entailed in work with families with psychological difficulties will be to discuss the two types of approach that are adopted by the social worker at the child guidance clinic—who by tradition, though not always in practice, has been a psychiatric social worker.

THE COMMUNITY SOCIAL WORKER

The principles by which the clinic social worker provides her psychological help are usually put into effect on a deeper and more intensive level than is practicable within the context of community work; but amongst these principles are to be found universal guidelines that relate to all levels and forms of casework, and ones on which the community social worker may usefully base her own. Later we shall also look at the work of the educational psychologist, and finally at that of the child psychiatrist, so that an integrated mosaic of the functions of the clinic as a whole can be obtained.

Although the dichotomy about to be discussed is far from sharply delineated and its components do not exist in clearly contrasting areas of black and white, we may for convenience divide the psychological functions of the social worker into two separate dimensions. There is her giving of insight through direct psychological explanations and advice on the one hand; and, on the other, her methods of providing insight on an indirect basis.

PROVIDING DIRECT INSIGHT

Taking the generality of families attending a child guidance clinic, a high proportion have problems in which the comparatively direct approach is indicated. Broadly this is the group with difficulties that have sprung from the ordinary hazards of bringing up children, to which anyone similarly assailed would have equally succumbed and often reacted with similar errors. Many such sets of circumstances, in which there was in fact no great depth of primary psychological aberration in members of the family, may have led up to the child's insecurity.

These family misfortunes include an early history of severe separation anxieties; sibling jealousy which intensified as a result of not being recognized, or occurring at a stage in family life when the parents were too preoccupied with other problems to cope with it; the growth of marital discord from unfortunate circumstances such as overcrowded or unsuitable accommodation, including in particular too close proximity between the generations; or the adoption of inexpedient forms of discipline owing to the absorption of false ideas during impressionable youth. Unfortunately, secondary problems arising from a subsequent degree of rejection of the disturbed child by the parents sometimes become grafted on to the primary difficulties experienced by the child.

When helping parents in this primarily non-neurotic group, the social worker will often find herself able to bestow great benefit by supplying direct explanations as to how the current situation arose during the child's earlier years. The factors in this group of cases, in contrast to those of the second group that will be described later, do not usually require her to invoke much material relating to the early-life experiences of the parents themselves. Psychotherapy can be largely confined to the here-and-now, with references only to the comparatively recent past.

It is unnecessary to reiterate the material that may need to be introduced in her discussions on this level, but if readers now refer to the relevant topics such as separation anxiety (chapters 2 and 5), sibling rivalry (chapter 2), and 'testing out' techniques (chapter 1), they will find themselves correspondingly equipped to fulfil the advisory functions.

By giving such insight with a skill derived from experience as well as from book knowledge, she will often enable parents to exonerate themselves quite rationally from the underlying self-accusations which they had previously been levelling against themselves. These direct perceptions she provides will often enable them to adjust to, and to rectify, any errors they may have made.

In other words here is an area in which the fact that self-acceptance leads to acceptance of others has a vital application. By coming to accept themselves the parents will be helped towards correspondingly accepting rather than rejecting the child. Since in this group any rejection of the child has arisen predominantly not from deep-seated emotional difficulties but from reactions secondary to family misfortunes, it will be found that on the whole these parents are comparatively 'undefended' and accessible to the direct explanatory approach. And when the child becomes more accepted by them, he too becomes disencumbered of the feelings of unworthiness and hostility that have contributed to his own rejecting reactions. The total situation may then start to go into reverse, even if the course towards recovery remains for a time a tiresomely fluctuating one.

One of the aspects of family difficulty in which emotions tend to run particularly high, in which reason has often ceased to prevail, and where distressing symptoms of emotional disturbance in the child have frequently developed in consequence, is that of severe sibling jealousy. It was touched on in the previous chapter. But it is also an aspect worth re-emphasizing in the context of management, since it can develop easily, lead in severe cases to disturbing and long-term effects, and can often be readily solved in the first instance if only its presence and significance can be recognized. Every child guidance clinic constantly encounters these jealousy situations where hardened if not intractable symptoms exist, but where in retrospect the starting point is easy to see. And they often create a strong impression that if timely and suitably informed intervention had only been available in the incipient stages of the jealousies the subsequent course of events would have been very different.

How can the social worker assist in the early management of sibling jealousy? First, she must recognize its presence. Secondly, she must be able to help the parents to accept it, understand it and comfort it away.

Even when sibling jealousy presents itself in direct forms, with the usual features of spitefulness recognizable as such by any impartial observer, the parents may be unable to perceive it, because of a blind spot in themselves. Parents strongly inclined to favour one child may well have a marked disinclination to observe the effects of this attitude on the other, for fear of being forced into relinquishing their favouritism or because of a reluctance to experience the pangs of self-reproach which such a realization would bring. But even when they are in fact prepared to accept its importance when recognized, they fail to detect its existence when it presents itself in forms which through sheer ignorance they are unable to recognize as indicative of this situation.

It is therefore important that the social worker should be on the lookout for the less obvious signs of severe sibling jealousy, and that she should be aware of their nature. These signs are in fact quite well-known in the relevant professional circles; but the more specifically she carries them in the forefront of her mind, the more likely will she be to think about them spontaneously when the occasions arise.

Amongst these disguised manifestations of sibling jealousy perhaps the commonest are those arising from the mechanism termed regression. By regression is meant the process of reversion into patterns of thought, feeling and behaviour that are more appropriate to an earlier developmental level. And it is a mechanism that can come into play at any stage of life.

It may be recalled that a lack of specificity between causes and symptoms characterizes much of child guidance work. And features of regression can result from states of insecurity as a whole, however the insecurity may have been caused. Regressive symptoms should therefore not be interpreted exclusively as pointing to sibling rivalry. Other causes of insecurity should also be considered. Nevertheless, regressive symptoms should always lead to an evaluation of the situation in terms of this particular possibility.

Even an adult may regress to some degree into the outlook of early childhood, with its changeability, petulance, peevishness, clinging etc., if subjected for too long to unendurable emotional burdens, or if assailed by the sudden impact of too acutely disintegrative misfortune. Even the most stable have their breaking point. In children, as yet only minimally solidified by the passage of years, this process occurs more readily; and sibling rivalry is one of the commoner stresses giving rise to it, the most frequent point of origin being at a stage when a child, too young to understand the essentially harmless nature of the situation, and already disturbed by the separation-anxiety consequent on his mother's disappearance into hospital for the birth of a baby, is faced with her return accompanied by an unexpected rival on to whom she lavishes a profusion of attention with an appearance of terse rejection of his own demands.

The child then regresses. Having been weaned, he may revert to the need for the bottle. Previously fully toilet-trained, he may lapse into incontinence. From the stage of normal independence, he may now become clinging and whiny. Hitherto capable of speech commensurate with his age, he may adopt an immature intonation and under-developed articulation.

Explanations of the significance of these features may be required. But even when their jealousy origin is perceived, the factor which so easily bedevils the issue is that because these features are obnoxious to the parents they automatically assume them to be a stance the child has intentionally adopted as a contrived form of protest. And the overtaxed mother is in no mood to cope with the recalcitrant behaviour of a child whose previous level of developmental achievement is naturally thought to indicate an ability for self-control and maturity which he no longer chooses to exercise. A campaign of understandable and often heated retaliation against the jealous child is therefore promptly mounted.

But it is based on a misconception. The retaliation is being directed against a child whose attitude, though containing a surface component of obvious hostility, is not predominantly that of an enemy. It is the product of the law of nature that is regression. If the mother were to engage in a little quiet reflection, which in the turmoil of her increased load of work she is often unable to undertake, she would usually achieve a different attitude quite easily. The social worker may play an invaluable part in helping her to do so. A moment's thought will reveal for example that an infant does not return to the bottle simply to annoy; and incontinence may occur during sleep. Whatever the anxiety lying behind it and any encrustation of hostility, the machinery itself is basically impersonal.

Another guise in which sibling jealousy may express itself without being recognized as such, even by the jealous child himself, is the adoption of a false front of independence in which he rejects affectionate advances from the parent by responding with an attitude, spoken or unspoken, of 'I don't need you'. If its true connotation, which in fact is 'I do need you', escapes detection by the parent also, then understandably this parent will feel hurt and may respond by a degree of counter-rejection that increases the child's insecurity and associated withdrawal. What began as an unconsious façade may finish as an intractable reality.

An alternative guise adopted by the child may consist, on the contrary, of an over-solicitous air of filial devotion. It too may obscure the presence of jealous hostility felt towards a sibling. The child who constantly acts out a monitorial role, assiduously reporting to the parents all the problems produced by his sibling, may be motivated by unrecognized attempts at compensatory ingratiation against the unfavoured position which he suspects himself of occupying. This undue 'goodness' may be over-valued by an otherwise perceptive parent receiving its advantages, and may mask the insecurity by which it has been prompted, leading the child to adopt patterns of similarly automatic obsequiousness in other areas of life, that bring further problems as well as leaving the basic situation unresolved. At other times it may be relevant to point out to a parent that a middle child is unknowingly jealous of the attention received by the younger child, while resentful of the elder child's privileges (or, essentially, what they appear to him to symbolize). And experience will gradually reveal many other patterns of disguised jealousy.

When the social worker has penetrated these various disguises in the child she will be in a position to explain the true situation, in direct form, to any parents who have been unaware that the problem has in fact been one in which their child has been seriously disturbed by his rivalry for their love and attention. Remedial steps can then be taken.

INDIRECT INSIGHT

So much for some of the material that may be involved when the social worker conducts her casework on a direct basis. The essence of the indirect approach, however, is to help clients who have more deep-seated psychological difficulties—be they parents, substitute parents, or any other adults in close family relationship with the child—to work through their ideas in such a way as to arrive at a decision based on reorientation of feelings as well as on this purely intellectual plane of understanding. The mother is gently led to look at her real feelings, in contrast to those which occupy the immediacy of her awareness, and relate them to the emotional experiences of her own childhood. This involves a procedure different from that of direct explanation.

To provide this indirect process of help, it is essential for the social worker to make it clear that she is adopting a non-moralizing view of the situation. Parents unlucky enough to be coping with a disturbed child have often been already subjected to condemnation, spoken or unspoken, by people less closely involved than themselves. While many people will have felt the unmixed sympathy which insight for those in difficulty can bring, others will have been too readily disposed to the easy task of jeering on the sidelines. And from the very fact that the parents have brought the child to the clinic it will be obvious to the social worker that they care, and that even the most well-intentioned of direct advice has been unsuccessful.

In relating her present feelings to those which she experienced in her own early life, a mother will eventually, if success is achieved, come to recognize that her present defence mechanisms such as repression, projection, etc., and the others discussed in chapter 8 no longer have their former relevance. They may have been necessary when she was an imperceptive and defenceless child. But she must come to see that they can now be safely modified.

When helping her client to acquire this self-awareness the social worker may have a very valuable part to play; but in order to do so it is essential that she has a clear grasp of the principles involved. Otherwise she may do more harm than good. By those unfortunate individuals seriously fettered by their own unconscious processes, the logic of reality is commonly ignored, rejected, or distorted. Too often the intellectual type of insight is not open to use by those whose underlying feelings cannot bear exposure to the light of day. And even when logical comprehension is present, it may not result in much useful change in practice unless it is accompanied by the processes that lead to the deeper reorientation of feelings. Indeed, recognition of the immediate logic is sometimes already present, and its reiteration to the client therefore adds nothing of significance. Laborious efforts of this sort may simply erode hope and confidence by the sterile nature of the repetitions.

Intellectual insight, therefore, sometimes needs to have associated with it a reorientation on the level of feeling, i.e., emotional insight. So we should now try to clarify this latter concept.

To be fully meaningful, and therefore to confer its fullest therapeutic benefits, the client's achievement of insight in this type of case—examples of which will be given later—must itself be an emotional experience. The caseworker can sometimes provide a medium through which the client may return in memory to her own childhood, where the origin of her difficulties will often lie. The term 'may' return should be emphasized, since in these cases any question of forcing the issue or pressing for an unacceptable rate of progress must be rigorously avoided.

Obviously the social worker cannot place herself in the position of a professional psychoanalyst. But she can listen with at least that degree of understanding which her own level of experience and knowledge makes possible. And she can understand with an insight that will safeguard her own feelings, knowing that the turbulent and hurtful emotions that may be directed on to her are often in fact merely symbolic representations of the client's repressed feelings towards significant people in her own childhood. Armed with this understanding the social worker will welcome rather than resent their development, being rendered immune from feelings of anger at any seeming ingratitude and being fortified against the sense of inadequacy that she might otherwise develop in reaction to a sense of failure to establish a relationship acceptable to the client. Similarly she will recognize the symbolic significance of the client's temporary demands for childish dependence, and the need for subsequent emancipation, which the course of the progress will entail. In other words, her specialized psychological knowledge will protect her against taking her client's reactions personally, so that her own self-esteem becomes neither unrealistically undermined nor unjustifiably inflated.

One of the factors that frequently limits the efficacy of the help given by those who have attained a certain amount of specialized psychological knowledge is an enthusiasm for premature presentation of underlying factors to those not ready to receive them. If correct psychological explanations are given with ill-considered prematurity, they will be rejected by the client in some form—by turning overtly hostile, by ridiculing the explanations, or by discontinuing attendance on any grounds that may conveniently be exploited for the purpose. Or the client may be rendered more pathologically disturbed. To give insight without the immediate means of remedying a seriously traumatic situation, at a speed too great to enable the client to come to terms with it, is apt, however well-intentioned, to be destructive.

Any social worker tempted to succumb to this impulse may help herself by keeping constantly in mind that listening is not in fact doing nothing. It is perhaps those beginning health visiting who form one of the groups most in need of remembering this principle. Members of the medical and nursing professions are naturally highly conditioned into dispensing direct information, and giving advice arising out of it. In psychotherapy, on the other hand, the art of listening with a restraint of comment based on an understanding of the patient's areas of need for protection is one that must be studiously cultivated.

In helping clients to look at their real ideas and feelings more healthily, the social worker may need to encourage them to relive and abreact their early childhood feelings. By their repeatedly doing so these emotions may become drained off, rather as a film scene loses its emotional impact through repetition. But this process is not necessarily sufficient to eliminate the secondary effects that have occurred on the basis of conditioning. Through habituation clients are liable to continue to bring old feelings irrelevantly into current situations. And because this reaction occurs automatically, it tends to take place without reference to the insight which they have now acquired. Nevertheless after each episode the emotional content tends to become less intense and eventually, if all goes well, hindsight becomes progressively easier to harness to needs. In successful cases, after these episodes—at least as a general trend—clients can more readily achieve an acceptance of their true significance, and even laugh tolerantly at themselves or manage to take themselves less seriously.

Although the need to avoid presenting psychological explanations often forces on to the situation a slow rate of progress, nevertheless beneath the surface intermittent flashes of insight may take place and momentarily rise up into consciousness; and on each occasion a little more acceptance and insight may be achieved. Thus even when the actual moment of seeing is sudden, the subconscious processes that have gone to building up the insight, release and self-acceptance have often been protracted.

The process of encouraging clients to talk about their own childhoods can often be accomplished with less difficulty than might be supposed, though areas of significant amnesia may exist within the total matrix of their childhood memories, sometimes pointing to emotionally charged material not yet ready for release. The shift of discussion from their particular child on to the subject of childhood in general is often a development that can flow naturally if good rapport has been obtained. And from there a narrowing of attention on to some of the more significant aspects of the client's own childhood experiences may also develop as reactions having a fair degree of spontaneity.

When talking about their early childhood and coming to see the relevance to the difficulties of their own children, parents will frequently arrive at a point where a little gentle leading is required. It should usually be provided in as tentative and oblique a form as possible, so that in laying down a bridge of insight between the past and the present the social worker in effect supplies only a drawbridge, which the client can draw up if protection against the onrush of unwelcome memories or inferences is required.

Another analogy—that of a sounding board or a mirror—may be helpful in remembering the basic principles of case-work procedure. In talking to the caseworkers about the sort of material we are now considering in general, and will shortly look at in detail, the client should in effect be talking to herself. It is on this basis that the social worker gradually provides such clients with the facility for proceeding towards self-understanding; but at the same time she cushions them, to the extent that it is desirable to do so, against the impact of too abrupt a recognition of underlying feelings and attitudes, affording the client a temporary protection against the distress which in many cases will flow inevitably from the dawning of realization. But when the parent's real feelings, in contrast to the attitudes occupying her immediate awareness, gradually come to light, together with the patterns of defence against them which she is adopting, the parent may begin to realize that emotions which were understandable and even necessary as a defence-less child no longer have their relevance and can be safely modified.

SOME PATTERNS OF TRANSMISSION
In the last few pages we have been talking about method rather than content. We have not yet looked closely at the psychological material itself. However, having seen these broad principles governing the procedures by which the material may be

elicited, we can now look at some of the actual substance that may be found in these cases.

To do so we are brought back to a consideration of the unconscious mind. And we must relate it to an important concept to which passing reference was made at the beginning of chapter 1, namely, that patterns of emotional disturbance may be transmitted from generation to generation through the operation of factors related to the unconscious mind.

The content of histories containing the more deep-seated type of material in child and family guidance work is endless in its variations. Nevertheless it tends to fall into a number of patterns of perpetuation from parent to child and onwards, which by their very nature can only be loosely demarcated but are often discernible as thematic entities, albeit with their infinite variations from case to case and their tendencies to intertwine and coalesce within any given case.

In extreme instances, the general progress and outcome in these sagas of family perpetuation can be predicted as having almost the inevitability of a Greek tragedy. But in the less heavily loaded examples the passage of time may introduce elements that dilute the force of the self-perpetuation. And in some cases the intervention of the child guidance team, or in the less severe instances the unaided efforts of the caseworker in the community, may serve to disrupt predetermined patterns and safeguard the future.

It must be realized that the sort of problems about to be described constitute only a minority of the cases dealt with in child guidance. Most situations are much simpler, having arisen on a basis of the less pathological types of circumstances already referred to. And although their management still demands specialized experience of disturbed children and their families, they are nevertheless suitable to be dealt with by the correspondingly superficial and less sophisticated methods that are based on direct explanations. On the whole these more superficial problems do not perpetuate themselves too significantly into the future generations.

However, we are concerned now, by contrast, to look at the patterns of those more deep-seated situations whose effects are liable to pass unremittingly from parent to child, through the operation of the unconscious mind. In chapter 8 we shall discuss the unconscious mind more fully, in connection with the part it plays in the development of the individual. At the present stage we shall examine some examples of how it may produce long-term effects on progeny.

When a child attends a child guidance clinic showing manifestations of insecurity—let us say a combination of stealing and poor concentration—it not infrequently happens that the mother gives the information that as a child she felt herself to be the 'odd one out'. Sometimes she uses this actual phrase; sometimes its relevance is obvious from her general description of her feelings and predicaments at those earlier stages of her life.

At the same time it is seen from the data she provides in describing her present attitude towards, and her management of, her child that she is—without realizing the origin of this management, and often even without awareness of its existence —using the child to extract from him as a compensation for her own early-life deprivations all the emotional 'juice' she can contrive to obtain. She is not to be condemned for doing so. She was not responsible for the compelling vacuum that developed within her in childhood which now leads her to cling unknowingly to her child. Nor is the child to be blamed for the fact that he reacts with neurotic failings and unacceptable responses. The die was cast twenty years or more previously.

The neurotically over-possessive parent with an excessive need to use the child for her own emotional support, thus preventing him from achieving independence, commonly reacts with a hostility that is alarming to the child, or with a display of martyrdom that instils into him a morbid sense of guilt that may be lifelong, whenever his expression of resentment asserts itself. And another element is often present. Frequently the mother has married a man whose own attributes are destined to lead to marital discord and mutual rejection. She then finds herself involved in a situation of emotional deprivation in her relationship with her marital partner in the present, in addition to the deprivations which existed in her childhood relationship with her parents. A double motivation, from both past and present, impelling a compensatory over-attachment to her child, will then exist.

A second pattern of morbid transmission that we should briefly discuss is one which though of different origin also involves mechanisms operating outside the individual's awareness. It is seen from time to time in child guidance practice when parents have been subjected in their own childhoods to a handling that was excessively rigid.

As was observed in the previous chapter, long-term responses to severely rigid handling may be the result of conscious and intended deliberation. The mother may, for example, intentionally decide that her own child shall not suffer the same fate as herself. But when the unconscious mind is involved, a different set of factors may come into operation. When a mother has a history of having been subjected to extreme rigidity of management in early life, it is sometimes found that on reaching adult life she has become a parent who either demands impossible high standards, or alternatively is afraid of imposing any limitations; or thirdly, that she vacillates between both these attitudes. Either of these extremes, or the third possibility, i.e., inconsistency, will be damaging to her child. And on reaching adult life he too will therefore lack the necessary emotional foundation for sound parenthood and will mishandle his child in turn. Hence the thread of this form of morbidity too is transmitted environmentally into the next generation and beyond.

On the surface it would seem paradoxical that two such widely divergent reactions as the demanding of impossibly high standards of conformity on the one hand, and the inability to impose limitations on the other, should emanate from the same source, namely inordinate rigidity in childhood. But reactions have their logical explanations in the unconscious as well as the conscious sphere.

The essence of this explanation, then, is that the child with a history of being subjected to extreme rigidity in early life has been left with a continuing but unrecognized problem over his aggression. For the intelligent person with a conscious knowledge of his problems, the means of dealing with them, or at least of attempting to do so, is to take thought about them and then adopt any steps that may be possible on this basis. For people who are unaware of their essential difficulties, however, this solution is not available.

We may consider the situation of a little girl caught up in this predicament and too young and inexperienced to come to terms with it on a sophisticated level. The sequence of events may be as follows. Without knowing she is doing so, she may push her aggressive feelings towards her parent out of her awareness because they run too heavily counter to the feelings of affection mixed with them. These aggressive feelings have become too painful to be allowed to remain within the field of conscious recognition. Consciously she retains her feelings of 'uncontaminated' love, though with a vague sense of uneasiness that renders her less than well adjusted and sometimes even afflicted with severe symptoms of insecurity whose origin is not immediately clear.

Being now outside her awareness, these subconscious aggressive feelings remain unresolved and consequently unchanged in their intensity. And from the very fact that it was necessary for the child to exclude them from her awareness in the first instance, it logically follows that even the possibility of their re-emergence into consciousness will in itself constitute a threat to her, at whatever stage in later life it may arise. In other words, it is logical to infer that these unresolved feelings will continue to cause her to have a fear of her aggression. If the aggression had remained present in consciousness it would have been more or less successsfully 'philosophized away' with the development of intelligence. But this process has not been possible, and the past events therefore persist unknowingly as a threat.

In these circumstances, on reaching adult life she may find that any normal display of aggression by her own child will be liable to produce in her a reaction of undue panic of essentially unknown origin. Any situation in which everyday and normal aggressive behaviour by the child might bring her own unwanted feelings of aggression to the surface is one that she cannot afford to entertain. Such episodes must therefore be stamped out in the child as soon as they arise. Hence her harsh reaction is essentially one of self-protection, though she often ascribes it to more conveniently obvious and palatable factors such as the need to instil good manners, self-discipline and social conformity.

From these facts it will be seen that if she adopts the opposite reaction, namely that of avoiding all clashes with the child, no travesty of logic is involved in the hypothesis. The paradox, otherwise difficult to explain, that two such widely divergent reactions as excessively suppressive measures on the one hand, and inordinate indulgence on the other, can both stem from the same causal influence—namely excessive rigidity of early upbringing—now takes on a comprehensible meaning. The severity of these responses, whichever one she may have adopted for self-protection, is out of proportion to the facts of the current environment. Sometimes also there may be vacillation between these two protective extremes giving rise to unpredictable inconsistency. And any one of these three reactions is in itself liable to result in damage to the emotional development of the child.

The long-term results on the child of parental attitudes arising from the unconscious mind will become progressively more obvious to readers as they reflect on them, and may become still clearer when they are encountered in the field of clinical experience. The child grows up without having received the sort of relationship necessary to permit normal emotional maturation; and so on reaching adult years he too does not possess the necessary qualities to enable his own child's development to proceed normally. A chain of morbidity has thus been transmitted through essentially environmental circumstances, though the subtleties involved have been more than are usually perceived by the average observer.

If the social worker now gives a little thought to this concept of repressed unconscious aggression in its relation to the ordinary reactions she has observed in her everyday life, she will soon realize that in spite of the fact that it hinges on the theory of the unconscious mind it nevertheless accords quite readily with her own common sense and experience. In effect the concept is merely an extension of the views she already holds. At times all people have experienced fears of their own aggression, and have felt impelled to walk away from situations rather than engage in an argument whose effectiveness is beyond doubt but which would evoke a sense of unwelcome inner turbulence. Moreover all people can recall occasions on which they have snapped out a remark with a vehemence that has surprised both onlookers and themselves by its seemingly unreasonable intensity. Such occasional incidents occur as the norm of the human scene. It is not difficult therefore to realize that in those whose previous experiences have been outside the norm these tendencies may occur with correspondingly greater frequency, severity and ill-effect.

The concept that the parents' own repressed aggression may operate as a source of mishandling the child is therefore one that is able to withstand the accusation of being unacceptably fanciful and automatically unworthy of belief. It has the merit of logic.

It is also possible to carry this concept further, and bring in related considerations which although admittedly more speculative similarly do not fly in the face of reason. There is a particular extension that can be invoked to supply an explanation of certain observations that are difficult to explain convincingly in any other way. It sometimes happens that when a child is brought to a child guidance clinic with a history of stealing in his home, his parents, who beyond any doubt are seriously distressed by this behaviour, are found on enquiry to be leaving temptation quite openly in the child's way. At first sight, therefore, the two areas of the picture appear irreconcilable. On the one hand, the parents are genuinely anxious about the situation, though sometimes with a greater display of turbulence than would ordinarily be generated by it; on the other, they are provoking the very state of affairs that is destined to lead to their own reaction. How may this discrepancy be explained? Clearly it does not exist for no reason.

It is the function of the clinic to try to elicit underlying motivations in order to help the people involved. In the circumstances of stealing that we are considering, an explanation which may sometimes have its place is that while the parents genuinely deplore the child's delinquency—a point that is likely from the very fact that they have come to the clinic for help—they must also subconsciously derive a form of satisfaction from the situation, in view of the fact that their own actions have been conducted in a way that fosters it. It would of course be absurd to ascribe such motivations to the majority of parents of erring children attending for help. But in relation to some it is a conclusion that may be inescapable.

The basic explanation appears to lie in the mechanism of identification and the consequent obtaining of vicarious release. One of the responses adopted by people with an excess of repressed inclination for delinquent outlet may consist of an attempt to obtain its release, not through giving vent to personally aggressive behaviour—which would violate their own standards and go against their conscious wishes—but rather by creating the circumstances in which such delinquency occurs, and in relation to which they can therefore obtain their own element of satisfaction through surrounding themselves with it. This concept may seem an unjustifiable indictment; but it is axiomatic that many ordinary and well behaved citizens derive satisfaction from witnessing the anti-social behaviour depicted in books, on the stage, and on the screen. If this conduct were wholly repellent to them they would not be attracted to the witnessing of it for sheer entertainment. In watching a play the audience may identify themselves with the characters portrayed. To the end of time there will be a market for crime entertainment, and it seems likely that at least an element of this principle of vicarious release is sometimes involved. Hence it is not unreasonable to suppose that parents whose backgrounds have engendered a strong need for release of aggression while depriving them of the means of consciously gratifying it, may sometimes unknowingly seek its release subconsciously through identification with their child's behaviour. This principle may sometimes explain ambiguities of attitude and behaviour that are otherwise seemingly inexplicable.

SOME PROBLEMS OF NON-ACCIDENTAL INJURY
A facet of parental harshness (chapter 2) on to which attention has become increasingly focused in recent years is the danger

of physical assault against a child, commonly in his infancy, by parents incapable of controlling their actions when assailed by these inclinations. The social worker's responsibility for assessment and management then lies in two directions.

On the one hand, such threats may not necessarily issue in physical action. In manipulative clients, for example, the inclinations may be more apparent than real. To place a young child in care under circumstances of unwarranted, if understandable, anxiety may be to condemn him unnecessarily to all the psychological hazards of separation anxiety (chapter 5). Usually, however, a parent's expressed fear, whether based on anxiety, presented as a disguised threat, or containing a mixture of each, merits serious attention which should include thorough evaluation in an effort not only to decide whether removal is necessary but also to formulate an alternative method of help if separation is not considered indicated. The psychological support to the family when the child remains there requires careful thought since, if the support is inadequate, a situation of physical danger to the child may develop, while if the case is conducted with a lack of reassuring self-confidence when the latter is in fact justified, these clients may then feed their own anxieties into social workers and other helpers surrounding them, reabsorbing these very anxieties with a resulting increase in their fears and turbulence.

Even if it has been concluded that long-term removal is not indicated, difficulty may be posed by the decision as to whether or not a child of potentially explosive and partially rejecting parents should be removed temporarily. Sometimes it will be felt that to remain with even bad parents will be preferable to placement in a foster home or a children's home. At other times a period of removal may supply a helpful cooling off phase whose restorative advantages will outweigh the feelings of guilt or anxiety implanted into parent or child. On occasions an offer of removal of the child in the event of need— into a paediatric ward for instance—may itself avert the need by reducing anxiety and diminishing the risk of explosive irritability. In addition, support by psychotherapy or calming medication at a psychiatric outpatient clinic, or attendances at a day hospital or a child guidance clinic, may help to prevent deterioration. Moreover, while some parents may have their self-image reduced to a severely low level by their child's placement on an 'at risk' register, others may possibly be rendered more secure by the support thus provided.

On the other hand, circumstances may exist pointing to a situation of untenable danger. Discord too acute or deep-seated for the necessary modification, in conjunction with a history of physical injuries of a serious nature perhaps previously concealed, may furnish an indication for removal which is unmistakable. Many grave and sometimes fatal injuries have in fact been recorded; and they have given rise to the terms 'the battered baby' and 'the battered child' syndromes.

Speculations on the causes of these syndromes are in continuous process, and constant attempts are being made to accumulate research data. Interest has become directed in particular on to the interactions within families, as well as on to the attributes of the specific individual who is suspected of potential assaults; and the possible significance of various circumstances in the child's earlier environment within the family, including the bonding processes between parent and child, have received attention.

Information is thus accumulating. But the common difficulty of assessing the soundness of the claims of research by those who have not themselves conducted it, but who rely on sound evidence for practical guidance, may prove disquieting to social workers involved in situations of possible gravity. Recognizing the existence of pointers to potentially serious violence, and assessing the weight of their significance, may sometimes go beyond the scope of the social workers unless aided by psychiatric opinion: attempts to penetrate the meaning of expressed threats, or to infer the presence or absence of unspoken intentions, may prove highly perplexing and disturbing.

In summary, while it is apt to be part of the pattern of history that hues and cries become replaced by substitute foci of interest almost year by year, there seems no doubt that in the past this problem has been insufficiently recognized. In borderline and obscure situations where the conflict between psychologically destructive action and risk of dangerous complacency are particularly acute, social workers may be well advised to consult a psychiatrist for assessment not only of physical danger but also concerning the broader aspects of a parent/child relationship and the significance of any courses of action envisaged. Fears expressed by relatives, neighbours or other wellwishers need to be fully noted; sometimes they may militate against the clear thinking that could be brought to bear on the problems in the absence of these considerations. A psychiatric consultation may then supply a usefully objective assessment.

THE CHILD GUIDANCE TEAM

In chapter 1 the members of the child guidance team were mentioned. It will be recalled that basically the team consists of the psychiatrist, the educational psychologist and the clinic social worker. The facts we have been considering in the meanwhile will have placed the reader in a position in which the functions of each of these members can now be looked at with fuller meaning.

THE CLINIC SOCIAL WORKER

The functions of the clinic's social worker can be summarized in the following terms. When the efforts of the social worker in the community would be insufficient unless backed up by additional forms of expertise—as for example when the child himself needs personal help in addition to the support and assistance given to his family, or when his disturbance has largely arisen in the school or has overflowed into that area from elsewhere—then it may be necessary for the assistance of the child guidance clinic to be sought. However, no further reference need be made to the social worker at the clinic, since the nature of her approach to casework activities has already been outlined.

THE EDUCATIONAL PSYCHOLOGIST

The next member of the team whose work we shall briefly discuss is the educational psychologist; and it may be of interest to the community social worker to learn about the background which precedes her psychologist colleague's entry into the child guidance team.

In contrast to the psychiatrist, who is in the medical profession, and the psychiatric social worker, who has passed through the field of social studies, the educational psychologist has been nurtured in the world of teaching. And in contrast to psychologists in other branches of activity, such as industry or mental hospitals, with whom she nevertheless shares the background of a university degree in psychology, the educational psychologist is at present required not only to have obtained an honours degree in psychology but also to have undergone teacher training, spent a minimum of two years in full-time qualified teaching, and to have taken a one-year course of post-graduate training in educational psychology and passed the prescribed examination qualification in this field.

Educational psychologists commonly work in two fields concurrently—the school psychological service and the child guidance clinic. In the main sweep of its professional activities and in its essential administration, the school psychological service lies outside either the jurisdiction or the supervision of the child guidance clinic, functioning as an independent entity without involving the clinic's opinions or its services in its routine activities. Its essential and ideal relationship with the child guidance service is thus one of amicable independence but mutual cooperation.

The psychologist's concern is not confined to children with backwardness in one or more of the areas of scholastic functioning. She is frequently consulted by schools about children whose emotional problems are causing anxiety there. Constantly meeting the psychiatrist in her work at the clinic she is in an easy position for consultation with the members of the clinic team if she considers it indicated; and after discussion with them she sometimes finds that she should use her influence in arranging a referral. Many children are in fact referred to clinics in this way, becoming the beneficiaries of the close though basically independent relationship that exists between these two services which nevertheless share a common member of staff and a common concern for the welfare of the disturbed school child.

In her second capacity—that of psychologist working in the child guidance clinic team itself—her functions are broadly twofold. One consists in giving children psychometric tests—a service that is usually provided routinely for each child attending the clinic. The other embodies a liaison function between the clinic and the school.

The psychometric tests for basic intelligence and current level of intellectual functioning consist of verbal and performance items. The verbal items are so constructed that material which could give an unfair advantage to those children from the higher educational backgrounds has been excluded from the tests when under the process of construction. Nevertheless the reader may feel that to eliminate acquired verbal information from these tests must in point of fact be a virtual impossibility. And it may be thought that by this token the exclusion of educational advantage must be merely relative.

We may usefully take a look at this criticism. Although some of the verbal items contained in the psychometric tests present words for definition, they concentrate mainly on tasks such as recognition of similarities and differences. The nature of this material is of general application, involving words and knowledge common enough to be within the range of almost everyone's experience. But as the tests 'graduate up' these common words become more difficult in what they conceptualize—though the tests are designed to avoid demanding any significant increase in the background knowledge required for successful answers.

What is being predominantly measured, therefore, is the child's capacity for understanding clearly what these well-known words mean in terms of the concepts they signify and evoke. It is his ability to comprehend meaning that is being elicited. The answer to the above criticism, then, is that the tests are rooted in the fact that everyone inevitably receives a certain minimal exposure to words, and that the majority of even the hardest words in the tests—though in some instances recognizably too hard for clear understanding by those of only average intelligence—can be reasonably assumed to have come within the testee's background of experience. However, one would expect a wide variation in their understanding by different individuals, dependent on the variations in their intelligence levels. This is in fact the case. The tests largely make their demands on the degree of understanding that can be brought to bear on known everyday words.

Performance tests for intelligence are similarly basic in their demands. Essentially they consist of an examination of the child's capacity to appreciate whether or not shapes relate to one another. Again, the concepts entailed in the recognition of spatial relationships will, up to the ceiling of the demands built into these tests, already have been amply instilled into the child by his acquisition of the common skills of ordinary living. Even the hardest performance tasks do not require special experience in the fields of manual manipulation or spatial comprehension. In summary, therefore, both verbal and performance tests should rest on a low ceiling of learning experience, but they should elicit increasingly high ceilings of innate ability. Hence while it is obviously impossible to construct questions whose answers will be entirely free from the influence of background knowledge and circumstances, nevertheless this aspect is kept to a level that in practice has minimal significance.

The only other area of the psychometric testing carried out by the educational psychologist to which we shall address ourselves before passing to a consideration of her broader communicative functions is her task of looking for psychometric evidence of brain damage. In chapter 4 we consider a few of the causes of brain damage and look at some of its grosser effects on behaviour. Often brain damage may be suspected because of the gross disturbances of conduct and attitudes to which it has given rise. But sometimes subtler evidence of its presence may emerge from the more finely calibrated data observed by the educational psychologist during psychometric testing.

The psychometic procedures designed to elicit evidence of brain damage in children necessarily rest on different principles from those that obtain in adult work, since the key to assessment of brain damage in adults lies in the comparison between observations about certain mental functions seen at the present time and those that are assumed to have been present at the time when the brain was undamaged. However, a child has not yet reached a stage of development at which any such comparisons can be solidly drawn. The time-scale available for assessment purposes while he is still in this early phase of life naturally does not provide for comparisons based on retrospective assumptions. Insufficient time will have elapsed to permit the use of this principle. In any case the damage may have occurred at the stage when the verbal knowledge that would have been evolved was still only being acquired.

That verbal knowledge should have been already laid down adequately, uninterrupted by brain damage, is an essential prerequisite in those methods of assessment of organic deterioration that are used in adult work. In children, for these reasons, different principles are required. A common and well known test that rests on these alternative principles is the Bender Gestalt test. This test, and any related procedures, have at their foundation the fact that damage to the brain, or at least to its surface area, the cerebral cortex, is apt to produce impairment of the sufferer's capacity for perceptual organization. This impairment may be reflected in a reduced capacity to copy spatial relationships, revealing itself by the testee's failure to copy correctly the prescribed diagrams. By contrast with the system for elucidation of brain damage in adults, here it is the child's capacity to comprehend and reproduce relationships exclusively in the visual field that is examined. And comparisons with previous levels of ability are not required.

The nature and degree of any inability for reproduction in this test may point to the presence of damage to the brain. But it must not be assumed that these findings necessarily provide a black-and-white answer to the question of whether or not brain damage is present. They carry inevitable uncertainties, which are broadly comparable with those relating to the findings of electroencephalography. On occasions they can be regarded as specific; in some cases their suggestive value is strong; and often their interpretation can only be a matter of considerable doubt.

These findings must therefore be employed only in conjunction with a thorough evaluation of the clinical and social circumstances relating to the problem for whose elucidation they have been used; and in the main they are confirmatory rather than unequivocally diagnostic in themselves. Nevertheless this confirmation can be very helpful. And in those borderline cases in which the diagnosis turns on uncertain clinical inferences, perhaps arrived at through inadequate evidence or personal predilection, psychometric features consistent with brain damage may tilt the diagnostic scales in the right direction, supplying a worthwhile addition both as a source of removal of misunderstanding of the child's behaviour and sometimes as a practical basis on which to provide skilled management for his difficulties—such as remedial teaching for any perceptual anomalies that may have been found. And, as always, the sooner the essential problem is tangibly uncovered and acted upon, the greater will be the benefits likely to accrue.

The educational psychologist's liaison functions between school and clinic are conducted in both directions.

It sometimes happens, for example, that the educational psychologist is able to bring to the notice of the members of the team the various points of diagnostic and therapeutic importance that have come to light at school. They might well have remained unknown to the family doctor or members of the clinic team if no such system for conveying this information to the clinic through the educational psychologist had been available.

Thus a timid child referred to the clinic because of poor concentration at school may deny any problems at home; and his parents too may not have recognized that he is cowed or withdrawn in the family. Indeed, they may have blamed the school for his poor progress, while understandably omitting to mention to the clinic those features of home insecurity which they themselves had not detected or had not recognized as significant. The school's observations, transmitted to the clinic via its educational psychologist, concerning for example the child's difficulty in facing up to situations at school, social as well as academic, can then be of considerable help to all concerned in recognizing the true nature of the difficulty and the most significant areas of its expression.

The realities uncovered by the psychologist's visit to schools vary. She may uncover the fact that a child is happy at the school though miserable at home; or miserable at school while happy at home. In the latter case, the school can be alerted to the need to search for possible sources of his insecurity in relation to its own environment. In the former, the factors within the family may benefit from re-examination by the clinic, in cooperation with the parents.

Many observations can thus be made from which the impressions previously gained can then be assessed more realistically, usefully complementing any history obtained from other sources. Parents may be reassured to know that the child is more successful and in less intractable difficulty at school than he himself, and they too, had supposed. On the other hand, they may be equally relieved to know, when his problems do indeed exist within his school life, that the school has now been made more clearly aware of his difficulties there and has thus become better placed to try to help. Often the psychometric assessment made as a result of a child's referral to a child guidance clinic will reveal him to have a lower level of ability than has been fully realized either at school or at home. Educational rearrangements and alteration of family attitudes made on the basis of this finding alone may lead to a striking improvement in his general insecurity.

When children are referred to a child guidance clinic the psychologist does not necessarily visit the school in connection with each child. Testing in the clinic often suffices. But every case needs to be approached on its own merit, and sometimes, with the parents' agreement, the educational psychologist may communicate with the school. The advice the psychologist gives the school may relate either to the academic or the psychological aspects of management, though in practice it is seldom that the two can be considered in isolation since they commonly impinge on one another actively, intimately and significantly.

A simple commentary on the educational psychologist's help in the psychological sphere has been given. In the academic sphere, the psychologist's advice rests both on data derived from the testing of intellectual functions, and also on any emotional insecurity found from special personality tests when indicated. She will need to assess whether any emotional disturbance is the cause or the effect of the academic difficulty. She will try to determine the duration of this difficulty, its severity, and the prospect of response to the appropriate methods of psychological help in those cases of academic underfunctioning in which emotional disturbance appears to be playing a causal part. If the latter influence seems likely, the views of the other members of the clinic team can be of considerable value, and may indicate a referral for fuller investigation at the clinic.

A wide range of scholastic failings may require the educational psychologist's special expertise. Sometimes there is a general poverty of academic grasp, reflecting a poor general intelligence subsequently revealed by psychometric test results and recognized by the psychologist to be a true indication of low basic ability. In the absence of these tests the full extent of the child's intrinsic general intelligence, or any specific disabilities such as forms of dyslexia, could not have been appreciated.

In other cases it may be felt that the test results are on the contrary an underestimate of innate ability, which has been partially submerged under emotional disturbances or has failed to fructify fully through cultural deprivations. Often a child has become severely 'emotionally blocked' in a particular subject, for instance as a result of having missed school or of having been psychologically disturbed during stages crucial to the further understanding of the subject in question; or indeed through having acquired for any reason an excessive anxiety about the subject and a consequent aversion to it. At times an academic 'block' may have arisen through a child's early difficulty in relating to a particular teacher—sometimes on a basis of predetermined factors of a symbolic nature originating elsewhere—with whom the scholastic subject-matter then became unpleasantly identified and therefore progressively distasteful and incomprehensible. The psychometric tests may then reveal hidden abilities.

In some instances the child will be found to have reacted to his failure by antisocial reactions that incited so much social and family disapproval that these secondary consequences added their own further force in precipitating a process of academic failures and disrepute. Intercession by the psychologist on behalf of the disliked child, backed up with appropriate explanations to parents and teachers of the origins of his difficulties, may then remove at least this factor.

Quite apart from any general psychological advice for management in the classroom that may be passed on by the psychologist, such as a child's special need for encouragement or his resentment of forms of approach which he has hitherto left unexpressed and which has remained unrecognized, assistance to teachers in devising remedial teaching schemes and educational techniques for children with difficulties in special subjects revealed by psychometric testing may help. Severe and incapacitating reading difficulty is an outstanding example.

Inexperienced teachers, perhaps in the first year of their work, may also be helped through talking to the psychologist, who will have years of teaching experience behind her, on methods of handling the remainder of a class in which a disturbed child has been creating problems of psychological 'infection'. And on occasions help may even be given in preventing difficulties in relationships amongst members of the staff themselves if they go awry as a result of the anxieties and uncertainties which emotionally disturbed children can so easily cause amongst those who have their interests at heart but who nevertheless so often find themselves frustrated at every turn.

It will now have become clear why a background of teaching is insisted on as an essential prerequisite for the educational psychologist's work at the clinic. Apart from the need for her to be conversant with the difficulties of children in relation to their school work, and with the attitudes of parents towards schools and of schools towards parents, the psychologist can only be accepted by members of the teaching profession as able to advise on the management of disturbed children in realistic terms if she herself has first served within their own ranks. Only by personal experience of the problems of schools attempting to cope with an emotionally disturbed child can the psychologist appreciate the practicability or otherwise of any recommendations she may make. And only by viewing these problems within the broader context of the psychologist's own frame of reference can the teacher become able to orientate herself to the fullest advantage of the child.

THE PSYCHIATRIST

We can conclude this short survey of the functions of the clinic personnel by reference to the work of the psychiatrist.

It is usually a psychiatrist who holds the position of director of the child guidance clinic, and it is on to the psychiatrist that the ultimate responsibility for both the overall assessment of the child's problems and that of the family will then fall, together with the task of coordinating a plan of therapeutic management in collaboration with the educational psychologist, the psychiatric social worker, and any other colleagues.

In addition, it is the psychiatrist's function, again in consultation with relevant colleagues, including those in the administrative spheres of medicine and education, to look at the clinic's resources and to present a reasoned case of need to the administrators when increases in staff and services are required. The need for cooperation between clinicians familiar with the local incidence and nature of the various clinical and educational problems, and the administrators who possess an understanding of factors such as projected population figures and the availability and deployment of finances is self-evident.

The subject of psychiatric resources is dealt with in chapter 5. All that will be remarked here, therefore, is that in addition to watching the likely future needs for staff and service increases, the psychiatrist is also concerned to ensure that the requests for them are made at an appropriate stage in the administrative and financial year.

In dealing with the problems of each child and family, ideally the psychiatrist should begin with the maximum information that can have been made available. Not only should the psychiatrist be acquainted at the outset with the features that gave rise to the referral, but this data should whenever possible be enriched and illuminated by information supplied by the educational psychologist, the psychiatric social worker, and any other worker whose contribution may serve to enlarge the clinical picture. The sequence of these contributions cannot be laid down rigidly; but in general the more information the team has available to discuss at the initial assessment, the better will be the prospects of achieving a reliable understanding of the problem.

In the discussions between the members of the team the good psychiatrist does not jump to a fixed conclusion, and is fully prepared when necessary to modify or even abrogate any first impressions in the light of observations or suggestions put forward by other members of the team. Any child psychiatrist unwilling to take full note of contrary views presented by others would drastically limit the value of the work done by the clinic.

Even the views of a very junior student of social work may on occasions have much to offer; and a change of opinion may well become indicated on this basis. Moreover, the psychiatrist's function vis-à-vis students is as far as possible to leave them feeling encouraged and not denigrated. There is no place for grandiosity in child guidance clinics. But in scrutinizing all the reports available, listening to the history, incorporating the findings derived from examination of the child, balancing the relative significance of conflicting observations and interpretations, and elaborating hypotheses of causes and effects related to the family constellation and the outside world, the psychiatrist finally fuses together the sum total of the available data to form a whole which is as coherent, meaningful and useful as the stage that has been reached will permit.

Direct work with the child

The psychiatrist may either deal with problems in the setting of the family group, or on a basis of individual interviews. With individual interviews, directions of emphasis vary from clinic to clinic. But traditionally there has been a tendency for the psychiatrist's endeavours and those of the educational psychologist to be concentrated more on the child, while the psychiatric social worker confers with the parents.

In its relationship with the child, the psychiatrist's own attitude must be as manifestly non-moralizing as that which is adopted by the psychiatric social worker towards the parents. In this relationship the child should have at his disposal a situation in which potentially he can feel entirely free from all the censoriousness, understandable though it may have been, to which he has so often been subjected in his relationships with those towards whom in other respects he is naturally far more fundamentally attached. Unfortunately at first, and sometimes even permanently, the necessary feelings of acceptability by the psychiatrist may be difficult for the child to acquire and for the psychiatrist to convey— sometimes because of a sense of stigma in relation to child guidance attendances that has been already implanted into the child. Also barriers may be raised by the symbolic position of parent-figures which psychiatrists are liable to find themselves occupying. Nevertheless, when such impediments have been removed this very fact of symbolic representation may itself be turned to therapeutic advantage if handled with suitable reference to the psychodynamics and the defence mechanisms involved.

In extreme situations, happily rare, the child's sense of individual worth and personal security may have become irretrievably pulverized by criticisms, explicit or implied, levelled at him incessantly and inescapably from all the most vital areas of his world. But in less severe cases, when once his confidence has been gained, he may become able to find, as a temporary requirement, a great deal of therapeutic shelter at the clinic.

This sense of relief experienced by children on feeling that at last they are receiving unconditional understanding commonly results in a benefit that more than outweighs any adverse effects that parents may have genuinely feared and perhaps defensively exaggerated. In any case a certain price in the form of a little loss of schooling or a little sense of oddity— which is already present in most clinically disturbed children of average intelligence in the school age-group, and is more likely to diminish as difficulties recede under child guidance than to become aggravated by the help—is usually a price that is well worth paying. Moreover, a sense of tangible reassurance that his parents care enough about him, revealed by the very fact that they have taken this step to help him, can come as a most therapeutic realization to a child who has hitherto had crippling doubts about the basic valuation in which he has been held.

In addition to this comforting inference that may have been drawn by the child himself, the psychiatrist can sometimes act as a further vehicle for communicating to him in more crystallized and convincing form the fact that his parents care for him more warmly and deeply than appearances in the past may have suggested. Parents' distress often leads them to adopt defence mechanisms whose effects can only have been interpreted by the child as evidence of indifference or active rejection. At the clinic, on the other hand, away from the provocative presence of the child, these same parents often express their affection for him with a sincerity that is clearly uncontrived and whose simple candour carries unquestionable conviction.

It may then be part of the function of the clinic, after suitable discussion with the parents, to exploit this situation therapeutically by relaying these feelings to the child. And if the child's belief that he is rejected has not become too impenetrably encased within his own reactions of withdrawal or counter-rejection, he may gain tremendous relief and benefit. Marked clinical improvement may well date from this point.

On the other hand, detailed reference to the parents' psychology with the child for the purpose of bringing him solace is highly inadvisable. The social worker must remember that apart from the general type of reassurance that has been mentioned, even passing references may carry their risks of misrepresentation.

In the first place, parents quite understandably do not relish being exposed to their children as the victims of their own difficulties. Secondly, a child's subsequent sense of lapsed loyalty can lead to guilt, anxiety, and ultimate resentment towards the adult with whom he is discussing his parents.

Thirdly, the stabilizing foundations of his faith in the strength of his parents can too easily be damaged. Lastly, the ability to grasp the concepts involved in psychological defence mechanisms is likely to lie far outside the scope of a child's intellectual development. But for the child to be told in a direct and simple manner that his parents have said that they love and want him may bring an improvement that could not possibly be achieved in any other way. No two cases are alike, but as a generalization it can be said that it is on this sort of level, and in these sort of terms, that any discussion about his parents should be conducted.

The task of communicating reality-feelings from one generation to another when misunderstandings exist may also need to be undertaken in the opposite direction. Sometimes when the child is away from the presence of his parents he too makes his genuine affection for them amply clear, indicating at the clinic his distress at his failure to have conveyed it to them. The turbulent hostility in a child who has generated counter-hostility in his parents is almost always only part of a state of mixed feelings within himself, and is accompanied by a counterpart of devotion that has often been rendered beyond his powers of expression through pride or as a result of the fear, often not clearly known to himself at that stage, that an intensification of his sense of rejection could ensue from any rebuff his approach might receive.

But he will sometimes express these feelings to the psychiatrist quite freely. And when this information is passed back to the parents they may be very surprised, touched, and relieved to discover that the child really cares. Again, improvement may be set in train with this disclosure. And as the child gradually unburdens himself at the clinic there may come the release of a previously inhibited ability to perceive the loving qualities that increasingly reveal themselves in his parents' attitudes; and a corresponding reduction of his sense of inadequacy—and any associated reactions of hostility, anxiety, incompetence and morbid attention seeking—may then occur.

Sometimes the psychiatrist approaches the child predominantly by conversational methods—though on a much more flexible and adaptable basis than that of the pre-determined questions of the psychometric techniques. This process must often be slow, since unwise attempts to force discussions of painful material, or to prolong an interview already stilted by over-contrived effort, may cause resistance or disturbance which renders future progress more difficult or impossible. But if these dangers are avoided, some degree of progress is usually achieved, provided that rapport is established and impatience restrained.

In other circumstances—if a child is too young or unintelligent or emotionally disturbed to engage in the relatively abstract concepts involved in verbal interchange—various forms of 'art' such as play or drawings may be employed. In play, for example, where family figures may be symbolized by the toys, much that is of diagnostic significance—perhaps even at variance with the child's stated feelings—may be revealed. The pressure with which a child plays may itself be illuminating, indicating the existence of underlying tension hitherto unsuspected in the light of inhibitions and inertia shown in all other directions. Moreover, play may serve as a medium for badly-needed abreactive release which cannot be made available elsewhere.

Work with the family as a group

In addition to the psychiatrist's direct involvement with the child, the system of interviewing family groups, sometimes run in harness with interviews with the family members individually, has come into increasing prominence over the years. Its exploratory and therapeutic advantages may not occur immediately, though they may be surprisingly effective. The strength of the group tends to be more than that of each of its parts, and thus encouragement may gradually become acquired within this setting when other methods have repeatedly failed to confer it.

Any distinction between the exploratory and therapeutic functions of the family group would be an artificial dichotomy. The insight which the family begins to receive about each member of the group may sometimes be used for further exploration, though often through questions spontaneously posed for group consideration by the members themselves rather than through direct references by the therapist to the facts and reactions observed amongst the group. Frequently the situation merely supplies a milieu within which the members obtain self-awareness without any formal information being imparted by the therapist; and it is this awareness—which arises as part of the general exploratory process—that is one of the therapeutic agents. At other times direct comments can usefully be made by the therapist, for example in drawing attention to a particular individual's reactions or in commenting on the contradictory nature of statements made by different members of the family.

An advantage of well conducted group treatment lies in the greater likelihood that the family's emotional drive may be retained within the family itself, there to be made use of in its own setting rather than directed outside the family on to the therapist and thus to some extent dissipated from its natural sphere. Within the family this drive may usefully act to highlight the patterns of relationship.

The number of patterns that may occur are as infinite as the uniqueness of the individuals comprising the group and as complex as the relationships between them. Yet a number of quite simple but highly significant findings often present themselves to the therapist, to other members of the group, and to those members who are themselves displaying them—initially sometimes without any awareness of their significance but ultimately with a useful development of insight and a valuable release of emotional tension.

Here are some simple examples. Family members may vie with one another for attention, and it may perhaps transpire that in earlier life serious problems of sibling rivalry existed. But in the process they may learn for the first time the arts of sharing attention, of tolerating the frustration that follows from the inability to obtain it, and of withstanding the trauma of being misunderstood. Their horizons may be widened by recognition of the different approaches that different people will bring to the same problem. Those members who at individual interview have adopted a front of belligerence may portray in the group situation a reaction of cowed docility that belies the attributes with which they previously misled both themselves and those to whom they talked on an individual basis; while those who at individual interview appeared self-effacing and quiet may in the group situation reveal direct evidence of self-assertiveness whose underlying presence could previously have been inferred only in terms of theoretical postulates.

There are many directions in which the family members' psychological self-awareness may be facilitated by the greater social self-consciousness due to the presence of a stranger in their midst, and in which there may arise an increased sharpness of many of their perceptions. They may come to realize that their normal mode of conversation is to shout at rather than to listen to one another. One member may repeatedly answer on behalf of another person, or may repeatedly belittle one or more of the family with an irrationality that will eventually dawn. A particular child may sometimes be found to be placed in the position of a mother figure, while the mother passively accepts, or perhaps overtly contrives to ensure, that the child takes over the role that she herself should occupy; or it may become manifest that the child enters into collusion to bring about this situation or another that is equally significant in the parent/child relationship. The attitudes of siblings in aligning themselves with or against a child who symbolizes the parent's function may then serve to declare the presence of psychological material that would not have come to light without the opportunity for group observation.

The existence of favourites or scapegoats not hitherto recognized or admitted, and on to whom emotions from other sources are being unknowingly projected, may come to light far more quickly and vividly than under other systems of exploration. Arguments between parents about methods of handling their children, previously only suspected, may need the presence of the children themselves to galvanize them into frank manifestation, perhaps additionally revealing a child's tendency to take sides with one parent or the other—even to the near-exclusion of a parent. And not only may rifts between the parents become clear. An unhealthy form of unity between them that comprises a psychological exclusion of one or more of the children may be adduced.

From observations made when the family are together there can thus emerge directly, or through symbolic manifestation, all manner of underlying difficulties significant to the surface symptoms. But other types of groups may also prove valuable in child guidance practice.

A good example is to be seen within a group of mothers all of whom have children with emotional difficulties, or who are likely to develop difficulties if these mothers' problems are not eased. These mothers may for instance gain harmless release of their tensions by expressing their feelings of anger against one another, rather than directing them on to their children. Moreover they may come to realize that they are not the only mothers with strongly hostile feelings towards their children and others, and thereby acquire an element of improved self-regard that can be highly beneficial. Sometimes they may then become able to accept criticism from other mothers—erstwhile 'failures' who finally succeeded—receiving useful insight in consequence, while still unable to accept such criticisms from any other person. They may also derive great encouragement from learning of these mothers' successes, which even if only intermittent were nevertheless achieved by parents who were previously submerged almost continuously under difficulties comparable with their own.

Any interest or admiration which other mothers express towards the children of their fellow group members at the end of the session may bring into the latters' own awareness their basically accepting feelings towards their own children, which under the impact of all their difficulties they had perhaps become prone to dissociate from their conscious attitudes of mind and behaviour. And whether group-work is with families, with mothers, adolescents or indeed with toddlers, and whether it is carried out by a psychiatrist or by a social worker with special understanding of this form of work—and whether by an individual alone or working with a co-therapist—its contribution to the relief of the emotional disturbances of childhood has stood the test of time and without doubt is here to stay.

Helping with adolescence

The terminal stages of childhood, like those of its outset, are particularly prone to cause difficulties. But in general they too can often be largely averted by timely understanding and a resulting good management. The adolescent age group often presents problems of its own because these young people are looking in two directions—backwards towards the childhood they wish both to abandon and retain, and forwards towards the growing up which simultaneously attracts and repels. At one moment the young adolescent may behave and feel as a child, while in the next he may emulate, and even to a considerable if embryonic extent embody, the qualities of an adult.

Parents irritated by the spuriously adult nature of some of the attributes of early adolescence often fail to recognize that in this transitional period there lies beneath the attempts to denigrate the older generation an anxious child. Each of these components requires support and understanding. It is important therefore for parents to respect the adolescents' underlying anxieties and foster his developing desire for adult attributes rather than belittle it because of its sometimes offensive or threatening quality and discard its value as premature because it violates their own sense of status. If able to cast their minds back to their own adolescence they will often recall that they too passed through a phase of similar anxieties and comparable mechanisms designed to cope with their own insecurities, including the very common mechanism of overcompensation.

As always, a useful role of the social worker may be to present either direct explanations or the less direct forms of psychological help. Many parents, who are free from significant psychological problems in general, experience difficulties arising from ignorance and from their own emotional reactions related to this particular situation. The 'identity crisis'— those disturbing though ill-formulated feelings of 'who and what am I?', which so frequently assail the adolescent groping towards self-understanding and fulfilment—sometimes forms a source of perplexity within him of which parents may usefully be made more clearly aware. It is in fact a problem for which he is commonly in need of considerable sympathy, both judicious and unpatronizing. In the development of his personality he looks at his parents and other adults with a disturbing uncertainty and an instability born of conflicting elements in his ambivalent feelings towards them, trying to decide which of their attributes should be embraced and which eschewed. And in the process of 'freeing' and discovering himself the adolescent often needs to put his parents in the wrong to achieve the 'breakaway'. But he has an equal need, however unapparent, to retain their goodwill and approval.

In the case of adopted children the identity crisis may cause still greater difficulties if a smouldering and long-standing need to discover the identity of their blood parents now erupts more acutely and produces its additional insecurity. This eruption can naturally be very disturbing to adoptive parents, who may need a social worker's help in recognizing that in large measure it is merely an exaggeration of an element of the normal developmental phase, and to appreciate that adolescents, being fearful of becoming mere copies of their parents rather than individuals in themselves, are prone in any circumstances to reject some of the help offered them. Reactions of misconceived resentment in the adults are likely to feed heavily into these difficult but usually temporary problems.

Another difficulty of the young adolescent, not always recognized as clearly as it should be, occurs when the need for social mobility of families leads to his becoming uprooted and puts him disturbingly adrift in the school into which he has been transferred. In the disruption of his school career he may find himself in considerable difficulty when trying to fit into a new social group and to adjust to the fragmentation of some of the academic subjects in which continuity of understanding is particularly necessary for smooth progress. And the general focus by the community on to academic success, frequently dictated by the increasing occupational demands for examination qualifications, often accentuates these anxieties.

In assisting their adolescent children to ventilate their feelings, adults may need help in assessing the problems in terms of the norms of today. The adolescents' comparative affluence, more advanced physical maturity, increasing social acceptance of sexual licence, and more ready expressions of the surface rebellion covering their perplexity, may all comprise strong threats to parents unless viewed realistically in relation to the changed social context. Today's competing philosophies and lack of clear-cut codes of conduct may be disturbing to both generations. But in making any adjustments it is also important to avoid well intended dishonesty. The adolescent needs reality in his parents. If parents behave, either in emotions or in mores, in ways flagrantly out of keeping with their own in-grained convictions, the deception is likely to be recognized. It is easy to underestimate the intelligence and perspicacity of the young. But judicious adaptation, which at times may even be facilitated by a frank mutual 'set to', though listening with respect, honesty, and when necessary an agreement to differ, will usually suffice to ensure an adolescent's healthy progres-sion from childhood to maturity during this phase of life which, like each of the developmental epochs, can offer its own rewards and satisfactions to the adults. And during its course, parents' anxieties may be relieved by the realization that the insecurities of adolescence, even if expressed through tempor-arily vexatious turbulence, seeming ingratitude, or distressing withdrawal, may still be preferable to these tensions persisting unresolved into adult life, when the era of family commitments will require as much freedom as possible from the underlying difficulties of the preceding phase of adolescent immaturity.

The threads of this and the preceding two chapters can now be drawn together by stressing the need to survey a wide panorama relating to the child's biography. For the social worker to bring into focus all this heterogeneous but inter-related material, she will need a skeletal framework on which to hang the details which her enquiries will elicit.

A format that can be usefully adopted, having the advantage of providing clearly classified and rapid reading, is to present the information under a sequence of headings comprising the family history, any physical illnesses—antenatal and post-natal—the standard milestones of the child's development, his general personality, phases of difficulty, moves of locality and school, separations from his family, details about the siblings, the general family relationships, and problems of the parents and other family members. Particular areas of history will require particular emphasis according to circumstances. Indeed this system may sometimes need modification in relation to the special areas of need required by any professional worker for whom it may be specifically undertaken.

A subordinate technique, which though not essential may be of considerably supplementary value, is to present some of this data in diagrammatic form as a family tree. Much may thus be seen at a glance. The construction of helpful genealogical tables requires a little practice; and it may be a useful exercise for beginners, after reading the following account of the procedures, to construct them for self-instruction, either as a series of hypothetical family trees based on their general understanding of family problems or in relation to individual cases with which they are familiar.

Male and female symbols are respectively ♂ and ♀. In normal married relationships these two symbols may be joined by two horizontal lines; but if the parents are unmarried the union can be represented by interrupted lines. Downward vertical lines can represent passage along the time scale into each of the next generations, with siblings then represented along a further horizontal line. With mixed families the presentations may become more complex. For instance, in families in which re-marriages or cohabitation exists, the children from any previous partnerships may be taken to live with the new partner who in turn may bring into this new family constellation the further children from a previous relationship. These situations may be usefully included in the graphical representations.

It may also be helpful to write brief synoptic comments against the various family members depicted, e.g. that a parent is kind and patient but feels trapped in a domestic situation for which she was not ready; that a sibling is attending a particular school, or that he has a history of special difficulties; that a grandparent was overindulgent to the child's parent; that an uncle had a depressive illness; etc.

Finally, although important in itself, this gathering of data about specific stages and events in the child's life for evaluation by the clinician is only a splinter activity within the general matrix of the social worker's wider psychological role. As a comparatively structured and concrete form of work it may come at times as a refreshing relief from the arduous function of assessing the less tangible types of material related to childhood disturbances, bringing a welcome sense of solid achievement. But it is her insight into the more nebulous factors, and her management of the more abstruse predicaments, that lie at the centre of her psychological work.

In other words, to take a formal and synoptic history of a child's background is relatively easy—almost a matter of rote when once the technique has been firmly acquired. On the other hand, to be able to recognize the existence of emotional undertones and cross-currents, to draw correct inferences about the origins and nature of psychological nuances, and to cope with them understandingly and in a manner averting the further problems which they so frequently foreshadow, will be the skills she will most need to cultivate in child guidance work.

In these three chapters a great deal of emphasis has been placed on parental mishandling as a source of childhood disturbance. It is very important, however, to keep in mind that natural vulnerability in a child may be the essential factor underlying his disturbance and that parental mismanagement may have played little if any part. Indeed workers at child guidance clinics frequently express great sympathy for the families as well as the children themselves, and feel a great deal of admiration for the efforts made by the family members, however ineffective. They recognize that without their own specialized experience they themselves would often have fared no better, if as well, in the same circumstances. Parents need not feel themselves under criticism. The essence of child and family guidance is to understand.

4

Some organic factors

In our discussion of causes of symptoms we have been concentrating on psychological factors. But naturally in children, no less than in adults, the whole vast range of the physical conditions that can undermine psychological health and happiness also have their place. Some will be dealt with in chapter 13. To these a few further conditions can be added at this stage, though the list will remain incomplete.

The intention is not to equip social workers to replace the role of other workers such as nurses, whose training relates more closely to the making of medical observations required for the detection of possible organic factors. But unless the relevant features are known, the need for medical advice may pass unrecognized.

Epilepsy (chapter 13) is a particularly good example of a physical condition, or rather group of conditions, that may have significant psychological effects. It can sometimes account for learning problems, for example. It is desirable that social workers should keep this possibility in mind, and if appropriate bring it into discussion when trying to assist parents and others to understand, help and accept the child, and to adjust their own hopes and cope most effectively with any learning difficulty resulting from the condition.

Some of the mechanisms through which an epileptic impairment of learning may operate are easy to envisage. Poor concentration may result from the emotional disturbance to which the child's sense of abnormality and personal isolation may have led him. When there is physical brain damage, of which the epilepsy is merely a symptom, this underlying damage may itself have reduced the intellectual capacity in its various directions. Sometimes it may be the changes in brain rhythms comprising part of a primary epileptic state that are responsible for the learning failures, because of the associated alterations in awareness, or the distractions of irritability may be the basic problem. At other times the medication received by these children may itself have dulled their mental faculties and led to or accentuated learning problems and irritability. This last possibility, of course, is a significant argument against an over-ready prescription of anti-epileptic drugs for states in which epilepsy is merely suspected but not adequately confirmed.

Physical defects may accompany epilepsy in a proportion of children, though they are comparatively uncommon. Special schools exist for epileptic children; but the vast majority of these children are rightly educated within the normal school system. It will be obvious, however, that if the epilepsy is associated with such physical misfortunes as impairment of hearing, vision and speech, or by slowness and clumsiness of movements that may include defective powers of coordination of hand and eye, then there may again be an associated backwardness in the related fields of learning on which the child's psychological as well as his educational welfare may depend.

In forestalling these difficulties the expertise of the school medical officer, teachers and educational psychologist may all be required. But it may also happen that the child's distress and struggles come to the notice of the social worker before they have revealed themselves in their full significance within the school or within the understanding of the parents. In that event she may, with the permission of the parents, supply a most valuable service to all concerned by drawing the facts and possibilities to the attention of the people responsible for his educational welfare, as well as through supplying psychological support to the family.

At a later date it may also be helpful, similarly with the parent's permission, if she discusses with the youth employment officer any aspects of the young person's social restrictions—and assets—of which her knowledge of the history may have made her aware. And in formulating her scheme of information for future planning it is important not only that she should remember the pathological features in his present and past history. She should also realize that the nature of this illness is such that the attacks may cease permanently, or subside and not recur with much significance for many years.

HEREDITARY FACTORS

The clinical features just discussed may have occurred as a result of factors that were either constitutional or which arose subsequently. In general, however, few psychological abnormalities in childhood can be automatically assumed to have an element of constitutional inheritance. Similarly, the vast majority of parents with disturbed children have no family history of psychotic illness. Any information about a known tendency that may exist in a nervous adult to develop mental illness on a hereditary basis is naturally worth placing before any child psychiatrist concerned to safeguard a child's future pattern of stability; and if parents in these circumstances agree that this information about their family history may be made available for the purpose, then it may prove of benefit both to themselves and to the family as a whole. Schizophrenic and manic depressive psychosis for instance (chapter 11) arise on the basis of a genetic tendency, though again only a minority of people with any such predispositions in fact develop these illnesses.

The mechanism of inheritance is broadly as follows. Within each cell of the body there exist minute structures termed chromosomes, consisting of string-like bodies formed within the nucleus of the cell during the process of cell division. These chromosomes are the carriers of genes, which are the factors by which personal attributes, including abnormalities, may be transmitted to the offspring. Defects that exist in the unfertilized germ-plasm, in the form of genes conveying illness potential, may therefore assume great importance in the study of human states. Indeed, when the geneticist looks through his microscope at the chromosomes he is looking at the basic stuff of life.

Facts determining hereditary transmission, and the details of their relevance to various types of mental illness, are matters that cannot be gone into here. But two points should be emphasized. Firstly, the social workers may sometimes be able to play a useful part in noting whether or not there is a history of mental illness in parents or near relatives. If possible she may usefully try to discover in more detail the nature of any such conditions that may have been present. Secondly, any insensitivity in putting these enquiries to parents who had been hoping for a comforting relationship with a social worker may produce an effect which from the very outset destroys the necessary rapport.

Such enquiries should therefore be made only with circumspection. On occasions genetic counselling may be of value, but a great deal of unnecessary anxiety may be unknowingly implanted by a social worker's portentous questions about macabre-sounding illnesses, or by ill-considered hints about abstruse clinical conditions that do not apply. The same principle naturally obtains when that part of the history is taken that concerns the other three areas of major importance—the antenatal period, the birth and the postnatal period.

ANTENATAL FACTORS

The hazards associated with the antenatal phase usually pass uneventfully. But in view of the tremendous embryological complexities that exist between conception and birth it is clearly possible that many sources of damage to the foetus, as yet unknown, may give rise to changes in the brain cells. Proper attention to the routine of antenatal care is therefore prudent on these general grounds. There are, in addition, a number of specific and clear-cut illnesses that are definitely known to put the foetus at risk. They can be highly significant in their effects; and they demand immediate medical attention.

Whenever a woman becomes ill, a social worker is liable to be called upon to help over the resulting practical problems—arranging for the welfare of children, assisting with continuity of claiming of social benefits, etc. There may be occasions, therefore, when the social worker can put to good use her knowledge of the effects on the foetus of a condition that has arisen during the antenatal period. Only two conditions will be described: toxaemia of pregnancy, and German measles or rubella.

TOXAEMIA OF PREGNANCY

Although not necessarily very striking in the severity of the feeling of illness it produces, toxaemia of pregnancy is highly significant because if untreated it can lead to dangers both to the foetus and the mother. It is therefore of great importance that it be dealt with at the earliest possible moment, and that all the measures prescribed to combat the condition are acted on unfailingly. Normally it responds excellently to treatment, and the mere fact that a woman has a history of this common illness certainly does not justify any assumption that she or her child have suffered any adverse consequences.

Nevertheless its dangers must be thoroughly forestalled. Of these risks, the most outstanding to the foetus is death in the womb; to the mother the main risk is of developing a particulargly dangerous form of convulsions. The latter development carries a serious chance of death; but with the emphasis on diagnosis and treatment it is seldom that such tragedies now occur.

The most obvious feature of toxaemia of pregnancy is the onset of 'waterlogging'. It commonly reveals itself in puffiness of the ankles, and, while in mild degree this occurrence may be consistent with a normal pregnancy, its presence should never be allowed to pass without medical opinion. A rapid gain in weight during pregnancy should be regarded as indicative of the condition until examination has proved otherwise. A rise in blood pressure forms part of the illness. Headache and disturbance of vision in a woman suffering from this condition should not be allowed to pass without prompt medical consultation.

The treatment necessitates rest and hence many implicate the social worker in the important function of arranging for assistance with ordinary domestic activities. Another aspect is the dietetic management. For the social worker to ensure complete observance of the prescribed restrictions may therefore be of

vital service to the client. Encouragement to attend punctiliously for examinations of weight, blood pressure and urine at the
correct times may also be of the utmost significance.

RUBELLA

It is probably well known to the majority of social workers,
though perhaps not to all, that rubella can sometimes have
devastating effects on the foetus. The virus of this condition
leads to an illness whose rash is dramatically striking but
whose course and effects on the infected individual are usually
so innocuous as to border on the trivial. But the effects it may
produce on the developing foetus can be very sinister. If it
strikes during the first sixteen weeks of pregnancy, damage to
the foetus may lead to maldevelopment of the brain resulting
in mental subnormality. Damage to other organs of the body
is also a very real danger.

It is always possible through ignorance—particularly if other
individuals known to have been infected by this condition
have been seen to have recovered uneventfully and with little
discomfort—that these graver possibilities will pass without
medical attention. Therefore if the social worker encounters a
pregnant woman who might have been pregnant at the time
of suffering from this illness, she should discuss the situation
with her so that immediate medical advice can be sought.

For this purpose she will need some acquaintance with its
symptoms. The rash of German measles is sometimes almost
the only manifestation of the condition, though on occasions
a slight sense of illness, headache or stiffness of the neck has
been present during the previous day. The eyes may be red-
dened, and a slight cough or cold may be present. A characteristic feature of the rash, which is often first seen on the forehead or behind the ears, is its pink colour whereas that of
scarlet fever is bright red and that of measles of a dull red hue.

From this brief description the social worker will have
realized that the serious aspect of the illness when it occurs
during pregnancy is paradoxically its very triviality. It is true
that while the rash lasts it is striking in appearance. But after
it has been present for two or three days it fades. Moreover

although there may be a certain amount of feeling of general ill-health during the illness, this aspect is usually far from being prominent. Yet if there is a history of these features, particularly if they were associated with enlarged glands in the neck or enlargement of those on either side above the nape of the neck, she should remember the possibility that an attack of rubella may have taken place, no less significant to the foetus if it occurred very shortly after conception. It may still have produced severe damage to the brain, with the risk of mental subnormality. If it is only suspected as a possibility, therefore, the social worker should take steps to encourage the mother to seek a medical consultation immediately.

BIRTH INJURIES

Antenatal abnormalities may not only damage the foetus while it is in the womb. They may sometimes lead to difficulties at the time of the birth itself.

Primary birth trauma is a tempting diagnostic scapegoat for the bewildered parent or even the puzzled psychiatrist. The known hazards of birth, the maternal amnesia apt to be associated with it, and the fertile but misleading psychological processes of retrospective embroidery to which it is consequently open in those so predisposed, can easily lead to near-dogmatic assertions by the mother that may contain more expressions of confidence than historical reliability. If the possibility of birth injury is seriously mooted, therefore, it may be felt that the only reliable account will lie in the original medical case notes relating to the birth and the condition of the infant at that time. It may then be found that there was little to substantiate the belief expressed.

Nevertheless, while as an explanation it can be invoked unjustifiably, the fact remains that birth injuries occur. Evidence from reliable sources may reveal, for example, that the child was born in a state of white asphyxia, in which case there may also be a history of protracted birth during which the baby's supply of blood was perhaps diminished for a dangerously long period. If there was severe disproportion between the size of the baby's head and the room provided by the mother's pelvis, the coverings of the brain may have been torn, or bleeding into the substance of the brain itself may have occurred.

Some of the most obvious effects of birth injury are to be seen in the development of spasticity—a condition sometimes termed cerebral palsy, in which paralysis and involuntary muscular movements may be prominent. However, although birth-injured spastics are commonly subnormal mentally, this complication is not inevitable.

One of the many anxieties the social worker may encounter relates to forceps deliveries. When forceps have been used to assist in a birth, it is sometimes assumed that they probably caused damage to the child. In point of fact this fear is commonly groundless and based on misunderstanding. Far from producing damage, their use may have forestalled the very problems which it is feared they have caused.

It is probable that nowadays forceps seldom cause damage. They are designed to fit safely against the baby's head and provide mechanical support without sharp pressure or crude force, and their use will often have speeded up the birth and sometimes averted the prolonged interruption of the brain's oxygen supply that might otherwise have damaged the brain. Removing the mistaken assumption that they caused rather than forestalled injury may relieve lingering though perhaps unexpressed anxieties that have haunted the parents for many years, and may in addition open the way to a scrutiny of factors in the purely psychological sphere whose belated recognition will then bring the sort of help really required.

POSTNATAL FACTORS

Now that we have briefly dipped into the spheres of heredity, antenatal life and the birth itself, there remains to consider the final dimension of existence within which the child's brain may sustain damage through some form of physical misfortune. The child's life history after his birth, which is naturally the area in which the social worker's interests and efforts will mainly be involved, contains a number of physical hazards of particular significance to the brain.

Amongst those which are rare but devastating are the severe processes of disintegration of brain cells, with changes in the structure of the tissues they form. Sometimes they are of unknown and irreversible origin. But sometimes a known cause may exist. Severe head injury, severe jaundice after birth, or occasionally sinus or ear infections spreading to the brain are examples of the latter group of possibilities. Rarely poisoning with lead, perhaps acquired through playing with objects containing this metal, may give rise to mental handicap. Exceedingly rarely brain damage may arise from immunization against whooping cough.

Two postnatal factors, though there are many others, are especially significant—convulsions of early life, and brain infections by organisms.

CONVULSIONS
Convulsions in early life can occur in association with common happenings such as teething or throat infections. Whether or not any particular child who has shown early convulsions will have any significant tendency to subsequent epilepsy is impossible to know without at least some investigation into the individual family history. Gratuitous and unsubstantiated predictions about individuals in these circumstances can be misleading. Sometimes an epileptic tendency may later reveal itself; far more often there will be no such occurrence.

In infants and young children convulsions precipitated by teething and infections are comparatively common and uneventful. Nevertheless, there is a very good reason why these convulsions in early life should never be disregarded. When promptly dealt with they should usually leave no residual defect. But the price for their neglect may be very high, since it involves the risk of brain damage. While they are in progress, prolonged convulsions will impair the oxygen intake required by the body as a whole, and therefore of the brain, partly by interrupting the normal processes of breathing. The brain can be very sensitive to such impairment. The temporal lobes are particularly susceptible to damage in this way, and the condition termed temporal lobe epilepsy may result as a long-term effect. Immediate medical action to prevent prolonged or rapidly repeated convulsions therefore constitutes an emergency.

BRAIN INFECTIONS
The brain is also open to attacks of a different nature from oxygen lack, some of which can be equally savage in their effects and leave behind a legacy of destruction that is equally disastrous. This sphere of danger to the child is the world of micro-organisms. And, of course, any perfectly healthy child, or indeed adult, may be quite suddenly struck down from this source, though fortunately the vast majority of children remain free from attacks by infections that bring risks of long-term brain effects. It is a fortunate fact also that most acute infections —however heavy and psychologically disruptive while their onslaught is in process—can be repulsed effectively by a combination of the natural body defences and appropriate drugs such as antibiotics.

The effects on brain functioning of the attacks by micro-organisms, therefore, at worst usually consist merely of delirium that is alarming when in progress but destined to pass without erosion of brain substance or long-term scar-formation. But at the time, in severe cases, a child or adult may become grossly confused, unaware of the true nature of his surroundings and assailed by feelings of intense terror and perhaps persecution. Misinterpretations of happenings in the environment, and even visual hallucinations, may result if the organism is sufficiently toxic. But the level of the confusion may fluctuate widely during the course of the attack, so that at times the sufferer becomes comparatively lucid, only to relapse into these features when clouding of consciousness reasserts itself.

These toxic confusional states, or phases of delirium, need

in themselves cause little anxiety about the long-term prospects. But there are some organisms that carry possibilities more sinister than those of the delirious episode itself. These organisms are those viruses that permanently destroy brain substance rather than temporarily poison its functions. The illness they cause is termed encephalitis.

In encephalitis the involvement of the brain is more profound. Its more deep-seated nature is sometimes revealed during the course of the illness by paralysis of muscles whose movements are innervated by the structures within the areas of the brain under attack. As a result the muscles of the eye, for example, may be paralysed, with such features as squint and double vision following in consequence. But even when these features form part of the general picture, it does not follow that mental damage will necessarily result, though the possibility is present.

Destruction of brain tissue may follow. Various types of virus may produce it. There is one well known form of encephalitis, produced by its own particular virus, known as *encephalitis lethargica*. This form is liable to have an extraordinarily disastrous effect on the moral capacity, destroying nerve cells in the brain that appear to subserve the function of moral understanding on its feeling level.

The extreme outcome, fortunately rare, is sad in the extreme. A child intrinsically endowed with warmth of feeling, sensitivity of appreciation of the needs of others, and fully capable of self-restraint in terms of the upbringing he has received, then becomes callous, cruel, delinquent and perhaps sexually precocious. Moral training cannot be instilled nor can social conformity be achieved, the situation remaining as sadly irreversible as the disintegration of the physical substance that lies beneath it—a disintegration that may be confirmed by electroencephalographic examination.

Many physical illnesses may affect the brain functioning and they may exist from the first day of birth or develop throughout any stage of childhood. Only a small number have been mentioned in this chapter. But at least these considerations may have served to underline the fact that no child with failing powers of concentration or adjustment should be regarded as automatically without need for medical assessment; and on occasions he may require recurrent review in this context during the psychological treatment, on the basis of the psychiatrist's medical understanding. The human organism, whatever its age, can only be reliably and safely viewed as a total psychosomatic entity.

5

Some resources in the community

In the life of the child, the earlier the use that is made of any resources required to produce sound psychological health the better will be the infant's prospect of successfully passing through the psychological hazards that may await him later in childhood. In the present chapter, therefore, we shall look at a few of the preventive resources available in relation to the vital pre-adolescent era, both for children of average basic ability and for the range whose intelligence is below the average. Again only a few examples of these facilities will be considered—nursery schools, schools for the educationally subnormal, classes for emotionally disturbed children, wards in which mothers can be in hospital with their sick children and boarding schools for maladjusted children.

NURSERY SCHOOLS

Nursery schools are designed to provide an environment in which a child can develop all his basic skills—physical, intellectual, emotional and social. Naturally therefore although these schools cater essentially for normal children they can also serve to prevent psychological maldevelopment, since they may help to supply a sense of security for those who are experiencing some degree of emotional disturbance. Of course they cannot serve as a substitute for other forms of professional help that may be needed for this purpose; but in any case some of the children attending a nursery school from families in psychological difficulty may already be known to the general practitioner, health visitor, paediatrician, community social worker or child guidance clinic.

Nursery schools set about implanting a sense of security in a number of ways—by supplying, though loosely, a framework of routine; by providing the companionship of other children; by giving the child the opportunity for conversation with adults; and by encouraging the use of stimulating play material.

THE FRAMEWORK OF ROUTINE

The routine of a nursery school can help to teach independence, for example to those children whose insecurity derives from parents who are so preoccupied with their own difficulties, material or emotional, that they constantly display a disturbingly disorganized state of mind to the child. In these circumstances the thread of predictability which runs through the school, leading him to acquire a reassuring knowledge of the expectations required of him, can supply a vital factor when it is partially missing elsewhere in the child's developmental life. In a nursery school such children learn about the need for routine social conformity, and broadly see the sort of matters to which conformity has its main relevance. Understanding and security may replace uncertainty. Self-reliance may supersede overdependence.

THE COMPANIONSHIP OF OTHER CHILDREN

The companionship of other children may also fill a developmental vacuum. Some children, because of geographical or psychological isolation, are deprived of opportunities for learning to communicate and share. In this group, behaviour disturbances are apt to arise from their inadequate ability to make constructive relationships. Later, associated learning disabilities can also develop, producing problems in the main school if the means for developing a better ability for adjustment has not been previously sought. As a forestalling recommendation, therefore, requests for nursery school placement may be made by a psychiatrist if subsequent maladjustments in relationship are anticipated. For an actively disturbed child to learn to improve his social adjustments before the age of main school entry may avert many distressing problems to himself, his family, and the school. Nevertheless in the nursery school itself such children are quite often found to be a much less disturbing influence than might have been assumed, not necessarily conforming in every respect but adjusting manageably with the help provided. In other cases the child may even prove to be overconformist, and may need to be encouraged in social experimentation.

RELATIONSHIPS WITH ADULTS

The nursery school's provision of the opportunity for increased conversation with adults can help to redress any relatively one-sided system of communication that may exist outside the school at this important stage of language development. When a parent has too little time, ability or inclination to answer a child's questionings, the child will at first often persist in his attempts, perhaps to a point rendering him almost intolerable. At the same time he may fail to develop normal language facility owing to lack of verbal nourishment. Eventually he may 'dry up'.

Within any of the intervening stages his essentially slow language development, poor both in its retarded verbal comprehension and in its restricted ability for self-expression, may lead him to severe and mounting frustration, because he knows what he wishes to say but cannot say it. This developing disability, which is also apt to lay the foundation of academic difficulties at a more advanced stage since words form so much of the internal currency of abstract thinking, may be reversed by timely help given from the general staff of the nursery school. But on occasions the headmistress may feel that the specialized services of a speech therapist are required; and after consultation with the parent she may then raise this possibility with the nursery school doctor.

A different form of communication difficulty may also afflict a child if he is subject to excessive rather than insufficient attention from a parent—whether that undue attention is exercised through overpowering talk with conversational interchange being heavily dominated by a parent's continuous initiative to the near-exclusion of the child's own participation, or through psychologically destructive interference in non-verbal directions. In the latter situation, if the child has not been encouraged to do anything for himself then part of the skill of the nursery school staff will lie firstly in helping him by direct instructions—he may not even know how to set about taking off his coat—and later by standing back and watching and encouraging, observing the point at which judiciously restrained but positive adult intervention may be indicated while keeping him in circumstances in which he can at the same time benefit from the example of other children.

PLAY FACILITIES

In many families adequate stimulation by play material is not available, if only because of restriction of domestic space and lack of a nearby public playground. The necessary facilities for development of physical skills may thus be denied to the child. In severe examples his activities may show a lack of co-ordination in the basic movements such as climbing and jumping, and also in the finer movements involved in picking up objects or carrying them. At the nursery school, by methods which include play with pencils and scissors for example, the child may be helped along the progression of these more finely calibrated developmental needs. At the same time the abreactive element in play may contribute a loosening element for those 'knotted up' children in whom the physical awkwardness is an expression of psychological inhibition.

The basic materials used in the play may include sand, water, clay, paper provided for cutting, glue, ordinary boxes (match-boxes, egg-boxes, etc., for modelling) and puzzles. Some of the apparatus is used specifically for constructive purposes, such as large and small bricks. Other items are for the domestic type of play—the wendy house, beds and bandages etc. in the hospital corner, and dressing-up clothes. Amongst the large apparatus may be found trucks, push and pull toys, a climbing frame and even a slide.

INVOLVEMENT OF PARENTS

Finally, involvement of the parents themselves in the nursery school system may be an important aspect. In nursery schools parents may be usefully encouraged to talk about their child and their expectations from the school. And because the nursery school is constantly caring for the child, and the mother visits the school regularly when collecting him, the school can often develop a special relationship with her.

Psychodynamics of the sort that come into the province of the child guidance clinic or the caseworker do not concern the school directly. But for a mother to spend five minutes talking with the staff from time to time can help her to put into much clearer perspective many of the doubts and anxieties she may have felt about an insecure child's present state and likely progress. Amongst the benefits to be obtained from such discussions are reassurance, advice on the child's general management, and an opportunity for the airing of domestic anxieties such as unemployment problems. Moreover, referral to useful organizations or to professional individuals, including social workers or health visitors, may be of great help when special problems are present. Even by introducing a lonely and isolated mother to other parents in her neighbourhood the school staff may contribute much towards her capacity to cope healthily and smoothly with a tiring and anxiety-provoking child.

SCHOOLS FOR THE EDUCATIONALLY SUBNORMAL

PRINCIPLES OF PLACEMENTS
Educationally subnormal children require education in special schools for the educationally subnormal.

In the official classification, educational subnormality is divided into two categories. Those backward children whose intelligence quotients are estimated as being between the figures of fifty and seventy-five are considered moderately educationally subnormal; those below fifty as severely subnormal. Two types of special school, corresponding to each of these categories, are therefore designed to provide the facilities most appropriate to the needs of each group.

The difference in the teaching methods adopted in these two types of school lies in their relative emphasis on, in the case of schools for the severely subnormal, those social skills bound up with the basic practical requirements; and, in the case of schools for the moderately subnormal, those methods more nearly approximating to the curriculum in schools for the normal population.

Schools for severely subnormal children therefore concentrate on activities that range from toileting and self-feeding at the lower end of the scale to shopping and the use of public transport at the other. In the schools for moderate subnormality, although the curriculum is often similar to that found in many non-special schools, the teaching is conducted at a slower pace and geared more closely to the individual child's needs within each class. Essentially schools for moderately subnormal children aim to provide each pupil with the capacity to live a comparatively independent existence. Those for the severely subnormal are geared to fitting them as well as possible for life in a hostel for subnormal adults and work in industrial units.

The manifestations of severe subnormality are obvious to the ordinary observer. But moderate subnormality may easily pass undetected. And because under ordinary social circumstances these individuals often appear normal, they are apt to find themselves in situations which overtax their capacities and sometimes trigger off states of instability that otherwise would not have arisen. Another difference between the two groups is that a high percentage of the severely subnormal are afflicted with physical defects. Unclear speech and sometimes even gross speech impairment are also very common. Physical defects amongst moderately subnormal children, on the other hand, are unusual.

In practice the intelligence classification figures of fifty and seventy-five sometimes carry the diagnostic uncertainties that are apt to exist in relation to psychometric procedures. Moreover, systems for planning the education of backward children cannot be based on the assumption that low levels of functioning are necessarily intrinsic or immutable. The intelligent child, perhaps not recognized as such in the first instance, who is seriously backward because of emotional disturbance may well be educationally inaccessible, if only temporarily, to the sort of school environment that would be correct if his good abilities were not immobilized by his disturbed emotional state. To deny him the teaching facilities relevant to his current educational backwardness, simply on the grounds that his basic intelligence is higher than that for which special schools for dull children are primarily designed, may do less than justice to his present and future needs. Whether his backwardness is inborn or due to emotional factors, the backward child may need teaching for a time under the circumstances that are only obtainable in a special school.

Because of the existence of borderline areas of ability—and because academic underfunctioning may fluctuate and become open to improvement under a specialized and slow regime of educational help, perhaps accompanied by psychological support for the family—special schools recognize the desirability of accepting children who fall into either the upper or lower end of the school's ability range on a merely provisional basis, with a view to transfer to a more suitable school if subsequent observations reveal the need. A child entering a special school will not necessarily remain there. But if his educational progress is badly enough blocked by his emotional state at a particular stage, such a transfer may be crucial to his interests.

Parents who are ignorant of these facts, and therefore fearful that their agreement to the child's admission will automatically lead to a fixed placement, should be helped to understand this element of flexibility in the system. At the same time, unrealistic promises of eventual transfer should not be inadvertently implied.

MENTAL SUBNORMALITY: RECOGNITION
The recognition of moderate subnormality is often dependent not so much on specific tests as on a familiarity with normal infants. If the social worker does not possess this breadth of experience she may usefully consult a colleague from an appropriate field who can provide it. The rate of development, rather than the static picture at a given point, will often be the most telling criterion. Moreover since any normal child shows uneven rates of development, proceeding in spurts, and also variations in the states of development of his various skills at any given stage, it again follows that adequate personal experience of young children, or access to it, are essential requirements. Guidance for health visitors about the features of the

various developmental stages is obtainable from suitable tables, a standard assessment system for example being provided in the Sheridan tests. The use of these methods is outside the scope of social workers, however.

If the social worker suspects subnormality, a useful procedure in the first instance may be to consult an experienced health visitor colleague, who will be able to advise about the steps for diagnosis and any subsequent measures. Assessment solely on the basis of any particular skill, such as walking, speech, or level of acquisition of bowel or bladder control, should not be made, though when in doubt specialized advice may be worth obtaining. Nevertheless subnormality may be suspected if an infant is severely apathetic, gradually reveals himself as badly lacking in capacity for rapport, is seriously devoid of a sense of curiosity—a psychological feature that sometimes leads to an unwarrantable suspicion of poor vision or hearing—or is outstandingly slow in developing coordinated and purposeful movements including a failure to play with the toys of infancy. Feeding difficulties, sometimes wrongly ascribed to maternal mishandling or milk failure, may also bring the situation to light.

As time passes these features may become progressively more obvious. But paradoxically the early apathy of a subnormal child may later change into excessive activity rather than inertia, and his absent inhibitions may then bring considerable danger to himself or others. Tangling with fire may be uninfluenced by previous experience; the ingestion of poisons whose prohibition he is incapable of understanding may cause tragic episodes if unforestalled. The continuation of general infantile behaviour into the later stages of life, perhaps with uninhibited and unendurable screaming, may render his management beyond the unaided powers of his family. And an inability to engage in even simple social relationships may necessitate a great deal of skilled attention in the special school.

Although the majority of moderately educationally subnormal children show no physical defects, numerous physical defects may be found in association with severe subnormality. Severe subnormality is commonly due to some form of brain malformation; and not infrequently malformations of other structures of the body then coexist.

Many permutations and combinations of these physical malformations occur. In some conditions they form specific entities carrying the names of the early workers who first described or investigated them. With other cases no such uniformity is found. There may be damage to the nervous system producing differing degrees of paralysis which affect various limbs, sometimes producing impairment of walking and perhaps slight jerkings or clumsiness. Abnormalities other than those of the nervous system may also be present, for example in the heart, spleen, liver, or bladder. The skeleton may be that of a dwarf, the skull misshapen in various ways, the eyes small or the eyesight damaged by malformations, the hands and fingers abnormal, and so on.

Obviously, such abnormalities do not necessarily imply the existence of subnormality. Nevertheless when associated with mental subnormality they may additionally carry their own special significance. Blindness and deafness—or lesser impairments of vision or hearing—as well as physical paralysis or uncontrolled movements can seriously mar the child's social relationships. An abnormality such as a squint, or a form of speech that is indistinct through partial paralysis or incoordination of the muscles of articulation, may be unattractive to potential friends and thus increase the difficulties of communication. A social worker's clearer awareness that problems of this sort may be destined to beset a subnormal infant can highlight from the outset his need for befriending arrangements at an early stage—a service without which a pattern of healthy self-acceptance may never become properly established. Other physical anomalies such as asthma, cystic fibrosis, epilepsy and cardiac and other organic defects also tend to occur.

One condition accompanied by physical concomitants in addition to the subnormality is the well known state of mongolism. This comparatively common form of subnormality may be revealed by the presence of a smooth skin, a minor degree of squint, eyes that slope inwards and downwards giving a characteristic appearance to the face, a tongue that is pointed, narrow, cracked and apt to protrude noticeably, and little fingers that curve inwards. In spite of their handicap these children, because of their warm and friendly natures, often endear themselves readily not only to their families but to people in general with whom they come into contact.

Amongst the physical defects that may accompany sub-normality, brain damage is liable to cause the greatest difficulty. It is commonly believed that it is only amongst the very dullest children that severe problems of educational and social management from this cause are found. This assumption is incorrect. Even the lesser degrees of brain damage, un-accompanied by the more obvious manifestations of organic damage to the nervous system such as spasticity or squints, may at times cause devastating difficulties within the family if unrelieved. The features with which the parents of a brain-damaged child may have to contend are outlined in chapter 4.

Expectation of length of life should be assessed if possible. Many children with even severe brain damage do not neces-sarily live less long, though mongols are notoriously 'delicate' and prone to infections which in the pre-antibiotic era were liable to be fatal. But other physical conditions may shorten life. Cardiac maldevelopment, for example, sometimes produces deteriorating health and a limitation of life span that may indicate attendance at a special school as near home as possible rather than lengthy periods away from home at a boarding school.

The health visitor, as the worker involved in the earliest stages and having the easiest access to, as well as the most ready understanding of, these more general medical aspects, may play the most natural part in advising both the parents and the local authority on the long-term planning. But social workers may also find themselves consulted, particularly if another educationally subnormal child in the family has previously caused social problems.

THE SOCIAL WORKER'S ROLE

Moderate subnormality

With children in whom evidence of brain damage is not present —and they constitute a very high percentage of those with moderate subnormality—a great deal of help may still be needed. Imperceptive parents without the benefit of guidance from a person with the requisite knowledge of moderate subnormality may fail to consult a doctor. In the absence of their doing so this condition may, in contrast to severe subnormality, escape notice until the child has started at a school for normal children. Occasionally even there it may remain undetected until the unfortunate child has perhaps reached eight or nine years of age or older, by which time a great deal of educational and psychological damage, possibly irreversible, may have ensued. The earlier the age at which the condition is suspected and the arrangements for medical and psychological examination instituted, the better for all concerned. Rarely the recognition of the psychological abnormality may also lead to the detection of a deteriorating physical condition not previously dealt with.

Gross overactivity may sometimes result from subnormality. But subnormal children who are not overactive can nevertheless impose severe strains on a family as a result of their very inertia and passivity. With either type of child it may be necessary for the social worker to ensure that the mother is given occasional opportunities for a break away from the child. The child may be temporarily placed in a suitable hostel, or perhaps arrangements for provision of baby sitters may suffice; or facilities for the parents to go on outings may render an otherwise impossible situation less difficult, preserving as a viable if precarious family structure one that would otherwise shatter into pieces under the weight of unsustainable burdens. Even visits by a social worker on only two or three occasions each year may prevent a mother over-reacting to the trivialities which loom increasingly large when her sense of isolation remains unrelieved, but which become seen in their truer perspective when she is supported in this way.

In some cases features such as incontinence, the occurrence of fits, and immobility increase as the child grows older. Under these circumstances the social worker should observe the family problems as an ongoing situation, if necessary arranging for the breaks to become more frequent and prolonged with the passage of time, remembering that conscientious parents may find themselves unable without prompting to admit to their increasing inability to cope.

In addition to the social worker's empathy, the arrangements she makes when necessary for a parent's relief from material pressure, and her psychological help in relation to the family psychodynamics, she can also provide parents with a great deal of useful information about the advantages and general ethos of special schools for moderate subnormality. She may also helpfully draw the attention of a reluctant parent to the serious difficulties previously encountered at the hands of another E.S.N. child in the family who did not receive the benefit of the early help now advised. And she can emphasize that even after being officially 'ascertained' as subnormal there will neverthe-less remain the possibility—mentioned earlier and embodied in the weight of official policy—for the child to be transferred to a school for average children if as a result of the work of the special school he eventually reaches a level of functioning suitable for this step.

As to the need to explain the nature of the particular school, after an exploratory visit there she will be able to convey—with illustrative points garnered from her personal observa-tions and discussions with the headmaster and other staff members—that the school, recognizing that it can only build on success, will not primarily seek out the child's disabilities but rather discover his individual assets, and that it will then try to help him to stand on his own feet in the context of any resulting improvement in his confidence. A good special school will try to nurture all his abilities. His physical assets as well as his most fruitful intellectual elements will be sought and developed as far as possible.

Thus in conjunction with the school the social worker aims to look at each child realistically in the light of all the data about his own attributes, the family attitudes and the social circumstances that can be obtained both from enquiry and from inviting the parents by prior arrangement with the headmaster to visit the school with her. With this full spec-trum of observations and reassurance in her possession, her attempts to advise, enlighten and modify anxieties will operate on a correspondingly sound and well-integrated basis.

Moderate subnormality in a child can give rise to forms of defensive difficulty within parents which are as undesirable as those generated by severe mental handicap. Indeed, since recognition of moderate subnormality may for a time be more easily avoidable than in the case of those children whose condition is severe and therefore unequivocal, lurking shadowy suspicions can produce even greater difficulties of acceptance of the situation, undermining parents' concentration over a prolonged period and leading them to call for social worker assistance because of their failures to attend successfully to the ordinary affairs of life.

To enable the parents of moderately subnormal children to abandon any defences of hostility, self-protective ridicule of recommendations, or unproductive indifference, the social worker will need a strong empathy with their reluctance to recognize distressing realities and an equally detailed knowledge of the resources available for the less dull child's welfare. Without these requirements she will be unable to use to its full extent her potential for advising parents who at this stage are enmeshed in their inhibiting emotions, floundering in their ignorance of available procedures, and fearful of approaching anyone more centrally placed than the social worker in the network of educational and medical 'officialdom'. Sometimes there is overt rejection of the child; sometimes parents conceal from themselves their own responses of rejection, and most often they have a sense of guilt about the general situation without any wish to reject.

For helping with these situations the social worker should see both parents. Often it is genuinely difficult for the father to attend, owing to his working commitments. But he may also fail to do so because he has even greater difficulty than the mother in accepting the problem. Whereas the mother's maternal instincts are often highly aroused by the physical contact and the intense caring in her relationship, the father's role usually involves these functions less strongly. But he may experience a disquieting violation of his sense of masculinity through having fathered a handicapped child. This outcome may not take the form of frank rejection. A partial acceptance of the handicapped child, but without playing with him or displaying the positive warmth extended to the normal siblings, may be his only outward expressions of these inner difficulties.

Severe subnormality

After the birth of a severely subnormal child the parents may not only feel shattered; they may feel left high and dry. The paediatrician explaining the nature of the problem may necessarily have been vague, since the causation, the variations in progress and the ultimate ceilings of ability can sometimes be very difficult to assess at that stage. When realization first dawns and parents feel very guilty, falsely accusing themselves of having been responsible for the plight of their child or defensively attributing the condition to negligence elsewhere, they may need to be reassured of the groundless character of vague fears, for example that minor deviations from the dietary norm, minor careless injuries sustained during pregnancy, or even their attitudes of mind, played any part in the causation. This reassurance is very important in safeguarding the child against the effects of the various compensatory mechanisms apt to arise when parents blame themselves, and which strongly alter their attitude to the child. And it should be provided early. When rejection occurs, it may start at the very outset, the mother occasionally literally walking out of the hospital. This sort of reaction is more likely to take place if the mother has not had the opportunity to handle the child; and, broadly speaking, the more she has handled him the less likely will she be to reject.

In addition to her part in alleviating irrational guilt, there are a number of other matters on which the social worker can assist. She may be able, for example, to impart the information that some degree of improvement, as in walking and feeding capacities, can be anticipated; and while hollow-sounding hopes should never be lightly expressed, nor doubtful realities overstated on the assumption that strong reassurance is needed as an emergency measure to combat the family's depression, nevertheless any information suitable for reassurance and obtained from experienced experts should be emphasized to the maximum extent justified. Facts given to parents in earlier interviews may have failed to register in their minds, or may have become distorted or submerged because of their numbed and bewildered mental state at the time when they were presented. Objective enquiries carried out subsequently by the social worker may help to remove misconceptions and clarify uncertainties previously crippling both to parents and child.

In some cases parents are even unaware of the existence of special schools for severely subnormal children, believing that permanent and continuous inpatient hospital care is the only system of help available other than management in the home environment. But the statement that nowadays such schools in fact exist may do little to relieve anxieties unless it is supported by concrete data about the particular school to which their own child may be admitted. The social worker should therefore visit the local school for severely subnormal children, discussing the problems with the headmaster and familiarizing herself with its work in general and its specific potentialities in relation to the attributes of the particular child. She should explain the nature of the family environment and the hopes and fears of the parents, in so far as it is proper for her to do so.

The information she may then be able to give the family— with the authenticity of personal observation—for example that the children are not herded together, that the atmosphere is calm and friendly, that the buildings are spacious and airy, and that dull and sometimes physically handicapped children are engaged in definite activities which include playing with toys designed to foster manipulative skills and games geared to the release of pent-up energy—can be of immensely good cheer to parents whose despondency has hitherto contained within it a hope for forms of civilized help which have always seemed too remote and vague for clear understanding or lucid expression. The points of resemblance of the school to schools for non-handicapped pupils can be usefully emphasized. Attention may be drawn to the high staff/pupil ratio, and the value of the specialized facilities available for speech therapy, physiotherapy, and other medical services for the percentage of children with physical handicaps. It may be found that in many ways the class in which a child starts at the age of three will be very similar to those found in an ordinary nursery school.

Counselling services may also be available from a worker who is associated with the school and has special experience with the problems of families containing a severely subnormal child. These services may include visits to prepare the family for the pre-school child's eventual admission to the school; and to this end the counsellor, or indeed any social worker who has suitably armed herself with the necessary data and given preliminary thought to its most effective presentation, may play a valuable part by introducing the parents to the headmaster at as early a stage in the child's life as may be thought expedient.

Long term supervision may also be required for the severely subnormal after they leave school. Normally at this stage they transfer to an adult training centre, formerly termed an occupation centre. A small percentage, however, are unsuitable for these units because of being either too bright or too dull. Those considered too bright may need to be placed into open employment; and the problem of competing on equal terms within the normal population may cause insecurity requiring social worker support and sometimes material help. Those who are too dull may require placement in a subnormality hospital if their parents are unwilling or unable to care for them twenty-four hours a day. A few industrial training units now provide facilities for adults who require constant attention; but it is likely to be many years before such facilities are generally available.

Borderline subnormality

Reference has already been made to the difficulties posed by the child whose abilities lie within the 'border areas', for example between the school for severe subnormality and the school designed to help those children with moderate subnormality. When in doubt it may be better for the child to attend the former rather than the latter. Not unnaturally, parents cherishing hopes that a child is as near normal as possible may express a preference for a school providing education for the less severely handicapped pupils, advancing arguments to lend the maximum logic in support of this hope. Their observations may be helpful, worthy of careful attention, and indeed convincing in themselves. But in the process of examining them a number of other aspects, which on balance may outweigh these arguments, can become seriously under-valued. Indeed, these aspects may themselves be so significant that to allow them to become eclipsed by considerations that are partly emotionally determined may act against the best needs of all concerned.

Schools directed towards the teaching of severely subnormal children, in contrast to those dealing with the moderately subnormal, of necessity have a much higher staff/pupil ratio—sometimes even amounting to twice that of the special schools for the less dull children. They are likely to be in a position to give more speech therapy and physiotherapy. And their smaller groups can shield a vulnerable and easily perplexed borderline child against the risk of becoming overwhelmed by larger groups relevant to the work of the type of school concerned with moderate subnormality—where the groups aim at pro-viding a level of stimulation that is essential for the children with ability suitable for its own form of approach but which is potentially confusing to those of lesser capacity or with serious emotional blocks. Shy children who thrive better with less competition may be more likely to flower and express themselves in the less demanding environment, free from those activities in which they too easily see themselves over-shadowed and hence become too readily bemused and re-gressed. Every situation needs judging on its individual merits, however, and in spite of all these considerations a hypersensi-tive borderline child may sometimes best be helped by place-ment in a school for moderate subnormality—particularly if infectious family distress would otherwise result. Again, there-fore, it should be emphasized that transfers in both directions, according to the developing and changing needs of the indi-vidual child, is one of the cardinal principles in the education of dull children.

Some home problems

The adverse effects that competition may bring to the sub-normal child, however, are by no means confined to his life at school. Inevitably the home provides an area of potential conflict in which equal or even greater problems may be generated. His sense of security within the family group is the most crucial of all his needs. Without it, the skill and facilities of the school may be virtually wasted.

Sibling rivalry constitutes a particular hazard for severely subnormal children. And its relationship to family size often seems more relevant than in the jealousies found between normal siblings. The only child also is apt to be hard hit, because so much of the family emotions become focused on to him. Normal children born later into the family can sometimes dilute these difficulties. But in a family composed of one child who is handicapped and one who is normal, parents may tend to expect too much of the normal child.

In such cases if the handicapped child screams, his sibling may be required to compensate by maintaining a commensurate degree of silence; if the handicapped child's appearance is untidy, a comparable level of smartness and cleanliness in the sibling is demanded in compensatory fulfilment of the parental needs. Hostility, guilt and insecurity can easily be engendered within the normal child if these demands are too excessive or if the parents' responses to his reactions are too adverse. This situation too may be relieved by the birth of further children. In this larger family group the mother then has less time to overindulge the severely subnormal child, there are more children to share the parents' tensions so that no one individual amongst the normal children is pinpointed for the role of providing parental fulfilment inimical to his own psychological interests, and the subnormal child receives more stimulation from the other children.

It will be clear, however, that general considerations of this sort, such as those relating to family size, cannot be applied to every situation. In many instances other factors will cancel them out or outweigh them. Hence categorical advice should not be given, nor should this question even be raised by the social worker with her client without prior discussion with the necessary specialists in this field. But their possibility may be worth recognizing in the process of total assessment—which in some cases may include a doctor's advice for genetic counselling—when the problems of any family experiencing serious difficulties that centre around a subnormal child are under consideration.

This discussion of subnormality has necessarily been designed to highlight the less desirable reactions. But most parents' reactions to their subnormal child are wholly loving and entirely realistic.

FACILITIES FOR REMOVAL FROM HOME

For a number of decades the potentially adverse effects of separating children from parents, pointing to the need to avoid such separation whenever reasonably possible, have become increasingly recognized. Nevertheless, circumstances can arise when removal from home may be essential, for example to a Local Authority Children's Home, a foster home, a hospital, or a boarding school for maladjusted children.

INDICATIONS FOR THEIR USE

Broadly the indications for removal fall into two categories. Firstly, physical circumstances may be too inadequate; secondly, psychological disturbances in the situation may render it untenable.

Of these two, the physical indications are often the easier to evaluate. They comprise such problems as homelessness due to an unmarried mother's incapacity to look after her child, family eviction following non-payment of rent, a demolition order, the closure of a caravan site, dismissal from lodgings, or parental separation for any reason. There may be insanitary conditions constituting hazards to health. Circumstances involving serious dangers of physical assault or neglect will require close observation and on occasions action for removal. Situations of moral danger to the child, of which incest is an obvious example, may raise the question of removal, though a commoner reason for a child's appearance before a court as being 'in moral danger' is to prevent promiscuity by the child —usually a girl repeatedly at risk of pregnancy.

THEORETICAL CONSIDERATIONS

To obtain the necessary understanding of what is involved psychologically at the time of early-life separation, and the reactions liable to follow years later, these situations must be viewed in relation to the normal processes postulated as part of early psychological development.

A useful frame of reference has been built from the basic tenet that the very young child, as yet incapable of clear thought and feeling, is inevitably at risk of believing (though in an unstructured and unlucid way) that his parents' emotions are as 'bad' as his own. At this stage his emotions have an intensity whose tremendous force can easily escape recognition by adults, because adults have reached a mature and integrated level of development and the emotions of their own infancy and early childhood have passed from memory. In ordinary circumstances because of the child's natural resilience his normal emotional hazards are passed through satisfactorily. Yet even normally, it is believed, his feelings entail inconsistencies which fill him with insecurity—inner inconsistencies unrecognized by adults and normally resolving themselves in due course without serious mishap but always carrying the potentiality for psychological difficulty if the circumstances of the child's life fail to provide the antidote of stabilizing adult relationships.

The 'badness' which the child nebulously though intensely imagines to characterize his own reactions lies in the ambivalence of his feelings, i.e. their contradictory nature in which love and hate, and aggressive urges and their counteracting fears and inhibitions all coexist without any mutual adaptation that is really smooth and safe.

The hostility which the very young child feels towards the parent who inevitably must to some extent frustrate his wishes is believed to possess a force out of all proportion to a similar situation as it would be experienced at a later stage of development. But since the intensity of these urges in a very young child is often not apparent to the adults, they tend automatically, but quite erroneously, to equate the relatively mild reactions which they themselves would experience in these circumstances with those which occur within the child himself.

The significant point is that many of the very young child's urges have the torrential strength of biological instincts for survival, which are as yet totally uneducated. Viewed in this light it is quite reasonable to assume that their frustration will produce an upsurge of anger, hatred and fear, which is of corresponding intensity. Fundamental frustration leads to anger, and anger to urges for retaliation. But in this early stage of life, when the child still cannot distinguish between fact and fantasy, or clearly conceive of the difference between the wish and the deed, if the mother disappears he may readily feel that her disappearance is the consequence of his own hostile wishes. According to the Freudian view it is at the early period of development that the seeds of fear of one's own aggression become sown—a state which according to this perceptive school of thought may persist as part of the unconscious feelings into adult life, where it can remain liable to exert a subtle but sometimes powerful influence on attitudes and conduct.

This confusion of fact and fantasy in the very young child is perhaps less difficult to appreciate when one realizes that even in adult life reactions may sometimes occur which have a general similarity to this process. It is a matter of fairly common observation that a person with significant feelings of hostility, though not unmixed, towards another may engage in irrational self-reproach after the latter's death, feeling that in some way, perhaps by neglect or by some other form of supposed selfishness, he himself could have prevented its occurrence. Feelings of this sort may develop as part of a bereavement reaction. In the more extreme cases those caught up with such feelings may even be haunted with the vague but disturbing feeling, which they nevertheless know to be untrue, that the death is a just punishment on themselves and is therefore in some way attributable to themselves.

Even in adults these feelings may not be experienced in lucid form and may be submerged in varying depths beneath the full reach of the reasonings of conscious deliberation. Nevertheless in adult life they are at least likely to be open, to a varying extent, to the dissuading power of adult intelligence. In the very young child, who is without the background of adult experience or power of clear reasoning, the situation may be more likely to develop and may prove more disruptive.

Hence the child at this early stage of development, caught between the untamed and compulsive demands of his murderous impulses towards his parents and the opposite need for their inhibition, may in a vague but frightening form anticipate a counter-reaction of severity equal to his own hostile feelings, which in his state of complete dependence and helplessness he will feel himself unable to withstand. Later, with the developing sentiments of love towards his parents a further element of guilt will be introduced into the already conflicting situation.

In this way the child's aggressive feelings at this very early stage of life, which he cannot help experiencing, form a source of threat to himself which may remain under control in the normal course of events but produce severely disruptive reactions if circumstance such as the apparent loss of his mother or the witnessing of serious marital discord enter into the situation.

When a somewhat older child is subjected to the experience of separation from his mother he may be less overwhelmed by the type of reactions described, but the general situation, though less traumatic, is still fraught with psychological dangers if he has not yet reached a stage of sufficiently clear understanding. The material contained in his misinterpretations may be less fantasy-laden. But the sufferings involved to the child may still be acute and even far-reaching in their effects.

If therefore a child at the age of, say, two is suddenly removed to hospital for example (or if his mother suddenly departs for any reason) the situation will inevitably be disturbing to him. It is postulated that in the young child the fantasy-laden conflicts already described may then become thrown out of their precarious equilibrium and come to dominate his feelings. In the somewhat older child a process of psychological regression, i.e. reversion to earlier modes of thought and feeling—which is a common response to stress in all age groups throughout life—may be the most obvious symptomatic result. Yet even if a reaction of regression does not occur, or if it is only minimal, it is believed that the situation of sudden removal, ill understood by the child, can become a source of both immediate and long-term emotional difficulties unless the most thorough and well-conceived measures are taken for reassuring the child at this stage.

HELPING SUBSTITUTE PARENTS

If separation is inevitable, the mother substitute should if possible not only be the person who is merely the most suitable choice in her own right, but obviously the one with whom the child is already the most familiar. Furthermore in her regime of looking after the child in the mother's absence the substitute mother should be encouraged to carry out the necessary activities, such as feeding, potting, and reading to the child, in the same general pattern and with as far as possible the same details of procedure as those ordinarily adopted by the natural mother.

Although when factors such as these are viewed in a state of detachment they are usually recognized intuitively, under the pressure of anxious emotions and the host of practical details requiring the mother's attention before her departure, she may easily forget to discuss them adequately with the mother substitute—with a train of unnecessary difficulties and perhaps long-term problems stemming from the omission. But some enlightened knowledge of the depth of her child's potential disturbance may help her to remember this need and act on the right system of psychological priorities even under the diverting influence of practical demands or simple ignorance of the realities.

If the child is of an age and intelligence to understand the meaning of words, the mother's task may be greatly simplified; yet the principle of ensuring continuity of pattern cannot be dispensed with merely for this reason. But she will be able to give the child an explanation in a more meaningful way about the experiences lying before him, such as hospital life or the nature of a Children's Home, better equipped to convey convincing reassurance. In other words her efforts can now be directed additionally towards making fuller use of the older child's more advanced intelligence—even though at times its underlying value may be discouragingly reduced by his preoccupation with anxieties about the ordeal before him.

The normal child who by these means has been successfully convinced of the fact that he is completely loved will usually derive sufficient strength to sustain him through the distress of hospital or other separation, and the discomfort of sickness or surgical procedures, even when the psychologically debilitating influences of these experiences appear for a time to have overcome his fund of emotional stability. With this provision of fundamental security the regression, in whatever form it has become manifested, will pass away in the fullness of time provided that its symptoms do not in themselves become a source of misunderstanding and resentment—for they are liable to persist after the child's return home and then alienate the adults' sympathies through the apparent lack of 'excuse' at this later stage.

This last problem needs to be emphasized to parents, together with the explanations of the nature of regression (chapter 1), because of its largely unexpected occurrence and its practical significance. In general the more psychologically mature and confident the parents, the less undesirable are their reactions to the child's appearance of rejecting them after his return. Yet even with the most well-balanced people it is always a risk to be kept in mind.

To summarize, at an early stage of his development a child has not yet established a secure view of life; with the passage of time it normally becomes built up step by step. But in the pre-verbal era breaks in relationships may be particularly destructive. Other things being equal an older child will often have a better chance of withstanding separations from his family, since having developed some capacity for the understanding of abstract concepts—a capacity which can only come with the acquisition of linguistic ability—he can then better understand those temporary and often in themselves innocent reasons for a parent's disappearance, e.g. a mother's admission to hospital. Furthermore, at a later stage the child's capacity for memory has become more developed, and the image of his departed mother, even with its disturbing aspects, at least exists as an entity possessing some psychological substance. This memory may act as a source of comfort and security because in these circumstances the loss is less absolute. The younger child on the other hand is left with nothing.

In addition to the age factor a situation which sometimes throws doubt on the desirability of recommending a child's removal from home arises when there is a serious likelihood that after he has left home the parents will vacillate over their willingness to continue to accept the recommendation for the separation. Experience suggests that if parents are unable to form, or cooperate over, a coherent policy for the child's care, rescinding their agreement when he is away from home with the result that he is returned to them, perhaps later to be sent away yet again (sometimes to a different foster family or children's home) if the situation again presents them with an untenable level of difficulty, then the child is liable to interpret the moves as repeated rejections and become distressed, perplexed and insecure. Often he becomes increasingly difficult to manage, progressively more unattractive, and creates the very conditions destined to compel continuation of the destructive process of frequent changes.

The effects on the other children in a family in which a member has disappeared from the home can be profound or comparatively slight, beneficial or disastrous. Whichever of these results flows from the move, however, one inevitable consequence is that the balance of emotional forces within the family will become reshuffled; and, in attempting to evaluate any benefits likely to accrue to a child whose removal is under consideration, a prediction of the final family situation should be made as fully as possible, if only because when the separated child returns home he will receive either the solace or the backwash of the situation which will then obtain.

These concepts have been outlined so that they can be recognized both in relation to the need to avoid separation whenever possible, and also in relation to the nature of the resources required to avert or minimize its effects if separation is inevitable.

MOTHER/BABY PAEDIATRIC UNITS

When a child is admitted to hospital, the situation is much less traumatic if the family are fortunate enough to live in an area in which facilities are available for the mother to go into hospital with her child. The question of providing facilities for mothers to stay with their ill children in hospital has received considerable attention from progressive-minded paediatricians, and useful observations on the subject have accumulated on the effects on the children, the repercussions on other children in the families concerned, and the difficulties found amongst the percentage of mothers who lack sufficient confidence in the system.

Dr Dermod McCarthy who, with his co-workers, pioneered some of the comparatively early work in this field, has recorded valuable observations on which the following points are based. McCarthy observed, for example, that the fretting behaviour seen in older infants and young children does not seem to be discernible until about the age of seven months, but felt that a mother wishing to stay with her young baby should be allowed to do so. And although it was found that children attending school are likely to accept the hospital situation rationally, nevertheless in the case of children of any age with cerebral palsy, mental subnormality, mongolism, or any handicap causing emotional dependence it was felt that the mother can usefully be encouraged to stay with the child in hospital, since these children are apt to be particularly vulnerable to separation.

The primary object of the mother's presence is, of course, to provide the child with emotional security. Sometimes, however, she can play a part in assisting with simple nursing procedures such as the giving of medicines or taking temperatures under supervision; and when the child becomes less ill she may usefully undertake some of the usual functions of looking after him, such as feeding, washing, changing napkins and in general anticipating the child's needs.

As indicated, an aspect to which thought and practical attention must be given is the possibility that her sudden departure from home may have serious repercussion on the remaining children of the family. Prior discussion is therefore required with mothers to try to help to decide whether it is the patient or another child of dependent age remaining at home who should be regarded as having the stronger claim on her presence.

One system that has been adopted for admission of mothers to paediatric wards is for each mother to be accommodated in a cubicle with her child, in a hospital emulation of the domestic atmosphere, each cubicle being glass-walled with curtains that can be drawn. In general these mothers do not object to being behind glass walls. In each room there may be, for example, an adult bed and a small easy chair, a folding table, a looking glass and a W.C. shared. Mothers may be given free use of a kitchen for making tea. A sitting room is also useful, and it has also been suggested that since mothers wishing to come into hospital may decline to do so because of another child whom they are unable to leave, children's wards should include enough space in the cubicle for this child also, considerations of infection permitting. Whatever the arrangements, however, any area containing a good mother/baby unit can undoubtedly perform a most valuable service to preventive psychiatry.

CLASSES FOR EMOTIONALLY DISTURBED CHILDREN

Special day classes for disturbed children, situated either within the precincts of a conventional school or within the general community, form a valuable source of help for suitable children afflicted with various forms of emotional difficulty.

THE GENERAL CONCEPTION

These classes are small and contain children of both sexes, usually four to eight altogether. A qualified teacher who has had additional training in the emotional disturbances of childhood is in charge, so that a certain amount of ordinary teaching can be provided when occasionally considered desirable. Predominantly, however, the class is geared to the achievement of psychological reorientation rather than to formal education. In the balance of this ratio, as in their other areas of emphasis, these classes vary. There are also variations in the administrative methods by which they operate. There are even variations in the titles by which they describe their work.

The community-based social worker may find herself involved in working with a family containing a child attending one of these classes—for instance, her visits to the family may have been ordered by a Court as a statutory condition in a case of child battering. Whatever the origin of her involvement, it may be helpful to discuss the relevant problems with the class teacher and become as familiar as possible with the principles and practice of the class concerned.

Children usually attend for one day each week, continuing to attend their usual school on the other days. They may engage in any of a whole range of play activities—with sandpit, bicycles, typewriters, climbing frames, musical instruments, clay and plasticine, jigsaws, cookery, dolls house, drawing and sewing materials etc. as well as with books for widening of general interests and, when appropriate, for more specialized tuition in subjects of formal education, though in many cases academic pressures are better avoided in spite of a child's manifest backwardness in his studies. At first the children may elect to play alone. But gradually they tend to move towards the adults, inviting themselves to be watched and later participating with them in, for example, craftwork or games such as draughts or monopoly.

In her general approach the teacher of a class for emotionally disturbed children is concerned to ensure that the child receives sufficient psychological freedom there. This concept is not, however, tantamount to total laxity of behaviour. Many disturbed children need a suitable opportunity to deal with their authority problems, because their previous authority experiences have been too heavy and rigid, too possessively stifling, or too indeterminate.

Psychological freedom can be provided by the relative absence of direction in play. Metaphorically the child receives a blank page on which he can symbolically write his problems. But although for the majority the choice of how they spend their time or use their facilities is their own, superimposed on this flexibility there is an element of predictable structure and functioning—perhaps, for example, drinks at 11 a.m., a fixed time for lunch, drinks in the afternoon and the routine of clearing up and going home. Rules for consistency of conduct may require that toys taken from a cupboard by a child are put back after use, or that the mess he is allowed to make is cleared up by him. The children have the necessary freedom to do what they wish; but they may be required to be responsible for what goes with it.

FACTORS IN SELECTION

Children chosen for these classes have sometimes—though by no means necessarily—been deprived of a warm, caring and sensitive relationship with parents or substitute parents. Their symptoms can include general withdrawal, elective mutism (failure to talk in some circumstances while talking freely at other times), enuresis, encopresis, psychosomatic symptoms, morbid aggressiveness, severe 'acting out' behaviour, interfering overactivity, and academic underfunctioning.

The grouping together of these children—different children attend on different days but remain in the same groups—requires careful forethought. For example if an undue preponderance of aggressively 'acting out' children are placed together, the resulting group can easily become unmanageable; similarly, groups containing an excessive proportion of non-communicating children may fail to provide the stimulant conditions to enable them to be 'drawn out'.

The history and circumstances of each child under consideration for attendance, as well as the nature of any resulting changes that may be anticipated within the group and the families of the other children there, must be scrutinized carefully by the teacher in cooperation with all the workers concerned. Thus while it is obvious that an aggressive child's behaviour can potentially cause a timid child to shrink further into himself, nevertheless inside every morbidly timid child there is the 'naughty child'—his alter ego—whose controlled release may be necessary. The presence of an aggressive child may help it to come out, since the very fact that in a small and more easily controlled class it may be possible to allow a child to act out his aggression more freely and safely than is practicable in a school devoted exclusively to academic education and character development can in itself provide the timid child with a situation in which he can relate to aggressive behaviour with a greater sense of protection and with psychological advantage. Also the teacher's comparative lack of denigration of the aggressive child may lead the timid child to develop a more ready acceptance of a certain amount of aggression— and bring him a more healthy and less guilt-laden capacity for self-assertiveness.

At the same time the aggressive child himself stands to gain valuable release of his hostile propensities by his controlled aggression being expressed in the class through permissible noise, through physical exuberance and through his behaviour with the inanimate play material and his facilities for receiving human relationships. He is now in a position to receive more reassuring attention for attributes other than those of the anti-social behaviour which has so often been his sole source of achieving attention in the absence of an ability to obtain it through healthy conventional relationships and standard scholastic achievements.

Age is another factor of importance when assessing the mutual suitability and potential capacity for reciprocal help amongst prospective children for one of these classes. But their chronological age is not necessarily the most relevant indication of suitability. Emotional age may be more significant. Indeed, it is often undesirable to mix children exclusively from the same age group. It can be hard, for example, for a child to be in frequent battles with others of his own age level. A preferable relationship may be one that permits opportunity for play with younger children, thus facilitating the process of regression when necessary. Some disturbed children already experience a surfeit of hostility from all directions, whose partial reduplication in the class must be avoided.

In other instances the need is on the contrary for the presence of older children with whom, in contrast to his opportunities elsewhere, he may at last find himself genuinely able to measure up. A still further advantage of a relatively wide age scatter and mixture of the sexes is the greater symbolic resemblance to a family group. The working through of sibling ambivalences, the expressions of symbolic jealousies, the associated manipulations against the parent figure, and the opportunity provided for young children to do what the older children do may all have their diagnostic and therapeutic value in well selected cases.

Within its obvious function of providing a 'safety valve' setting, in which disturbed children can let out emotions whose expressions elsewhere are impermissible, a vital element in the class is often the allowing for regression when necessary. In an environment in which he can regress freely, the child may be enabled to recapitulate and release some of the distorted emotions he felt at his earlier stages of development; when necessary he can receive the mothering appropriate to them, and thereby he can work through and pass beyond those stages at which his emotional development became arrested.

Fundamentally a child's underlying inclination for regression is met in the class not by contrived attempts to evoke it but by providing him with opportunities for spontaneously fulfilling this need if it exists. Play apparatus commonly forms the trigger, the child using any material conveniently available. Paint and water, for example, may be exploited automatically by the child for messy activities more appropriate to a younger child. A child of six or seven may put on nappies as an unsolicited act of play. Another may engage in infantile pursuits such as spontaneously using a baby's feeding bottle or licking spoons in an infantile manner. Children whose age would normally be far beyond that associated with an interest in the wendy house may proceed uninvited to play inside it on a regressed level of feeling and behaviour.

Their play with inanimate objects, however, is not conducted in a vacuum divorced from adult relationships. In some instances close adult participation is even forced by the immediate practicalities, as when a strong child's regressed disinhibition requires close control to prevent eruption of his aggression to a point that would threaten the psychological interests or physical safety of the other children. But with all the children the teacher aims to provide the form of relationship required by the particular stage of emotional development into which the child is currently regressed—and from this basis aims to build up a capacity for progressively maturing relationships.

OTHER DIAGNOSTIC AND THERAPEUTIC ASPECTS

The special ethos of these classes thus facilitates valuable diagnostic as well as therapeutic developments. In their comparatively free setting the child frequently reveals material quite different from that observed elsewhere. When the children realize their acceptability and their freedom from pressures for achievement they may proceed to present the hidden qualities which basically they wish to be seen, since it is in relation to these attributes that beneath the surface they feel the need for help.

Their real problems then emerge. The eldest child constantly implored to be a 'big boy' and set a good example can be a baby; the over-possessed child, forced to be a baby, can safely experiment in growing up. A child believed to be happy at school and at home, referred purely as a problem of educational underfunctioning, may disclose himself in the class as miserable and disgruntled there; but such a child may paradoxically claim at home that he loves going to the class, expressing pleasure to his mother about his constructive activities there. But his real satisfaction there may not be of the type his mother assumes. Being in fact miserable at the class may enable him to adjust more healthily at home and school, and then to express a real happiness rather than the previous façade, fortified now by the lack of immediate expectations and pressures at the unit.

In other words the metaphorical blank page is available there; and the child is encouraged to put on to it the material he needs to present, receiving enough structure to provide a sense of safety within which he can bring himself to do so, with relationships suitable for the purpose, and with the material equipment for his play providing its own medium for his symbolic expression of his needs. What lies behind his tempers, withdrawal, etc., is the essence that comes to light within the class, and with which the class helps him to cope. His problem cannot be removed—and occasionally not even modified—exclusively by help external to himself. Moreover ready-made answers cannot be fully given to the child. Ultimately he must recognize the need, and acquire the capacity, to adjust to whatever residual situations confront him.

But when he does so, as for example when he becomes more lovable and thus receives more family love in return, he himself may influence, as well as merely adapt to, the vicious circle into which his own difficulties had previously been feeding.

THE ANXIETIES OF PARENTS

Not unnaturally, parents often experience considerable doubts in the first instance about the value of these classes, whose methods seem so foreign to those conventionally adopted for scholastic progress and character formation. Points commonly advanced by parents, and indeed sometimes by teachers, are that a child who is already backward inevitably requires more, not less, teaching; that a child needing to talk about his difficulties may in fact already have a sympathetic and understanding teacher prepared to listen and advise; that children should be taught to respect, not argue with, authority; that a child may become 'contaminated' by the presence of aggressive and ill mannered companions; that the child will feel himself singled out as an oddity.

All these anxieties are understandable; and unless the facts relating to each are presented cogently to those raising them, who may include teachers, they may withhold a readiness for the child to attend. For this purpose the following further points may be helpful for presentation.

If a seriously disturbed child has shown himself incapable of concentrating at school on a full-time basis, to continue with this manifestly limited process is hardly likely to use time to good advantage. The system has already proved itself ineffective for the child in question. A child unable to concentrate cannot benefit from any increase in, or even the continuation of a teaching system which, however skilled, is inaccessible to him. Moreover even though a teacher, however understanding, may devote extra sympathy towards a child in difficulties, nevertheless, with a fixed timetable and a disturbed child who throughout the day becomes progressively less relaxed, this teacher's sympathy and help will often have only limited opportunity for expression in an ordinary school setting and will commonly meet a child too tense and anxious to absorb and respond to it. Furthermore, this service alone cannot supply the sort of peer relationship situation necessary for a lifting of defence mechanisms and the working through of the more deep-seated psychological needs essential for those children requiring a special class based on the non-educational approach.

Seriously disturbed children lacking the capacity to respect authority frequently cannot tolerate a regime of discipline suitable for undisturbed children. Often for such children to be able to cooperate healthily they must first feel themselves acceptable. The class for children with emotional difficulties does not aim to give them a system of values at variance with those of the general community. But it aims to render them more self-accepting, so that they can then proceed gradually to look outside themselves. But to do so they must first be enabled to look inwardly at themselves without the tempestuousness or withdrawal that impedes the ordinary methods of educational assistance or even renders them sterile.

A parent's understandable fear that the child may imitate or absorb antisocial attributes seen in the class may be assuaged by several observations. As already indicated, disturbed children often have limited capacity to respond with benefit to standard situations; and to be deprived of some of the time that would otherwise be spent in an ordinary school will therefore involve little loss. In addition, a degree of delinquency seen by the child to be associated with particular problems, and only experienced in a special class which is psychologically supervised and attended on a minority time basis, is unlikely to take the imitative, timid or overcontrolled child too far downhill. On the contrary, useful tolerance and understanding, rather than serious mimicry, may well result.

By these explanations parents and teachers may be helped to accept the value of the work of the class and come to recognize the advantage of the loosening up processes, the dilution of the disturbing pressures, the abreactive release, and the various other factors of value provided there. It may nevertheless be important to emphasize that attendance for a number of terms is often essential. The group of children may need to be together for a substantial period to enable the class to become sufficiently integrated to supply its maximal therapeutic benefit; its members will often need time to find their feet and work through the challenges to be met. Ultimately, however, the child should gain in happiness. And even if his welfare is measured by the parents only in terms of his academic success, they can usually recognize on discussion that a happy child is likely to learn with more success than is an unhappy child, and that he is likely to feel himself progressively less of an oddity in his ordinary school environment when he becomes more successful there both in his work and relationships.

BOARDING SCHOOLS FOR MALADJUSTED CHILDREN

INDICATIONS FOR TRANSFER

Occasionally it is felt necessary that a child be transferred to a boarding school for maladjusted children. If a suitable placement is available, and if the problem is considered to be of sufficient severity, the local authority education department meet the necessary fees as far as possible.

These schools, however, are not those—formerly termed approved schools and now Community Homes—to which delinquent children are sent by operation of law. Nevertheless misunderstandings and unfounded inferences of 'them and us' are apt to arise, parents sometimes even using the term 'put away' in connection with the child's placement. It is true that in some cases the children have shown delinquent tendencies; but often the children in these schools suffer from different symptoms of insecurity, such as a tolerance to frustration which is only that of a much younger child, a mixture of inadequate clinging and resentful hostility, various features of severely excessive attention-seeking, a precociously ponderous manner, or a morbidly anxious overconformity; and the more crippling effects of the defence mechanisms discussed in chapter 8. Moreover children cannot be sent to these schools without the consent of their parents.

The essential indication for the transfer of a child to a

school for maladjusted children is that the emotional disturbance, which often includes learning difficulties in spite of normal intelligence, is sufficiently severe and cannot be eased satisfactorily while the child remains at home attending a local school. But for the purpose of this assessment the severity of the child's insecurity is not the only consideration, though it is obviously of great importance. The basic question is the likelihood or otherwise of achieving the necessary reversal of the symptoms and causal factors if the child remains continuously at home. This is an equally crucial aspect, for it sometimes happens that even although a child exhibits acute symptoms of insecurity, nevertheless the environment may, with suitable help, improve sufficiently to provide the degree of relief necessary for the child's recovery—remedial teaching for the child, for example, or casework with the family. And, by contrast, a child with far less acute symptoms may be destined to remain set in an intractable and perhaps ever-hardening state of educational stasis or emotional insecurity if the environment is beyond the necessary aid. This underlines the principle that consideration must be given not only to a child's symptoms themselves, but also to the essential origin of any insecurity at home and to the accessibility of the child and family to effective help.

We should now look more closely at some of these indicative factors. Of all the children for whom transfer to a boarding school on psychological grounds may be helpful, it is the emotionally 'rejected' child who on the whole is in the greatest need. Rejection by parents is not the commonest reason for a child's need for a boarding school for maladjusted children. Many of these children are from loving families, genuinely saddened by the plight of their child, of whose difficulties they were not the primary cause and for the solution of which they would make any possible sacrifice. But if on the contrary the child is rejected, not only may he or she benefit directly by removal from the home pressures, but since the child's disturbance so often forms a psychological irritant within the family setting there may be a reasonable prospect that in his absence the tensions there will become reduced to an extent that will make him more acceptable during his holiday periods at home—with the object of eventual reintegration. Naturally, however, any contrary factors must be taken into full acount, such as a possibility of reinforcing feelings of rejection or of precipitating an increased withdrawal of the family during his absence. Moreover, since periods of return home during the school holidays may re-impose considerable strain on the family emotions, the caseworker concerned with the problem should whenever possible take steps to provide the necessary support to the family at these times. Simultaneously the child guidance clinic may usefully see the child to assess his own reactions to the changing situation since his departure, and try to help him through the difficulties which he may be facing on his period of return, or reinforce the advantages gained.

The statement that the 'rejected' child is in need of help calls for some amplification of the meaning of this term. A neat and succinct definition cannot be given. As indicated already, rejection is seldom absolute; and since it is usually only partial, with the rejecting parent simultaneously having protective feelings towards the child, the use of the term will be misleading unless this fact is borne in mind. However, when the home has for any reason become a battleground in which the child's presence is tacitly resented or in which the resentment expresses itself in more overt actions or attitudes producing insecurity, then a serious or at least a significant degree of rejection may be said to be included within the family attitudes.

This does not necessarily imply the need for separation, but it does comprise a situation in which a skilled evaluation of the nature and origin of these emotions is required. Tact based on experience and knowledge must always be the keynote of any attempt at amelioration, since the risk of inflaming sensitive emotions is always inherent in these situations.

A degree of rejection may be suspected when the child's confidence and self-esteem is continuously or frequently under attack. And the very existence of this situation, however unrejecting the parents' basic feelings, may render the child so likely to misinterpret it as one of true rejection that he develops symptoms of insecurity which may prove intractable if the situation cannot be sufficiently modified.

Some specific situations which the child can misinterpret

all too readily as rejections are worth mentioning. For example, when loving parents are by temperament nevertheless so obsessed with the need for perfection that they are driven to exert excessively high and incessant moral pressures against the child, they may have great difficulty in convincing him that he is loved and accepted in spite of the fact that this is indeed the case. He may easily conclude that he can never be good enough; and sometimes with this lack of emotional freedom he cannot pass through the stages of childhood imperfection which are necessary for healthy emotional development. In consequence, a paradoxical mixture of sombre precociousness and immaturity is liable to characterize his outlook and demeanour, with poor general adjustment and failure of personality development. This naturally is often of great distress to the parents, whose genuine intention has been to help the child towards an achievement of the best that is within him.

It must be emphasized that this picture is to be distinguished from that of the home which is merely well organized and healthily and insightfully encouraging of good work from the child. An environment with good standards, securely organized and in which the expectations are kind but where the boundaries of permitted conduct are clear-cut and firm, has the basic ingredients to make for a secure and happy childhood. Judicious encouragement of a child's capacities can obviously help tremendously towards self-respect; and it is incorrect to equate a parent's devoted conscientiousness with an unhealthy state of obsessional rigidity. The former is a stabilizing influence; the latter can produce effects that are severely disturbing. Occasionally it can even constitute grounds for transfer to a special boarding school where the acceptance of lower moral and scholastic standards will provide antidotal encouragement and reassurance to the child, diminishing his tension and releasing a capacity for smoother social adjustment.

Parental inadequacy of personality, if severe and resulting in maladjustment in the child, may constitute another reason for recommending placement in a suitable boarding school. Severely inadequate personalities very easily become dependent on welfare services; but with a certain amount of concrete support from these sources they can often be kept precariously afloat materially, though sometimes their emotional inadequacies require additional help of a psychological kind even when their success in meeting the demands of ordinary citizenship—though at great cost to their narrow reserve of strained capacity—is sufficient to maintain them at a satisfactory level of financial solvency and law-abiding conduct.

Within the family setting a number of features associated with inadequacy are frequently seen in relation to the children. One is the inadequate's poor capacity to think ahead in terms of the child's needs, and in relation to our present theme its significance also lies in the likelihood of situations of inconsistency of management. Thus the child may be unable to predict whether he will be sent to bed or into the street. In severe cases of inadequacy—as may also be found in families where parents lack good health or material means—the children commonly receive too little home security for their social development or educational progress.

Hence an older child may be subjected to such traumatic experiences as refusal of service in shops because of his parents' unreliability over payment, or the ostracizing withdrawal of other children from his company in play and friendships. To the extent that his parents may possess the insight and the capacity to provide him with fundamentally compensating advantages within the home, these disturbing effects will be minimized. But when this fortunate situation does not obtain the child may be subjected to the combined impact of both spheres of misfortune. The results can be devastating to the child, whose maladjustment may become more and more ingrained by the mutually reinforcing and endless processes of stimulus and response.

A most valuable contribution may be made by any good school whose staff have the necessary perception and time to give the child at least some of the support of the kind he lacks. Yet teachers in conventional schools are commonly burdened with heavy work-loads, and are often functioning under a degree of pressure which is far from conducive to a contemplative, or even an objective, attitude towards delinquency or towards the academic backwardness that arises from emotional disturbance. With the inevitable pressures on most teachers to produce scholastic success and social conformity, it is only natural that they may sometimes feel more drawn to those children who are successful, clean, well mannered or well spoken.

A particular legacy of inadequacy sometimes passed to children through an associated attitude of inconsistency is a psychoneurotic over-attachment by the child to the parent fostered by the process of erratic rewarding. Abortive and transient approval of the child by the parents may repeatedly but falsely raise his hopes of maintaining their acceptance. And although these parents may in fact have little solid core with which either to accept or to maintain rejection of the child, the hope of gaining evidence of more lasting acceptance inspires within him the attempt to do so. At the same time the risk of failure appears to him to require a redoubling of his efforts to maintain a satisfying relationship. This cat and mouse situation may lead the child to develop a clinging and over-attached dependency—a state which is bound to colour his outlook and impede his progress towards the healthy emotional independence which should be the ultimate destiny in any child-parent relationship, and the one towards which every parent should gradually work. In intractable circumstances of this sort it may be necessary to seek a supplementary environment designed to instil the character training which would otherwise be lacking, and to emancipate the child from the conditioning effects of uncertainty which would otherwise result from these incessant struggles in the home sphere.

There are various other family patterns which may at times be so intractable that when the child has developed signs of severe emotional disturbance it is felt that the additional influence of another environment would be to his advantage. It should again be emphasized that circumstances are infinitely variable and each of these situations must be thoroughly assessed on its own merits. Any blanket recommendation for removal of a child in relation to any of these circumstances would be incorrect in principle and misleading in practice.

Another indication for boarding school may arise in a child of a broken home, one of whose parents has been granted custody and the other access. The overall interests of the child may well have been served as satisfactorily as possible by this decision, and the possiblity of associated disadvantages to the child may have been rightly accepted as an inevitable and justifiable risk for the achievement of the best balance of his interests. Yet he may then find himself in a position in which he is repeatedly subjected to cross-examination by each of his parents, afraid of disclosing confidences or fostering discordant emotions, and thus incapable of enjoying his parents or relating to them. Inwardly he may feel undeserving of either parent, since if he pleases one he cannot please the other.

When the 'ding-dong' of these fundamentally disturbing emotions clatters unceasingly within the child he will often fail to achieve a basic sense of security, and even with the passage of years will be at risk of remaining immature. A good therapeutically-orientated school for a child disturbed by these circumstances may be of considerable help, by diluting the disturbance through providing a respite and an understanding of his basic difficulties, while the parents, being less frequently thrown off balance by the presence of one of their sources of mutual hostility, may have better prospects of at least gaining some improvement in their own individual emotional equilibrium. On the other hand, the transfer to a boarding school can sometimes raise more psychological problems than it solves and cannot necessarily be regarded as desirable.

Another problem which may occasionally raise the question of a possible need for transfer to a boarding school for maladjusted children arises when a sensitive family is severely ostracized within its neighbourhood. Obviously this may occur in a variety of situations, and these may stem both from the primary circumstances of the environment itself or from the particular personalities of the members of the family.

Thus, in addition to the problems posed by those delinquent or severely inadequate problem families who will excite condemnation in any area, a potentially well-adjusted family may find itself living, predominantly through force of events, in an area composed of neighbours of different educational backgrounds; and these families with an outlook and code of manners which elsewhere would be accepted as an essentially healthy norm may then find themselves so much at variance with their immediate environment that they can gain little worthwhile acceptance from the group. An example might be found in the case of a woman with a streak of Bohemian indifference or a scholastic preoccupation, who allows her children to appear habitually in public in a dirty or untidy condition—particularly if she happens to regard bridge as a waste of time or is unacceptably lacking in concern about the condition of her garden hedge. Here one may have admirable parents whose scale of values nevertheless differs obstrusively from that of the equally admirable people who set the culture pattern of the environment concerned.

The possible effects on children resulting from severe isolation of the family, for whatever reason, will depend on many factors, the most obvious of which are the age of the child, the security which he receives within his own home, and the completeness or the severity of the isolation—whether it is presented in an acrimonious manner or as the less overtly rejecting reaction of indifference. The significance of the child's age lies in the fact that when he is young he is least dependent on the responses of outsiders, so that these effects will be mainly indirect, flowing from the disturbance caused to the parents. On the other hand, with the passage of time he becomes more sensitive to the innuendoes of his increasingly recognizable environment.

Many other psychological factors—severe over-possessiveness for example—may lie behind the recommendation for a suitable boarding school. Sometimes parents comply with the advice; sometimes they refuse their consent; sometimes they themselves exert pressures for the transfer.

Any of the possible reasons for parents' wishes for a child's removal from home require assessment on the basis of as clear an understanding of their own psychological backgrounds as can be achieved within the limitations of time and available data. The process may require repeated interviews, involving the need to try to look at their real feelings in contrast to those emotions which may be the most immediately apparent to themselves. Parents' feelings and motives on this matter are seldom unmixed. Even the most 'rejecting' parent usually has associated regrets, which though eclipsed by other emotions towards the child sometimes reveal to the experienced observer that the rejection is essentially more apparent than real. Moreover, even when rejection is strongly present it is often found to be a reflection of unrecognized attitudes that predominantly spring from factors other than basic feelings for the child himself and which may therefore be open in some cases to modification through psychotherapeutic insight conferred by casework.

EFFECTS ON THE FAMILY

It is an obvious truism that parents have different feelings about their different children; and parental happiness, resentments and depressions may be related to the presence or absence of a particular child. To mention a simple type of example, if the mother has been, or is thought by the father to have been, instrumental in the removal of the father's favourite daughter from the home he may then turn against the mother. When apparent to the other children this type of reaction will cause them distress by witnessing their parents' discord. Or they may subconsciously suspect that they too are, or are likely to become, a similar source of parental disturbance; or they may wonder whether they too would be missed as much by the parent concerned, or whether their own absence would perhaps be equally welcome.

Thus a sensitive child remaining in the home may, without clearly realizing his own reactions, experience the situation as one that casts a disturbing doubt on his own acceptability. A warm enthusiasm given to his rival's homecoming may reinforce his own feelings of insecurity and even engender uncertainties in him about his permanency in the home. He may feel guilty if he has contributed to his sibling's problems by having effectively blamed his own misdeeds, or transferred his parents' resulting hostility, on to the child who has been removed; and so the removal of this child towards whom he has felt jealous may bring not only its satisfaction but also its self-reproach. And with the removal of the 'object' which has hitherto served to 'draw the parents' fire' an element of anxiety about his own exposed position may at times be added to all the other disturbing emotions.

Other effects on the family will be seen when we discuss the factors involved in presenting the recommendation.

THE NATURE OF THE SCHOOLS

Schools for maladjusted children vary in their size, the nature of their facilities, and the forms of education—in its broadest sense—in which they principally specialize. To discuss in any detail the various techniques by which these schools attempt, often with a high degree of success, to remodel the outlook and salvage the capacities of their pupils would go beyond the scope of the present chapter. However, it may be said that one of the most important common denominators to the majority of these schools is their emphasis on small classes. Another is their use of the system of house parents. Small groups with a warm friendly atmosphere in which the child can develop form the keystone of their approach.

Children suffering from emotional disturbances are frequently incapable of fully exercising their capacities to learn. Indeed some degree of learning disability is usual even in the presence of average or superior intelligence. Hence comparatively individual teaching is commonly required, and a high staff/pupil ratio, in addition to good teaching skill, is a prerequisite for restoring these children's academic functioning.

Yet even with the greatest of skill, in explaining the rules of mathematics, grammar, etc., the teacher's efforts will fail to reach their full fruition if the child has an emotional block against receiving them. And until the emotional barrier—which may be complex and firmly established—can be removed, the child will at best remain only partially accessible to the more academically educative approach, in however specialized and expert a manner it may be presented. Some of these inhibiting factors will present difficulties of a challenging variety; others will be open to fairly simple management.

Because problems arising from failures of personal relationships in earlier life play such an important part in the difficulties found with many of the children in these schools, the teachers are themselves oriented towards placing a special emphasis on constructive relationships for teaching purposes. The general psychological environment in the school outside its classrooms is also directed towards the achievement of good relationships. To fulfil this need for 'out of class' rehabilitation the system of house parents is widely adopted.

'Out of class' activities arranged by the house parents may be organized on a formal basis or they may be relatively un-structured. Many factors will determine the system used in a particular school, such as the age of the children, the predilec-tions of the individual house parents, the particular facilities available at the school, e.g. the presence or absence of extensive grounds for open-air activities, and the range and type of emotional disturbances in the children catered for. In addition to the social activities the house parents carry, of course, much of the responsibility for practical tasks like ensuring that the children are safe, fed and physically comfortable.

Whether the divisions between organized and unstructured social activities are evenly balanced, or whether there is an emphasis in either of these directions, the overall principle is always to try to build up happy and sound human relationships as the basis on which mental health is to be built.

Thus the two major services in the remedial work at a board-ing school for maladjusted children are those provided by the teachers and those provided by the house parents. But since the psychological needs of the child exist as a total compound built of numerous elements many of which cannot be con-sidered in isolation, the work of these two groups of services will necessarily overlap and involve the need for interchange of information and joint contributions to the planning of policy, both in general matters and for the most suitable management of particular children. Indeed in some schools there is no hard and fast division between the teachers and house parents. Teachers often carry out extraneous duties after school and at weekends and are as much involved with the children out of school as in the classroom. This closeness of the teaching staff is even greater when, as often happens, they have residential accommodation within the school. Further-more in some schools there is freedom of choice for the children to seek out those adults with whom they feel most able to relate at the particular stage of development which they happen to have reached.

Even with small classes and children of inherently average intelligence, the teachers will not necessarily find themselves in a position to follow conventional educational practice. A child's emotional disturbance may render him currently unable to feel, or to force himself to feel, sufficiently interested; the disturbance may have deprived him of the necessary confidence and brought about a sense of inadequacy so ingrained as to make him temporarily inaccessible to the encouragement that usually flows from tangible demonstration to a child of his own capacity or from direct reassurances. In severe cases it may even deprive the child of some degree of his contact with reality.

When disturbances of this sort exist the teacher clearly cannot remain exclusively concerned with immediate academic results, although as a member of a profession whose aim is to impart knowledge the ultimate attainment of academic progress will always occupy its place in his scale of values. But for the teacher to put into temporary abeyance the immediate demands of scholastic progress may at times be the most effective means of achieving this very object. In some cases a direct and practical approach to learning may be required in the initial stages, without the situation being tied to a rigid curriculum, while in others a more theoretical approach may be indicated. With some children the encouragement of a relatively abstract level of thought may be possible; in others, learning may need to be related more closely to real-life situations in order to engage or maintain the child's interests.

It is obvious that the relationship which a maladjusted child forms with his teacher may have a profound therapeutic value which far transcends the confines of its purely academic implications, valuable though such a relationship may be in this sphere also. But it is to the house parents that the child will turn in his attempts to gain the more broadly based security supplied by the family setting. It is for this reason that the house parent system is the cornerstone of the boarding school for maladjusted children. And as in any family, or in any classroom, the needs both of the individual child and of the group of children on whom this child is reacting require careful balancing one against the other.

A maladjusted child's therapeutic need to 'act out' his difficulties through aggressive behaviour may need recognition, together with the provision of facilities for doing so. One therapeutically valuable situation for the management of pathological aggression in a maladjusted child may be the opportunity for him to display, at least temporarily, a degree of hostility in his attitude towards an understanding house parent who, unknown to the child himself, symbolizes another adult towards whom he already has feelings of aggression, recognized or repressed. These feelings may thus become released, accepted and worked through to a healthy conclusion.

Yet in the same group there may also be a timid child who at that stage is unable to witness situations of aggression without further detriment to his own psychological health. It is clear that in these circumstances the interests and progress of both these children will need to be carefully thought about, balanced, and kept under frequent review. Obviously their conflicting interests may require the curbing of the aggressive child for the sake of the other. No two cases are alike, however, and there may be occasions when the timid child can be actively helped by exposure to some degree of banter in a situation combining tactful protection and the opportunity for helping him to adjust to this type of impact. This can be a valuable step towards the regaining of confidence and self-regard.

In concentrating on the need for security that permeates the emotional makeup of a timid child, the aggressive child's equal or even greater feelings of insecurity can easily be lost sight of. But the perceptive house parent will be alive to this pitfall and will realize that although the aggressive child needs to be given a sense of security he may well have experienced innumerable and cumulative incidents of rejection in varying degrees throughout his lifetime which will have rendered him temporarily incapable of receiving this necessary help. Although requiring management which often varies widely in its detail, both the aggressive and the overtly timid groups have the same basic requirements for their improvement—the need to be helped to feel themselves genuinely acceptable and worthwhile.

A 'structured' environment has its part to play in helping both groups; a set-up in which credit is given for general smartness and for the acquisition of improved self-control supplies an opportunity for the development of feelings of self-esteem which were previously lacking, provided that the various other elements necessary for healthy self-regard are not neglected.

Beyond broad general principles, any scheme for correlating the various types of personality disturbances with the corresponding types of requirement in the school environment can only be undertaken with reservations. The reason for this difficulty is that very many factors have contributed to any individual case. The resulting personality disturbances, while to some extent falling into broad general categories, are therefore so variable in many of their attributes that attempts at this type of prediction become too far removed from the principles governing reasoned prognostic precision. Similarly the therapeutic environments themselves, composed of such varying types of children and acted on by adults of varying temperaments, orientations and skills, cannot lend themselves to much classification that is either clear or useful.

Within these fundamental limitations, however, certain reflections of a general nature can be made. At least in theory, the anxious, obsessionally conforming type of child for example may stand to benefit from an environment which while securely ordered nevertheless has a marked element of flexibility leading him to realize that there are many types of acceptable conduct, and that he can safely be himself. Again, the child with a better-integrated personality may be able to cope with 'freedom' with considerable benefit, while the child whose personality is more disintegrated is likely to benefit from a relatively 'directed' system of management.

For suitable children there is no doubt that a school with an artistic bias, and a strong emphasis on creative activities and 'gentle' pursuits, may prove to be their salvation. However, a possible danger—which would nevertheless be recognized by any skilled and intuitive staff member—may occasionally arise if an adult in a school in which there is very little formal punishment expresses disapproval on a large number of different matters. This well intentioned 'restraint' may constitute a situation in which feelings of unredressed unworthiness or fears of tacit loss of approval can develop in the child, and subtly undermine his emotional development. This danger of passive erosion is one which every wise teacher and house parent will keep in mind.

PRESENTING THE RECOMMENDATION

Whatever the parents' reasons for wanting or acquiescing in the child's removal from home, whether desirable or undesirable and whether comparatively narrowly-based or widely multiple, the particular feelings evoked in them by a recommendation for the child's departure will have a profound influence on his own well-being, either reinforcing any benefit achieved by the boarding school, Children's Home, foster home or other environment, or detracting from its effects. For example, parents may sometimes feel, quite incorrectly, that they have become 'written off as useless', with the result that they cease communicating with the child, or do so with a lack of enthusiasm which misleadingly implies to the child that through his symptoms or misdeeds he has lost his family's support. He will then feel himself rootless; and with his previous suspicions of rejection thus apparently confirmed the results can be serious.

Sometimes it is clear that to raise the question of a boarding school at a particular time would be so disturbing to one or both parents that the subject should be postponed until attempts by casework have been made to render them less vulnerable. At other times it is evident that they need to take an immediate decision, though afterwards there is usually a prolonged waiting period before a placement can be obtained. It may sometimes be anticipated that parents' insight and objectivity will have fallen to an irreversibly low ebb by the time the question is raised if the matter is shelved. An important part of the adviser's function then is to balance these considerations and pinpoint the most desirable time for discussion and recommendation.

If this assessment of the time factor is badly made and the parents consequently commit themselves to a firm refusal, not only may they remain set in their unwillingness to give consent, but any prospect of achieving a satisfactory therapeutic relationship with them is apt to become correspondingly threatened. As a result of a premature suggestion that their child might usefully spend some of his time away from the home environment the parents may feel guilty and one may blame the other, with the result that pre-existing embitterment becomes intensified. Even the risk of marital breakdown may be precipitated. The very recognition of this possibility may deter parents from accepting the recommendation; and they may require timely reassurance by the psychiatrist or case-worker that they are exaggerating any such danger and will be supported through the phase if it forms a serious threat.

Many other disturbances in family alignments may arise when a child is recommended to leave on the basis of professional assessment. Sometimes the most easily anticipated are repercussions from the grandparents; and at times this conflict about the desirability of agreement may almost take the form of two armed camps. Equally commonly, however, the shifting of intra-family constellations may occur in forms that are less obvious but which can still produce family barriers against accepting the recommendation.

It is, of course, entirely healthy that parents should be hesitant over expressing immediate and unquestioning agreement to the suggestion that their child be sent to a largely unknown destination and to a form of educational and social life that is often entirely unfamiliar to themselves. It is usually an indication that in spite of the stresses to which they have been subjected by the difficulties in the situation they have nevertheless retained their natural sense of protectiveness towards the child. It is often a response to be welcomed. But at other times less desirable motives, not necessarily clear to the parents themselves, may play a part in their hesitancy.

They may feel keenly, for example, that they have failed; and they may then wish to continue the struggle for successful parenthood until they finally meet with the success which they regard it their duty to achieve. In allowing their child to go away for remedy of the situation elsewhere, they may see this hope fading from their reach, and may dread the feelings of guilt within themselves which they foresee as the inevitable consequence. Often, however, in talking through these difficulties with the psychiatrist, the clinic social worker or the educational psychologist they come to realize that although these fears of impending self-reproach were well founded, in that they prove on discussion to rise to the surface, nevertheless the fear that they would permanently remain as a source of constant distress was unjustified and false. And when these parents are helped to see that the very manner in which they will handle the child during his holiday periods at home will be vital to his future welfare, and that his progress at school will turn on their letters or visits, then their sense of irremediable failure will often subside, giving place to a determination to play their full part in the concerted efforts now being made to help their child.

A particularly difficult position exists when their sense of failure is bound up with an underlying suspicion that as parents they have not merely been ineffective but seriously rejecting. This state of mind violates far more deeply and destructively than the mere sense of failure itself, and is prone to lead to an emotional disturbance that is more intractable and less easily and safely dealt with by direct forms of discussion. To imply inadvertently that this type of need for self-protection may lie behind a parent's reluctance to agree to a child's transfer to a special school is clearly likely to produce a thoroughly undesirable effect. At best it is likely to be fruitless; at less than best it may evoke reactions leading to further deterioration in an already unsatisfactory situation. Furthermore the assumption itself may well be incorrect.

In these cases in which the parents believe, rightly or wrongly, that they themselves have contributed to their child's insecurity by a process of rejection—and since all parents at times have degrees of feelings of rejection it is clear that those who are deeply prone to self-accusation may easily exaggerate the part played by this process—their aversion to the child leaving home may contain strongly rooted elements. They may fear that by agreeing to the need for the recommendation these worst suspicions about themselves will be proved. To demonstrate to themselves that this is not so, these unhappily placed people may resist the recommendation—in the process losing sight of the interests of the child. Or there may be an element of unrecognized self-punishment, impelling them to preserve their distress and attempt a form of penitential reparation by maintaining the status quo—again without awareness of their motivations and again without full regard to the best interests of the child.

The solution of such problems must often be undertaken by an indirect approach, which calls for an understanding of the principles and practice of casework (chapter 3), and often presents a heavy challenge to the worker concerned. In general it may be said that if these parents can be helped to feel safe enough to face their underlying thoughts and emotions, they will emerge into clearer consciousness. In successful cases the individual will then gain the capacity to travel beyond them, recognizing that he does not basically wish to adopt a rejecting attitude and that in so far as he may have done so the emotion arose out of natural difficulties, parental disappointments and disturbing stresses. This insight may lead to a healthier and happier footing, with restoration of an outlook which even if brittle from the influence of a long process of conditioning may still permit of improvement in the relationship with the child. Once re-established this improvement often becomes progressively self-consolidating.

We may now turn to some of those anxieties in parents which are more straightforward and on the whole more easily dispelled. Nevertheless even these less subtle anxieties may sometimes present stumbling blocks serious enough to jeopardize the child's prospects of being allowed a suitable boarding-school placement by his parents. They include the fears that in a school for maladjusted children their child will be under a stigma, that he will deteriorate through lack of stimulation, that he will be dubbed an oddity, will grow away from them by receiving an education superior to their own, or will be brutally treated.

A few remarks about such points will often help to assuage unnecessary fears, which of course may not be openly expressed and may exist in quite a formless state. It must always be remembered that these fears are fully understandable and reasonable in themselves, and are based on misconceptions deserving of sympathetic and patient discussion. When they are dealt with on this basis the anxious parent usually feels sufficiently reassured to agree at least to investigate any proposals made in this way. More often than not agreement to the resulting recommendation is then obtained.

When the objection is raised that in a school for maladjusted children the child may deteriorate through lack of learning-stimulation and healthy competition from companions drawn from the ordinary run of children, it is important to recognize, and to emphasize, that the child has in any case already shown himself incapable of deriving enough benefit from day-school management. Therefore he is likely to lose little or nothing educationally by removal from his present educational environment; on the contrary, he will usually have the great advantage of much smaller classes and, at least when he has improved, this situation should provide the best means by which he may regain time already lost. For this reason it follows that in the selection of a suitable school full regard must be paid to the child's educational potential, and the selection should not necessarily be restricted by consideration only of his currently poor performance. Reports based on psychometric examination by the educational psychologist can yield information of great value in finding the most suitable placement in relation to the obscured potentialities in his inherent capacity.

Another common fear is that the child will fail to obtain employment because of a supposed stigma through having attended a special school. In fact, however, because of careful liaison with careers departments, the employment prospects of such children may be higher than those of many children leaving 'normal' schools.

Even more understandable is the anxiety that the child will be subjected to bad influences from the friends and companions by whom, it is feared, he will be constantly surrounded in the new school environment. Here three points may be of help. Firstly, the staff of a good school will be alive to this danger, and by their training will have become oriented towards providing a framework of psychological support designed to supply the security that obviates a child's tendency (commonly arising from his lack of self-respect) to seek self-satisfaction through delinquency. Bullying will be watched for, and the selection of children into the school will have been based on the need to secure an admixture of personalities and maladjustments appropriate to render these problems reasonably manageable and free from serious potentialities.

Secondly, these schools have a relatively high staff/pupil ratio. Thirdly, in spite of the parents' understandable fears that the children may exert a mutually adverse influence, it should be recognized that on the contrary they may be of considerable help to one another. Children who with the help of a psychologically skilled teacher have gained some insight into their motives and reactions, and have therefore to some extent travelled past their difficulties, may themselves proclaim to their friends, with pride in their own perspicacity, their own newly-found insights. For example, those asthmatics in whose attacks there was at one stage a psychogenic component may become aware of it, and then describe how they had previously used their symptoms to escape from difficulties but had later come to see for themselves that the illness and its consequences were far more unpleasant than the situations from which at that time those symptoms were unwittingly used as a means of escaping.

The fear that stigma attaches to education at a school for maladjusted children is, like the fear of stigma from a mental hospital, a notion which though still tending to linger is becoming progressively less valid. With the decline of the contempt and fear in which psychiatric patients in general were formerly held, there has also been a blurring of the boundaries of status which previously existed between children receiving special forms of eduction and those passing through the standard educational channels.

Finally, in practice there is usually little or nothing to demarcate these children from those of the population as a whole. The schools have ordinary names that carry no misleading flavour of abnormality, the uniform is conventional, and there is no widespread dissemination of the child's problem in official circles—no automatic involvement of police, for example. Of course the education department will receive the necessary information about the child and the circumstances of his insecurity (which will be treated confidentially) since it is the ultimate agent instrumental in organizing and supervising the child's most suitable transfer. Local authorities, however, will not lend themselves to transfer of children to schools other than those which have been formally approved by the Department of Education and Science.

Part Two

The psychiatric hospital

6

Admission to a mental hospital

To anyone working in an admission ward of a busy mental hospital, where almost every day brings one or two new cases, the spectacle of patients arriving distressed by their own misconceptions of the nature and functions of the hospital vividly highlights the need for preliminary assistance to be given them before their admission. The social worker may be well placed to give it.

Frequently it is at this early point that the information is most necessary. The social worker should be able to present it with confidence and as much detail as possible. And it should be imparted spontaneously rather than have discussion limited to those questions specifically raised by the client.

The social worker may usefully carry out this function almost as a routine duty if her involvement in the situation can be smoothly and acceptably achieved, unless the patient is known to have received all the necessary information already and to have grasped it as realistically as his mental condition will permit. These clients are liable to be tormented with fears of the unknown which need to be assuaged; and it will be worth devoting the next few pages to some consideration of how the social worker may set about doing it.

In the first place, her freedom from the authoritarian aura that so often surrounds the doctor's position confers on her an advantage which at times can supply an essential element for persuasion, usefully and perhaps even indispensably supplementing the endeavours directed on to the problem from other sources. Indeed, when as a result of her influence the patient decides to accept hospital admission, clearly her efforts will have been as much the architect of his recovery as those of any of the psychiatrists or other workers involved in the case.

When a patient's steadfast refusal for admission has led to despair on the part of everyone who has failed to persuade him, I have myself had cause to be grateful to the social worker who has eventually secured his agreement and confounded the pessimists.

THE IMPROVED MENTAL HOSPITAL ATMOSPHERE

To equip the social worker with as much knowledge as possible to undertake this role, a few points about the history of mental hospitals, though history of comparatively recent date, may be illuminating. The middle-aged psychiatrist—unless his sense of sympathy has become exhausted by the constant drain imposed on it, or has been badly eroded by the inevitable ingratitude of a small number of patients, or has been swept aside as a defence against the poignancy and at times intractability of human predicaments—will usually derive a deep satisfaction when comparing the conditions of some of the chronic wards of twenty-five years ago with the far more civilized state of those of today. In this respect perhaps the experience of his general social worker colleague of comparable length of service has contained contrasts that are less striking.

The difference between the mental hospital scene of a quarter of a century ago and that of today is more sharply demarcated and makes a more vividly contrasting impact than do the changes and evolutions witnessed in the sphere of the social services. Chronic wards and corridors echoing with the shouts of hallucinated and deluded patients, the sights and sounds of patients glaring ferociously or vacantly through the slit-like grills of side rooms in which their violence made it necessary for them to be incarcerated almost continuously, the pungent and institutional smell of the widely prescribed paraldehyde, and the spectacle of patients sometimes exhausting themselves in frenzies of activity in padded rooms, have given place to a relatively calm and orderly life that could hardly have been imagined in those earlier days.

It cannot be denied that even today the admission wards

sometimes contain a few noisy or temporarily violent patients. From the very nature of psychiatric illnesses such situations are inevitable. But often they are much less distressing than might be thought. And they tend to prove readily susceptible to skilled and experienced management.

Patients admitted with these features commonly respond well to the appropriate level of medication or other clinical measures such as E.C.T. Often within twenty-four hours or so, acute problems have either been reduced to quite acceptable proportions or have been brought under full control. Nevertheless it sometimes happens that a patient continues in this vein. Perhaps for example an hysterical patient is implacably determined to create a disturbance; or a noisy patient may be suffering from a physical condition that precludes the use of psychiatric medication in a dosage sufficient to achieve the desired effect.

Measures may still be available that can go a long way towards solving the problem. Acute hysterical behaviour is often short-lived. Also a psychopathic personality (chapter 9) may be discharged if it is felt that no worthwhile benefit can be achieved by further efforts on the part of the hospital. The noisy patient may be nursed at nights in a side room while other patients are moved into a dormitory more distant from the source of the noise. Patients needing to be temporarily in bed throughout the twenty-four hours may be transferred to a dormitory out of earshot. Those patients already up and about, who will always constitute the majority, will in any case mainly be engaged elsewhere in the hospital during the day or will be in the ward sitting-room probably well away from the noise. And, arising from the principle that troubles shared are troubles halved, a sense of camaraderie often develops amongst the other patients, who accept the situation with an equanimity that can be remarkably goodhumoured. Even during a phase with a noisy patient, admission wards are by no means necessarily the upsetting environments that might be imagined. And often for long periods they are entirely free from seriously disturbing factors.

If troublesome episodes happen to occur, therefore, they may be somewhat vexatious but are usually a small price to pay considering the benefits which accrue from the treatment. They do not alter the fact that there has been an enormous change for the better in the atmosphere and services of our mental hospitals today compared with twenty-five years ago.

The detailed course of events that led to this rapid metamorphosis need not be gone into here. It will be more apt for the social worker to dwell on the features of present-day hospitals, and particularly on those of the mental hospital in her own locality. But in an increasing number of areas the general hospital too contains a unit admitting psychiatric patients. So she must acquire the relevant knowledge of this hospital also. However, usually it is the mental hospital which tends to inspire the greatest fear and aversion in prospective patients, though doubts and uncertainties are commonly felt about entering a psychiatric ward wherever situated.

REASSURING THE PATIENT

How then can a social worker dispel these fears? First and foremost she can make a point of visiting the hospital concerned, repeatedly if necessary, with a list of items clearly in her mind on which she intends to obtain enlightenment. She need not feel any diffidence about asking questions of members of the hospital staff—doctors, nurses, administrators or workers in any other branch of the organization. If she has difficulty in obtaining the information she seeks, and works within a system permitting her to do so, she should have no hesitation in writing to the medical director or hospital secretary, asking for an appointment to see a suitable person there to discuss the workings of the hospital as a whole or of any particular department about which she feels the need for a greater understanding. The benefits can be reciprocal.

Many hospitals supply a booklet as a guide for their patients and relatives. The social worker would be well advised to possess herself of one before her visit. Naturally these booklets have to be brief and succinct if they are to meet the purpose for which they are designed. For the social worker they are no substitute for a personal visit to clothe the skeleton of the data they present. Only this can give the necessary clarification and make for the necessary ring of conviction which her mere quotations from the written word can never convey to a client when unsupported by the testimony of personal observation and experience. She should also remember that such booklets may sometimes have fallen behind current events. They need periodic revision as staff members change and new techniques develop.

Amongst the many aspects of the hospital life to which she should address herself, a good starting point is for her to discover the average length of stay of patients in the hospital, and the numbers of patients discharged home annually. The hospital secretary will have this information. Often the prospective patient will then be agreeably surprised to learn that many people remain only a few weeks, and that the hospital discharges home hundreds of its patients annually. But it must be kept in mind that many clients, even when told that they are not rarities singled out by a cruel fate to be submitted to an ordeal of hospital admission, are still liable to be unconvinced by vague assurances. Figures, even when approximate, are often more telling.

THE ROLE OF THE NURSE

Next, or at any rate early on in the discussion, the subject of the nurse in the hospital may be usefully raised, since a word is often desirable to remove a patient's misconceptions about the nature and role of the nursing staff. While this profession is widely recognized to be a benevolent, dedicated and indispensable body of people, there is also occasionally found, particularly amongst the older generation, a lingering notion of hard and grimly efficient ward sisters and of very young nurses passing on these qualities in their own turn to their patients. Ill-founded visions of entering this supposedly forbidding and turgid atmosphere can easily tip the scales of a patient's decision against accepting a recommendation for admission.

Arduous routine and satisfactory responses by nurses to the

directions of ward sisters are essential if any ward is to be happy and viable. But there is no doubt that in the past all this was apt to be overdone. Today the general change of climate has brought with it a sharp scaling down of nursing authoritarianism. Undercurrents of resentment and overtones of unnecessary servility have become recognized as undesirable, and productive of poor rather than good work in the pyschiatric field. The centre of gravity has shifted to a point at which great store is set on a happy as well as an efficient atmosphere. Clearly, the two are inseparable.

In accordance with these principles nurses are taught that the ward should radiate warmth and friendliness, and to realize to the full that this state or its converse will largely derive from their own attitudes and efforts. And the ward sister, by the time she has achieved the seniority necessary for appointment to this post, will have come to know that if the nurses are happy, and can establish good relationships with the patients and with each other, the ward will have gone a long way towards its aim of becoming a therapeutic environment, capable of containing without destruction of its essential good cheer a percentage of patients whose illnesses would otherwise present a threat to the emotional welfare of those with whom they mix. Out of this philosophy there emerges a ward environment that provides an experience which in its own way can be enriching, inspiring forward-looking rehabilitation rather than comprising an alarming or debasing picture of incarceration.

SOME ANXIETY-PROVOKING MEDICAL TREATMENTS

Uncertainty about nursing staff attitudes, however, is usually only one anxiety amongst many. Fears about the medical treatment itself can loom very large. Amongst this group of anxieties the commonest and most potent centres around the possibility of receiving electric convulsive therapy (E.C.T.). (Chapter 6.)

ELECTRIC CONVULSIVE THERAPY
Patients often have a horror of this treatment. Every psychiatrist

who has been concerned in outpatient work for any length of
time is only too familiar with the anguished and sometimes
panic-stricken tones contained in the question, 'I won't get
electric shock treatment, will I?' Frequently these patients stand
in desperate need of convincing that they will not be called
upon to endure an ordeal to be dreaded as physically painful
or mentally destructive. Usually they feel unwell—often more
than is realized, since the extent and nature of their distress
frequently exceeds the diminished powers of self-expression
imposed on them by the illness. Commonly they are hyper-
sensitive, sometimes tormented by excursions of imagination
as a result of which every pin-prick takes on the pain of a knife
thrust. At times they are deluded with the belief that they
deserve punishment, and therefore occasionally ascribe to the
treatment a morbidly welcome quality of punitive violence
from which they nevertheless recoil in fear and revulsion.

From these considerations, combined with a childhood
conditioning, which many of us share, which makes for automatic avoidance of electric shocks with their dangers of injury
or death, it is easy to understand a patient's immediate resistance when the merest possibility of this treatment has been
raised. But it may not be easy for the psychiatrist, working in
the conditions of hectic tempo and overloaded timetables that
exist in the average outpatient clinic, to counter these anxieties
unaided. On the other hand, in the more familiar surroundings
of the patient's home, or in other suitable circumstances away
from the dauntingly clinical atmosphere characterizing many
outpatient departments, a leisured talk with a knowledgeable
social worker may achieve the desired effect.

The letters E.C.T. stand for Electric Convulsive Therapy—a
phrase liable to be quite unnecessarily distressing. Usually therefore the process is best described to the patient as 'electrical
treatment'.

The very word 'convulsive' has a chilling ring. It is true that
it remains included in the initials of the official medical
designation of the treatment, but it should be eschewed when
conversing with the patient or his relatives, except perhaps to
be mentioned, when reassurance is required, as being entirely
obsolete in its significance. In the present era, and indeed for

decades now passed, the word has been unrealistic. Convulsions simply do not occur in this treatment; or when they occasionally do so their force and significance are negligible.

Prior to the turn of the 1950s the situation was very different. The production of convulsions was an intrinsic part of the procedure, and at that time they were believed by many psychiatrists—incorrectly, as was subsequently discovered—to be an essential element in the therapy. But these same psychiatrists, while recognizing that on balance the treatment was overwhelmingly indicated for patients suffering severely from illnesses largely inaccessible to other measures, nevertheless on one level of their reactions often themselves found it repellent.

But history was to proceed along a more fortunate course, and today this situation belongs to a former world. It may be of some interest to look back at it. The original concept, largely erroneous but destined to bear a therapeutic offshoot of incalculable value, was that the production of convulsions might confer benefit on schizophrenia. This concept arose from the notion, also incorrect, that a 'biological antagonism' existed between schizophrenia and epilepsy. It had been considered by psychiatrists that the two illnesses coexisted less frequently than could be accounted for by chance, and, on the basis of the supposed 'biological antagonism' put forward in explanation of this belief, it was further assumed that to induce epileptiform convulsions in schizophrenic patients might therefore exert a fundamental effect against the illness.

False in its premise, it nevertheless opened the way to a brilliant outcome, of which today's patients are the long-term beneficiaries. Unfortunately, along the road to this achievement suffering was engendered. In order to induce the convulsions the techniques adopted, which were the only methods for the purpose known at the time, were found to inflict distressing psychological discomfort on the patients during the treatment sessions. At one stage in history camphor, and at another a drug called Cardiozol, were injected into the patient's vein, because when they had been carried to the brain by the blood-stream their action was found to induce the convulsions sought for. Unhappily, during the latent period between injection and loss of consciousness these patients experienced horrible feel-ings of impending dissolution, which like so many subjective experiences are difficult to imagine but whose unpleasant nature the nursing staff of the period were confidently and universally able to confirm from their own observations of the patient's reactions during the treatment. Nevertheless an im-provement in the mental state, albeit temporary, was sometimes achieved. It became clear that in this situation there might be the stirrings of exciting new possibilities for the future.

Modifications of principles and practice gradually followed. One was the observation that patients suffering from certain forms of depression obtained better and more lasting benefit than did schizophrenics. It resulted in a shift of emphasis on to the depressive group of patients as the most suitable candi-dates for convulsive therapy. Another advance was the replace-ment of the chemical methods of induction of convulsions by the use of electricity for this purpose. Thirdly, the convulsions associated with the procedure were virtually eliminated by the discovery of muscle-relaxing drugs for intravenous use. Now-adays the only muscular response to this treatment, therefore, consists merely of twitching of the eyelids, facial muscles and sometimes other muscles. In former times the convulsions were very strong, and resulting fractures were quite common though they usually occurred only in vertebrae which healed with no more effect than a passing backache. Neverthless, fractures of limb bones were not unknown. Today none of these episodes occur.

Various machines, in general showing progressive refine-ments, have been designed from time to time to provide the passage of the electric current. They exist in the form of com-paratively small boxes. It is not necessary to enter into the scientific aspects of their workings or the techniques of their use. However, the essence of the procedure is that a current of extremely small electrical strength is given for at most a few seconds. After being wheeled into the treatment room, usually well sedated, the patient is put pleasantly to sleep by injecting an anaesthetic into a vein—most commonly in the arm. A small electrode is then placed on either side of the forehead, the current is switched on and within a few minutes the patient

194 The psychiatric hospital

is ready to be wheeled out of the treatment room. The whole procedure lasts only a minute or two, and the patient is usually soon awake again, although occasionally up to about half an hour, or occasionally a little longer, is required to 'sleep it off'.

It is not intended to enter into theories about the mode of action of the treatment, or to discuss at this point the types of syndromes for which it is indicated. However, the patient can be reassured about its level of safety. Amongst medical operations involving the administration of an anaesthetic it ranks very highly indeed as a safe procedure. Even a simple dental extraction has occasionally resulted in an emergency situation, and as minor a matter as taking an aspirin can lead to severe reactions—even collapse or death. But such episodes are extremely rare, and many thousands of electrical treatments are also carried out every year entirely uneventfully. When recommended and given by experienced doctors, who will of course pay regard to the patient's physical condition, the patient need have small anxiety in accepting the recommendation. It does not produce brain damage in clinical practice; and the amount of electric current used is minute. The nature and effects of treatment will, however, in any case be explained to him in the hospital by the doctor dealing with his case.

It will be seen that this account of E.C.T. has been presented both for the general interest of the social worker and also to furnish her with enough knowledge to help her in persuading an unwilling or wavering patient to accept the treatment or not to be deterred from agreeing to admission because of the possibility of the treatment being given. Nevertheless it is important to emphasize that she herself should not initiate suggestions as to any treatment that her client should be given.

This statement may seem unnecessary or even derogatory in its implications, but it refers to a situation that can occur more easily than might be supposed. Anxious and imaginative patients are sometimes unsuspectedly liable to misconstrue their interview with a psychiatrist, and an inexperienced social worker may easily be misled into believing that she is supporting a psychiatric recommendation when in reality it is the opposite situation that exists. Only when she has ascertained unequivocally that the psychiatrist has made his views crystal clear should she exercise her supportive function of persuasion. But in these circumstances she may play a useful part in confirming the efficacy of any treatment recommended to her client which in her experience has conferred benefit on any patients personally known to her or about whose progress she has heard.

There are times when the course of a patient's illness in hospital takes an unexpected turn. It may then be that a change of therapeutic intention will become indicated. To implant into him preconceptions about the management of his case may lead to disappointment, frustration and hostility. And this forfeiture of his cooperation, which can too easily develop into a permanent state, can also impose a disservice on a long chain of other individuals whose welfare, both emotional and material, is dependent on his recovery.

BEHAVIOUR THERAPY

A treatment given very much less commonly than E.C.T. is the technique known as behaviour therapy. It has been carried out increasingly for a number of years for the small minority of patients who stand to benefit from it, and since its principles and practice are little understood outside the small circle of those who prescribe and undertake it a brief outline of this field will be worthwhile.

Behaviour therapy, primarily the function of the clinical psychologist, is a very scientific form of treatment. It rests on factors specifically pertaining to physiological conditioning. The two main processes involved in behaviour therapy techniques are classical conditioning, as described by Pavlov (chapter 8), and the complementary form of conditioning known as operant conditioning, which was developed subsequently.

An important process in behaviour therapy is known as reciprocal inhibition. This term denotes the conditioning of an incompatible response which inhibits the maladaptive state for whose alleviation it is being undertaken. Various methods can be used, each requiring preliminary decisions resting on practical experience of the technique. But the overall aim is to bring into close mental association a state of therapeutic relaxation and the anxiety content of the condition whose treatment is being attempted. This technique of 'specific desensitization' sometimes offers a hope of improvement for a variety of phobic anxieties.

The relaxation may be induced by various methods such as rapidly-acting drugs (chapter 10), by hypnosis, or by using a machine which feeds the sounds of the patient's muscle tension through earphones into his own awareness for his guidance, thus helping him to relax his muscles. At the same time the phobic stimulus is presented. Thus an association of this phobic state with the state of pleasant relaxation, rather than with the unpleasant tension and the panic of itself, may be engendered. Clearly, however, too powerful an anxiety stimulus will militate against successful achievement of relaxation. A 'graduating up' process is therefore used, the initial situation being of minor anxiety but being then increased by gradual stages, during which the patient's accommodation to their effects will serve to avert the full impact that would arise if the initial phobic stimulus were as strong as that which is reached finally.

There are various techniques by which the phobic stimuli are aroused. Sometimes the patient is led to imagine the anxiety-producing situations for himself; sometimes they are presented to him in pictures; sometimes they are given directly. (In other words he imagines the situation, he is supplied with pictures portraying it, or he is put into material circumstances of the sort which at the same time produce his morbid reactions.) The construction of the stages of increasing intensity that will need to be gone through is a task that requires a great deal of prior discussion and reflection if it is to be related adequately to the patient's individual history and needs.

In the form of treatment known as 'aversion therapy', on the other hand, it is the association of an unpleasant stimulus which is used as the conditioning mechanism. The original application was for the treatment of alcoholism. Now discredited for this purpose, and seen as anachronistic in the distance, it regressed with little compensating advantage towards the features that characterized the dark ages of psychiatry;

its acceptance nevertheless persisted into the second half of the present century.

An injection of Emetine or Apomorphine, drugs used to produce vomiting, was given at the same time as the alcohol was pressed on to the patient at frequent and regular intervals during the treatment, in the hope that the association of the unpleasant state of the drug-induced gastric upset with the pleasures of the alcohol would result in a cancellation of any inclination for the latter. But with the hindsight of follow-up observations it was eventually found that in general little lasting benefit had accrued. And the nausea, retching, vomiting and exhaustion, together with the retention of the vomited material in the patient's vicinity to assist in the process of aversion, and the vigorous continuation of treatment that was required until it sometimes neared the critical point of physical danger, all combined to render this treatment unacceptable to many patients. Moreover it could not be relied on to be effective, because the timing of the aversive stimulus needed to be within seconds. This timing was not practicable, since it was not possible to predict when the patient would vomit.

The unfortunate history of this particular technique of aversion therapy should not be carried over into influencing one's view of other examples of the concept to a point that would automatically lead one to discourage the patient and thereby deprive him of the advantages from the treatment which he might reasonably seek. Time has brought other types of aversive stimulation, safe and much less unpleasant, in the form of mild electric shocks induced from a battery and ad-ministered on the arm or leg. Unfortunately alcoholism has proved resistant to these also; but other psychiatric conditions —most notably sexual deviations including transvestism and certain forms of homosexuality characterized by inhibition against, rather than a history of basic lack of interest in, the opposite sex—have shown some promise of at least a tempor-ary improvement and an increased accessibility to psycho-therapy that was previously found impracticable.

In the light of the unacceptability of the vomiting technique for aversion to alcoholism, which is clearly a fully justifiable conclusion, those with influence over a client's decision may reasonably question the ethical validity of the modern technique which makes use of electric shocks. However, the unpleasantness is incomparably less intense, and provided that the patient is willing to undergo the treatment there seems little ethical objection. Moreover because the treatment can only succeed if the patient wishes to cooperate, there would in any case be no clinical point in undertaking it against his will.

An important duty devolving on the social worker, both from the ethical point of view and in terms of the pyschological medicine concerned, may nevertheless arise when court proceedings are impending against a patient who might perhaps benefit from this treatment. She must appreciate that in view of the deterrent quality inherent in the treatment it will be necessary for her to avoid putting forward any implication that it should be used on a basis that could be misconstrued as judicially punitive. Furthermore, if she has any reason to believe that this recommendation might be made to the court from other sources, she should take any reasonable and proper steps to ensure that a prior discussion is held between those contemplating suggesting this possibility and a consultant psychiatrist able to advise on the case.

We should now briefly look at another constituent of behaviour therapy, namely operant conditioning.

This form of conditioning is a process complementary to the classical conditioning of Pavlov. In operant conditioning, steps are taken to substitute the patient's or animal's passivity by a process of his own active participation. In this form of conditioning he engages in an active 'operative' part as well as in a receptive role. His activity is stimulated by the use of rewards or incentives, these being made use of on a scientific basis.

We can now think about a few simple examples of operant conditioning. Situations designed to canalize random movements into constructive activity have been set up both in experimental animals and human subjects. It has been found, for instance, in the case of certain animals that if a particular movement by the animal activates a pedal that leads to the appearance of food, then the probability that this action will be repeated is increased. By a comparable process in the human sphere, the random arm and hand movements, for example, of severely mentally subnormal patients (chapter 5) may become directed into channels of practical learning value such as self-feeding in those cases open to this form of approach.

SOME OTHER ANXIETIES

Disproportionate fears of the unknown other than those concerned with treatments and matters which are often quite trivial in themselves may need alleviation. An outline of admission procedures may help. Simple explanations about circumstances to be anticipated on arrival at the hospital, together with the reassurance that the patient will be adequately directed, befriended, and not expected to act too spontaneously or merely on the basis of prior information given by the social worker, may assuage much unnecessary anxiety.

Knowledge that the hall porters at the reception desk are ready and pleased to give information and guidance may relieve unspoken fears of wandering around unaided, and may thus console the patient who is afraid of his own shyness or in painful doubt about his own competence. Instructions on personal effects to be taken—night clothing, dressing-gown, toilet requisites—with the information that if anything is forgotten the nursing staff will be pleased to arrange help with the situation—may similarly serve to set his mind at rest.

Discussion may be necessary on measures to be adopted relating to finance and personal possessions. Explanations about the handing in to the ward sister or charge nurse of those valuables which cannot be left at home, and the information that a receipt will be given, may diminish uneasiness about loss of possessions and reduce reluctance to cooperate. Clarification of the procedures for obtaining national insurance medical certificates for sickness or injury benefit, and for their transfer to the local office of the Department of Health and Social Security and the subsequent return to him of a draft that he can cash at the hospital shop or any post office, can give him an improved sense of safety and personal responsibility stemming from the knowledge that he can buy stamps, luxuries, etc. while in hospital. He may also bank the money with the hospital authorities until he needs it. Alternatively, he may prefer to leave these matters in the hands of his relatives.

Any other pieces of information designed to help him to cope with the as yet ill-understood new demands of hospital life will be worthwhile. But in addition to these demands, which will be foreign to his past experience, there are many aspects of hospital life which can be comfortingly familiar but which are so commonplace that they are often out of the fore-front of the mind of a patient who is anxiously peering into the unknown and preoccupied with assessing the nature of the unaccustomed experience to which he may be subjected.

Often therefore they will not receive his consideration. These commonplace aspects are to be identified with the routine of life around which he has habitually orientated him-self and which cannot be broken without a disturbing feeling of tension ensuing. Unfortunately, since the tension generated by this possibility arises from feelings engaging only his marginal awareness, it is indeterminate and its origin and nature may escape his clear recognition. Obviously this vague state of unease, which may tip the balance against his decision for admission, will not be dispelled by any discussion confined simply to his acute fears centred around the more unusual experiences confronting him.

The social worker should not neglect the importance of these cardinal points of life's personal and social orientations when talking with the client before admission. Their simplicity does not denote a lack of significance. They can supply the security of an accustomed frame of reference. So she can use-fully familiarize herself with the details of the facilities for obtaining newspapers, receiving letters, making telephone calls, and any other aspects relevant to this provision of a sense of continuity of life routine about which she has learnt from her own visit to, or enquiries from, the hospital. And it may be very helpful to mention this information to the patient.

Many prospective patients have serious anxieties and guilt feelings about the sort of fellow patients with whom they will come into contact. Though commonly exaggerated, and often essentially erroneous, these misgivings are understandable.

Not only do patients frequently have a sense of failure, but they may be beset by the fantasy that in mixing with people afflicted with serious mental illnesses they too will become 'infected'. The minor fears of grave mental illness that lurk within the minds of many normal people who are unlikely to be destined for psychiatric breakdown may assume gargantuan proportions amongst patients about to enter a mental hospital. To the patients' haunting suspicions that they have already started to slip down the slope leading to insanity there now becomes added the dread that they will further acquire these attributes beyond any salvation if they allow themselves to become contaminated by those more severely afflicted.

These sufferers believe that they are more ill, or potentially so, than is in fact the case. But other patients, grossly lacking in insight into the serious nature of their illnesses, bitterly resent and repudiate any suggestion that their thinking processes are in any way disordered. When such a suggestion is made they commonly commit themselves to a refusal of admission, which once made they become progressively more unable to retract even if their lack of insight is not met with any further threat of challenge. However, the realistic comments that they are tired, or that they need treatment for their loss of appetite, insomnia or loss of weight, and that it may be well provided in a mental hospital designed to supply a regular and comparatively restful routine, make an argument that will sometimes secure their cooperation.

Patients who are deluded cannot (chapter 11) be disencumbered of these delusions by attempts to persuade them of their irrational nature. Nevertheless they will sometimes agree that the state of their nervous system—caused as they believe by the anxieties arising out of their alleged problems—does in fact merit a period of rest and treatment in the hospital. For example, a patient suffering from delusions that he is persecuted by neighbours will not accept that he is wrong in his belief; but he may accept that he needs help over the state of insomnia etc. which he thinks has followed as a result of the supposed persecutions.

Between the two extremes of fear of non-existent insanity or an unjustified belief in its impending development on the one hand, and a refusal to accept its existence on the other, there is a wide range amongst patients in their interpretations of their states. To explain to clients that no two cases are the same is to make a statement that is both correct and often of good cheer. Some patients lack confidence in their capacity for work, some have difficulty in forming friendships, some are plagued with insomnia, some cannot bear to be with other people.

It can be fairly said that just as in a general medical ward the patient's illnesses will vary from, for example, pneumonia to leukaemia, similarly if one patient in a psychiatric ward witnesses another patient's illness it carries absolutely no implication that it is the illness from which he himself suffers. They may or may not have some features in common—the same symptom of shortness of breath can occur in conditions as different as pneumonia and leukaemia—but this fact is irrelevant. In causal situations too a similarly wide variation obtains. Poor living conditions, financial stress, anxiety about relatives are all varying examples which may be readily seen by the client to point to the comforting principle that no two cases are alike.

From these facts it follows that the treatments to be given will be correspondingly various—and of course they may include attempts to alter whatever social conditions may be thought to have contributed to the illness. Not only does this variation of management apply to the more traditionally medical measures of drugs and E.C.T. The communal forms of psychotherapeutic help (chapter 7) will likewise be applied with a judicious selectivity. The majority of patients benefit by attending the occupational therapy department, for instance; but it is recognized that it is unkind and clinically unwise to force a patient to attend group activities if his anxieties would become undesirably raised or his powers of adaptation overtaxed. Again, patients may gain in socializing capacity, with a resulting improvement in fulfilment and therefore self-esteem, by attending traditional hospital entertainments like the dances, cinema, visits with friends to the hospital canteen, or participation in games such as table tennis, football, cricket or tennis. But although they will be encouraged if indicated, they will not be unreasonably coerced into doing so.

It was emphasized earlier that, subject to psychiatric confirmation, the client should often be told that he is unlikely to
remain in hospital for a very long period. This information is
partly based on statistics relating to the average length of stay
of patients in the mental hospitals of today. Such figures should
not be quoted in detail, however, since in the event of his
remaining in the hospital for a different length of time he may
tend to view himself unfavourably and possibly react with
discouragement in relation to this background of comparison.
Nevertheless when presented in general terms these encouraging figures can be usefully reassuring to patients who have had
forebodings on this score.

It will be obvious that little more than broad approxima-
tions about anticipated length of stay can be given to the
patient or relatives. On the whole, these periods range from a
few weeks to a few months; but obviously it is only the psychiatrist dealing with the case who can provide any comprehen-
sively reasoned estimate. Moreover, the patient should be encouraged in advance to resist any tendency to compare the
apparent rate of his progress with that of other patients, in spite
of any similarities in outward appearances that may seem to
characterize the illnesses. Another aspect of the patient's stay,
and one which the social worker may be well-advised to raise
spontaneously, is the likelihood of his having periods of leave
from the hospital during which he may return home while
under some of his treatment. This possibility may not have
occurred to him. He should be told of it.

The potential value of periods away from the hospital receives high priority by medical staff in the planning of his
management, and he need not fear that he will be under the
necessity of pleading for the facility as a privilege to be sought
in automatic opposition to the inclinations of medical or
nursing staff. Of course they will oppose the suggestion if it is
seen to be clearly against his clinical interests; and naturally
they will be reluctant to give their acquiescence if to do so
would involve the running of unwarrantable risks. But the
interests of the patient predominate in the eyes of everyone
concerned with his welfare. The benefit to his happiness, the
clinical value of a report from the relatives about his condition

while at home, and the stabilizing value of his maintaining contact with ordinary life and its routines will all weigh very heavily with the doctor when the request is made. As soon as circumstances have become suitable, and when the application has been made by the relatives or friends to whom he will go, the patient will commonly be encouraged, not deterred, in his wish for a period of a few days or even a few weeks away from the hospital environment.

Doctors in mental hospitals are busy people, and it is often both impracticable and undesirable for them to interview a patient with the frequency that he or his relatives may regard as his need. Usually each patient is under the overall care of a consultant psychiatrist, with a psychiatric assistant who looks after his day-to-day medical and psychological welfare. The latter doctor often carries out the majority of the psychiatric interviews considered necessary. But whichever of these doctors may be the more intimately involved in the details of the psychiatric help given to any particular patient, there is no doubt that in some cases an excess of attention is not only unnecessary but may indeed bring its own clinical disadvantages. Generalizations cannot easily be made, but with the wide variety of illnesses under treatment in, for example, an admission ward, there must necessarily exist a correspondingly wide disparity amongst the intervals between the interviews, and in the duration of the interviews themselves, required by the various patients. Some will be seen comparatively often; others less so. Some will require prolonged discussions; in other cases more rapid assessments of the progress will fully meet the need.

The patient who is seen less frequently than some of his companions in the ward need not for this reason feel any sense of neglect or abandonment. It is a common practice in such wards for the consultant psychiatrist, his assistant, the nurses and others concerned in the patient's management to meet together frequently and regularly to discuss the treatment and progress of each patient under their care (chapter 7). On this basis the patient's interests are unlikely to be lost sight of under the pressures of work on the doctors, even though they may sometimes see certain other patients more frequently.

Finally, a word about a principle that is of paramount significance in modern psychiatric thinking. It is axiomatic that in
the community no patient can be validly considered except in
his relation to the family and social setting within which he
has his existence. Similarly in hospital, to try to help any
patient without full emphasis on this fundamental principle
would be to cut at the roots of one of our most basic conceptions. Direct contact with relatives, or with others on whom
the patient may depend, is therefore an indispensable element
in the social worker's approach to the patient's admission if
his interests are to be served within their most meaningful and
fruitful psychological context. Relatives too should therefore
be told of all the considerations we have discussed. They should
be asked to write to him and if possible to visit as regularly as
his condition permits, ensuring continuity both with his basic
home relationships and also with the general foundations and
framework of his life. They should be requested to observe his
progress and report about it to the hospital staff. They should
be encouraged to enquire, by letter or telephone, about his
present condition and his future mode of life.

Those who work in mental hospitals and psychiatric outpatient clinics sometimes tend to lose sight of the practical
difficulties and the searing conflicts imposed on a patient and
his relatives by recommendations for hospital admission. The
heat of the job may prevent the necessary time and patience
being available for full explanations. The burdens of responsibilities may pull against the relaxed state necessary for smooth
and effective persuasion. And the number of outpatient book-
ings often precludes follow-up appointments early enough to
consolidate any preliminary success towards agreement.

Often the social worker can help in problems of a practical
nature, such as the management of children while a mother is
in hospital or by assistance with financial arrangements while
a father is away. Without such help these problems can too
easily form rocks on which a recommendation for admission
may founder. The social worker often has a uniquely useful
portal of entry into areas in which she can contribute much
that is valuable both psychologically and materially to the
patient facing hospital, and to his relatives. It is hoped that the

information touched on in this chapter will be helpful to her in her efforts to do so.

LEGAL ASPECTS OF ADMISSION AND DISCHARGE

The majority of patients entering a psychiatric hospital or the psychiatric ward of a general hospital do so on a voluntary, or as it is nowadays termed, informal basis. These patients have all the legal rights of any other citizens. A patient of informal status cannot be detained against his wishes, nor can he be brought back to the hospital if he was there on this basis. He may be strongly advised to remain or return, but cannot be forced to do so, although for circumstances of a serious nature the Mental Health Act 1959 still provides, under Section 30, that the medical officer in charge of the patient's care may recommend a period of compulsory detention lasting up to three days. At the end of this period the Order lapses and the situation must be reviewed.

In spite of all efforts made to help a patient to accept admission, through indicating to him the nature of hospital life and explaining his rights of self-discharge as an informal patient, his anxiety sometimes remains unassuageable and his lack of insight into the fact that he is mentally ill persists as an insuperable barrier against obtaining his cooperation. In these circumstances the help of the law is available for compulsory admission.

For this minority of patients requiring compulsory admission, three sections of the Mental Health Act 1959 are mainly used—Sections 25, 26 and 29—though a relatively small number of anti-social patients required by Courts to enter hospital compulsorily will, if accepted by the hospital (and all hospitals except those specially designated for this function have the power of refusal) be placed there by the Court Order. In some instances (Section 65) the Court incorporates in its requirement that in the event of discharge or leave from hospital coming under consideration, approval from the Home Office must be obtained before these measures can be granted. In other instances (Section 60) no such restrictions are imposed.

The Mental Health Act on which all the procedures for compulsory admission are based is a rather complex and detailed publication. Access to the information contained in it, and to any interpretation that may be required under circumstances of particular difficulty, is a necessary facility for the social worker. It is a facility which she should unhesitatingly use when in doubt. But it must be remembered that its provisions do not apply to Scotland, which has its own system of laws for mental illness.

It would not be appropriate here to discuss the numerous provisions contained in this Act. They range widely over many aspects of mental health in addition to those relating to admissions and discharges. However, Sections 25, 26 and 29 will be outlined, after which it may be helpful to point out a few of the practical difficulties and pitfalls sometimes encountered by social workers in relation to them. For an adequate knowledge of even these Sections, the data contained in a handbook cannot suffice. However the following information, while far from comprehensive, may serve to simplify and clarify the social worker's task when consulting the Mental Health Act itself.

It must also be stressed that the points described here only apply to the law as it stands at present (1977). Since its inception this Act has already been amended on a number of occasions, and further amendments will no doubt be made (chapter 9). It is therefore very important that everyone concerned in mental health matters which involve legal procedures and definitions should take steps to ensure that they are familiar with the law as it stands at the time of their involvement.

SECTION 25

Section 25 empowers a patient's compulsory detention for twenty-eight days. It requires the written confirmation of need by two medical practitioners and is intended for use for those patients whose clinical condition is not so acute as to require admission within the period liable to be involved in any delay in obtaining the two medical practitioners. Whenever possible one should be the patient's usual doctor. But when this is impracticable the point can be waived. Any registered medical practitioner is legally acceptable under circumstances of necessity. The second doctor, on the other hand, though not necessarily a psychiatrist, must invariably be on a list of practitioners officially approved for this function. It is the responsibility of the social worker to ensure that this requirement is complied with.

Each of these practitioners, one but not both of whom may be on the staff of the hospital to which the patient will be admitted, will complete either a separate Form 3A or a joint document (Form 3B) naming the date of his last examination of the patient, stating whether or not he was previously acquainted with the patient, declaring that he has been approved under the Act as having special experience in the diagnosis or treatment of mental disorders, and testifying that he is of the opinion that the patient is suffering from mental disorder of a nature or degree which warrants detention in hospital under observation for at least a limited period, and that the patient ought to be so detained in the interests of his own health or safety or with a view to the protection of other persons.

If either of the last two circumstances does not apply, the doctor deletes that particular statement from the form. The form also requires him to state that informal admission is not appropriate in the case. Finally, since Form 3A is used both for Sections 25 and 29, it contains a clause, to which further reference will be made under Section 29, indicating that delay would be undesirable. In completing a Section 25, however, this clause must be deleted, since unlike Section 29 it is not a Section relevant for situations of acute emergency. It is also important to remember that it is illegal for the patient to be removed to hospital before both practitioners have completed the forms. They sign separate forms which are identical. Moreover whatever Section is used for admission this legal prohibition against removal until completion of the forms invariably applies. It is thus the social worker's responsibility to ensure that they are presented to the hospital at the time of the patient's arrival there.

When involved in the possibility of Section 25 the social worker should whenever possible consult the next-of-kin. But while their views will usually be helpful and will naturally be accorded their full weight, no relative has the power in law to prevent or rescind a compulsory admission under this Section. However strong the opinions expressed or the pressures exerted by even the nearest relatives, they can neither incriminate those drawing up the Section nor absolve them from proceeding with the admission if it is indicated on adequate clinical grounds. Knowledge of these points can be helpful to a social worker under criticisms or moral pressures from hostile relatives distressed by a compulsory detention whose validity they themselves may be unable to recognize. Commonly, however, relatives perceive the advantages of admission to hospital, and welcome rather than resist it.

Section 25 only empowers a patient's detention for twenty-eight days. The law requires that at the end of the twenty-eight day period the patient be either discharged from hospital, regraded to informal status, or, if further compulsory detention is required, that he be regraded for detention under Section 26. Throughout this period neither he nor his relatives can obtain his discharge if in the opinion of the doctor in charge of the case, termed the responsible medical officer, such action would be clinically wrong. But it is not permissible for the responsible medical officer to have omitted to take one of these three courses of action by the end of the twenty-eight days covered by the Section 25. He may, however, remove the patient from the Section before that stage if he regards it as indicated.

SECTION 26

When it is considered that twenty-eight days in hospital would be too short a period for the clinical needs, a Section 26 may be invoked—either for the initial admission or to ensure continued detention when the patient is already in hospital detained under another Section. This Section, which is used comparatively rarely, empowers compulsory detention for an initial period not exceeding one year, although again the responsible medical officer may rescind it at any point, however early, if in his view the full period proves unnecessary.

For Section 26 a Form 5A must be completed by two registered medical practitioners. Again, one must be on a list of approved practitioners and the other should be the patient's usual doctor if possible. By contrast with Sections 25 and 29, the consent of the next-of-kin must be obtained. If it is withheld, this Section cannot be used. Nevertheless, the Mental Health Act also states (Section 27(2)) that the nearest relative must be consulted unless it appears to the mental welfare officer that such consultation is not reasonably practicable or would involve unreasonable delay. When all these conditions are fulfilled, and provided that the clinical indications are present—such as perhaps a failure to have improved satisfactorily while already detained under Section 25, or a history indicating the likelihood of such a failure—the Section has the advantage of empowering detention for a period more likely to achieve therapeutic success.

As with the Form 3A for Section 25, the Form 5A relating to Section 26 requires each medical practitioner, who once again signs a separate but identical form, to state the date of his last examination and his previous acquaintance or otherwise with the patient, his status of approval under the Act and his opinion that the patient is suffering from a mental condition of a nature or degree which warrants detention in a hospital for medical treatment within the meaning of the Act.

But on this form there is the additional requirement of inserting whether the relevant condition consists of mental illness, severe subnormality, or subnormality and/or psychopathic disorder. Furthermore the grounds on which the opinion for compulsory detention is founded, in addition to the confirmation of need, must be stated by the medical practitioners; and they must also indicate whether other methods of care or treatment (e.g. outpatient treatment or local authority services) are available and if so why they are not appropriate and why informal admission is not suitable.

These last items of information are also required for Section 25. But the reader will appreciate that for detention under Section 26, fuller and more explicit information is required. Moreover, since twelve months is a long period for potential deprivation of ordinary liberty, under the provisions of this Section (though not Section 25 or 29) the patient has the right to apply for his case to be reviewed by a Mental

Health Tribunal. However, he must make the application within six months of his admission under Section 26 or his sixteenth birthday, whichever comes later.

This request must be acted on by the hospital. The tribunal consists of three members—a lawyer, a layman and a consultant psychiatrist not on the staff of the hospital concerned. It can scrutinize case notes, interview all concerned in the management of the patient, or subpoena any witness. It has the power to order that the patient be removed from the compulsory detention if the indications for such detention are thought by the tribunal to be lacking. The liberty of the individual can thus be rigorously safeguarded. It should however be noted that the patient may not make another application during the twelve months from his admission date.

SECTION 29

For cases so urgent that very speedy removal to hospital is essential, or when a second practitioner is not available for purposes of Section 25, the use of Section 29 is indicated. The form for this purpose (Form 3A) is the same as that used for Section 25.

It will be recalled that when used for Section 25 one of the clauses in this form must be deleted. This clause, to be deleted in a Section 25 but retained in a Section 29, states that in the opinion of the practitioner it is of urgent necessity for the patient to be admitted and detained under Section 25 of the Act, and that compliance with the requirements of the Act relating to applications for admission for observation other than emergency applications would involve undesirable delay. Naturally the form states that this clause should be deleted unless the medical recommendation is the first recommendation in support of an emergency application under Section 29. In other words, under the emergency circumstances of Section 29 this clause indicating the urgency must be left undeleted. Under Section 29 only one medical practitioner is required, the consent of the next-of-kin need not be obtained, and again although the usual doctor is preferred it is permissible that any registered medical practitioner sign the form if necessary.

Section 29 empowers compulsory detention for three days.

As with Sections 25 and 26, at the time of its expiration the patient must be discharged from hospital, regraded to informal status, or compulsorily detained. If the last action is needed, Section 25 or 26 are available for use, subject to the individual conditions relating to each. But whatever section is decided on, it must in law be completed within the period of three days covered by this emergency section.

SOME AREAS OF POSSIBLE MISUNDERSTANDING

It may now be helpful to draw attention to some particular points about which social workers are apt to be unclear, but which may require their direct action or involve them in circumstances where explanations may be helpful to clients or relatives perplexed by the situations in which they find themselves.

Section 29 requires that the actual time as well as the date of admission to the hospital be recorded in order that a patient admitted on Monday at 5.10 p.m., for example, will have become regraded by Thursday at 5.10 p.m. (not 5.15). The organization of these tasks does not fall on to the social worker but on to the administrative and clerical staff of the hospital. Also, it is not always realized that a Section 29 needs only one other doctor to convert it into a Section 25. The second doctor involved in this procedure is commonly one working in the hospital, and no action to obtain another practitioner is required from the social worker. It is sometimes wrongly assumed that the additional doctor needs to be obtained by the social worker.

A few points relating to detained patients on leave from hospital are worth keeping in mind. If the condition of such a patient deteriorates to a point at which the responsible medical officer considers that he should return to the hospital, the procedure laid down requires that a letter be handed to the patient, or to the person for the time being in charge of him, by an escort. This letter explains that he must return. If he fails to comply with the requirement he may be escorted back to the hospital. In the event of need he may be taken into custody, and returned to the hospital by any social worker, any officer on the staff of the hospital, any police constable or anyone authorized in writing by the managers of the hospital.

Patients detained under Section 26 may be granted leave from hospital for a period at the discretion of the responsible medical officer. If he is required to return to the hospital, the responsibility for the prior notification of this requirement to the patient rests not with a social worker, but with the hospital administrator on the recommendation of the responsible medical officer. His condition while in hospital will then be reviewed by the responsible medical officer, and if his clinical state is found suitable he can be given a further leave period. If, however, any six-monthly leave period would continue after the expiration of the period of twelve months' detention provided by the Section 26, and the responsible medical officer envisages the possibility of continuing detention being required, then he must see the patient on an outpatient basis with a view to renewing the compulsory order in the event of the clinical findings confirming the need. Any such order can of course be rescinded later by the responsible medical officer if the patient's progress justifies his doing so. But it is not always realized that no routine action by the social worker is statutorily required in relation to any aspects of leave, though on occasions the hospital doctor may make a request for information from her to assist in evaluating the patient's condition, prognosis and life circumstances. Also, the patient ceases to be liable to be detained at the expiry of a period of six months from the beginning of leave of absence.

If a patient is transferred while under an order for compulsory detention—under whatever Section he is detained—a signed transfer order and the original documents relating to the detention must accompany him to the receiving hospital, copies being also kept at the transferring hospital. If this transfer order and these documents, correctly completed, do not accompany him on arrival, he must for compliance with the law be sent back to the transferring hospital without admission to the receiving hospital, whatever the other circumstances

In acting in accordance with these principles it may be supportive for social workers to realize that, in order to minimize any possibility of error, it is usual that the detention documents are scrutinized after the patient's admission by two persons in addition to those who have signed them. One will be a consultant psychiatrist at the admitting hospital other than the psychiatrist under whose care the patient will be observed or treated. The other is the hospital secretary, the latter being concerned to safeguard against inaccuracies in such matters as names, addresses and dates. Any errors then discovered must be rectified by the relevant person and the document returned to the hospital within fourteen days of the patient's admission. It should be added, however, that neither of these procedures, though commonly carried out, is a legal requirement.

7

Further aspects of hospital life

That we exist in relation to one another is clearly a basic law that we ignore at our peril. And if we happen to break down into mental illness or emotional ill-health, disturbances in these relationships inevitably ensue. It is only within a well-considered setting of human relationships, therefore, that psychiatric treatment in hospital can be logically and effectively carried out.

All the communal treatments adopted within the hospital rest firmly on this premiss; and we may usefully give some detailed consideration to the most important. It is perhaps formal group therapy, both as it was originally conceived and also as it is now practised in relation to the more sophisticated concepts and techniques of today, that embodies the most direct example of the category of treatments in which the setting of personal relationships is exploited specifically for its therapeutic value. But certain other activities—occupation, art, drama and music—all use the basic principle of the value of the group.

From time immemorial each of these fields of activity has, of course, made its own contributions to personal fulfilment and alleviation of suffering. But as therapeutic agents these contributions have usually operated on an unstructured basis. Only in relatively recent times have attempts been made to channel and concentrate the material of group discussion, art, music, etc., into methods specifically designed to provide situations of formal therapy and rehabilitation. In this chapter we shall examine not only the more established forms of communal activity, such as hospital entertainments and the work of the occupational therapy department and the industrial units. We shall look at three of the less common therapeutic activities—music, art and self-catering flats—some of which are as yet available in only a minority of hospitals.

WARD MEETINGS AND GROUP THERAPY

The better preserved category of patients, and indeed many of those whose difficulties are dispersed more diffusely over their personalities, can sometimes benefit from techniques of group discussion. In addition to individual psychotherapy, psychotherapeutic help may sometimes be provided by suitable ward meetings, if time and staff are available for this technique in addition to the other forms of treatment demanding staff attention. A system of ward meetings can also help to ensure that, as in general hospitals, the progress of patients remains under the fullest review possible.

These meetings may be conducted in different ways. They may be large or small. The frequency with which they are held varies, being determined by factors such as the type of ward and the anticipated length of stay of the patients. In some the doctors, nurses, occupational therapists, psychologists and other staff involved—which may also include community social workers, probation officers, disablement resettlement officers, art and music therapists—may all attend regularly. Sometimes individual patients are invited into the meetings to discuss their problems; or it may be felt preferable for the discussions to be undertaken without risking distress to the patient by his attendance, though the necessary information about his progress will be available for discussion by the staff members themselves. Alternatively, selected groups of patients and staff may meet together. Again, there may be a meeting for all the patients in a ward, together with all the staff.

Hence in those hospitals in which emphasis is placed on group methods, a wide range of methods may be adopted. But all these approaches try to provide an opportunity for ventilation of feelings, which may include discussion of the day to day ward management and bring about the building of relationships and a sense of community between patients and staff.

The basic group processes through which insight is achieved, guilt feelings assuaged, and sometimes in which the pressures of the group ethos may act usefully on individual members to effect changes of attitudes, vary in their subtlety and depth. But even the relatively superficial and unspecialized approaches may have much to offer. Patients compulsorily detained under the Mental Health Act, for instance, may gain a useful feeling of having a voice in the management of the ward's affairs. Anger or fear of authority may be mitigated. And therapeutically valuable self-acceptance, and the acceptance of deviance in others, may develop. Some group discussions may usefully follow on the direct supervision and semi-formal teaching already carried out at the more elementary level of need, as will be discussed later in connection with rehabilitation. But the necessary levels of sophistication vary. Sometimes formal group therapy of the type designed to help people to understand, modify, and come to terms with their own behaviour and its deeper implication is the primary aim. In other instances group discussions directed at the simpler levels of psychological and practical functioning may suffice in the first instance, or even remain the only type of group technique required or possible

ENTERTAINMENTS

The fact that the nursing staff are so well aware of patients' needs for general entertainment is a testimony to the therapeutic efficacy of these activities, and their existence has often given a sense of comfort to prospective patients contemplating admission. Sometimes there is a specially appointed entertainments officer; or this function may be included as an important branch of the work of a rehabilitation officer or committee. Whatever the organization of the entertainment system, however, there are usually included within it films, concerts, dances, bingo, table tennis, outdoor sports, and outings of patients to coastal areas, sometimes lasting a week, or to local swimming-baths.

The departments of the hairdresser and the beautician give

ample confirmation to the adage that people often feel as good as they look. In some cases, by the time a patient has visited the beautician, attended the hospital dance, and mixed socially with members of the opposite sex it will be clear that these elements have produced as much, or even more, of value than have the formal psychiatric treatments or occupational therapy. And any informal or loosely organized activities on the ward itself, such as scrabble or simple card games, perhaps with nursing staff participating, may go far in stimulating attention, raising morale or even on occasions removing clinical symptoms or at least reducing their impact.

OCCUPATIONAL THERAPY

Among the most important of the treatments in any mental hospital is occupational therapy. It is not merely a system to pass away the patient's time or release nursing staff to attend to their duties. It is intended to be a medically prescribed activity—or rather a large group of activities—tailored to the needs of the individual patient and carried out in careful association with the other forms of treatment. It specifically aims to help the patient to resume as normal a life as possible.

OBSERVATIONS

In occupational therapy the patient's work may serve as a useful indicator of progress or relapse. The occupational therapist may find that changes in its quantity, quality, and aims all correlate with the clinical evidence; or her observations may give reason for modifying any assumptions made in the absence of this information. These observed changes may point either to an improvement or to an incipient deterioration which can then be forestalled by prompt alteration of the clinical treatment or adjustment of the social circumstances. Modification of the occupational therapy itself may also be required, for example to avoid overtaxing a patient's fluctuating capacity or to provide a greater stimulation towards alertness. For all these purposes the occupational therapist must be well versed in the symptoms of psychiatric illnesses and the psychodynamics of interpersonal and intrafamily relationships. And passage of this information to the G.P., psychiatrist or social worker may be necessary.

TREATMENT

Therapy too is not haphazard. It is based on definitive and meaningful principles. When a diagnosis has been arrived at, a scheme of rehabilitation for the client is formulated to include the clinical, social, psychological, physical and occupational aspects, with free interchange of observations among the workers concerned with these various areas. In this way cross-fertilization of understanding and the avoidance of reduplication of effort can be achieved.

As clear a definition as possible is made of the aims to be sought and the hazards to be avoided in relation to any particular patient's mental state. Thus a patient suffering from an endogenous depression (chapter 11) may need stimulation of a kind that is free from the complexities that might overtax his diminished concentration or feed into his depressive self-reproach. Only tasks that can be achieved easily should be aimed at while he is hampered by the slow pace of work imposed by the psychomotor retardation. Failure to recognize this symptom can lead to a prescription of work which can even aggravate the illness. Hypomanic states may require tasks that are quickly achieved; and the material may need to be free from parts and processes giving scope for morbid distractability or rapidity of association. As improvement occurs, however, work with more facets on which the patient can associate may reveal whether normal or morbid reactions are still occurring.

In schizophrenia the aim is commonly to bring the patient out of himself, purposeful activity replacing the long periods of sitting and immobility that can reinforce inertia or a sense of isolation and undermine his general physical condition.

Occupational therapy has an important part to play in the management of the psychoneuroses also. In anxiety states, for instance, a housewife whose anxiety renders her unemployable outside the home may need work and hobbies motivating her not only to look outwards from herself but also into the world beyond her home. At the same time anything that increases her anxiety or leads to boredom, with its sequel of anxious speculations, is avoided.

The hysterical personality may, if insufficiently occupied, develop or continue in disturbing symptoms, physical or mental. The motivations are often to escape from a situation forcing premature and intolerable self-inspection of inner conflicts. Areas of inner distress or emptiness may be thus rendered less destructive by the opportunity for suitable diversionary activities. The work prescribed for this purpose, which if well chosen and supervised may make a worthwhile contribution both to the community and to the patient's sense of fulfilment, can be strongly therapeutic, the activities increasing confidence and encouraging a mature sense of responsibility. The relatively low tolerance to frustration afflicting many of these sufferers may require that work activities be carried out with material that will not readily fall apart and thus lead to frustration or symbolize to the clients their own lack of sustained integration.

In obsessional personalities the necessary aim may be to strike a happy medium, the activity being designed to comprise something meticulous enough to accord with the obsessional personality's need for perfection while avoiding opening the door to activities leading along paths of self-perpetuating and interminable 'progress'.

All the activities have as their common denominator the aims of assessing and improving work potential, encouraging personal expression, helping patients to mix and relate together, of facilitating healthy verbal communication, of encouraging them to look outside themselves, and ultimately of surrendering some of their more crippling defence mechanisms. If these aims are successful, the patients' confidence is built up, their concentration improved, their sense of responsibility increased, and a readiness for decision-making acquired. And as a result of any reasonably solid gains in these directions, an enhancement should then take place in their ability to put into healthy perspective the stresses of ordinary life.

The occupational activities conducted in the occupational therapy department or on the wards are too numerous for full mention, but they include clerical work, filing, typing, sorting, gardening, many craft activities such as dressmaking, soft toy-making and woodwork; also light assembly work like packeting, e.g. Christmas cards, or the counting of objects and placing them in packets. The activities fall broadly into a number of categories—projective techniques, the encouragement of projects, and many other pursuits, group, domestic or recreational.

PROJECTIVE TECHNIQUES
Projective techniques are activities that make use of various media such as art, drama, music and pottery, for diagnosis and therapeutic self-expression, in symbolic, form of personality attributes and psychoneurotic problems. The intention is that the patient should project these atttibutes into the particular medium. In projective technique the patients are unaware of how their responses to the stimuli will be interpreted, and so with their attention directed away from themselves and on to the stimulus, they communicate more freely.

Modelling—very relevant for creative release through non-verbal expression—can be conducted with advantage in a group setting. In the group each person, including the therapist, is given a lump of clay for expressing emotions. An invitation such as 'We are going to explore with clay how we see things' may lead to revealing productions.

One patient may make a model of a head—ugly or beautiful, revealing how she views herself or others—which can be easily done without any marked artistic skill through the simple creation of ears, teeth, nose, etc. Another may produce a little house containing either a solitary person or a few people representing a family group. A third may produce disintegrated pieces of amorphous clay, perhaps symbolizing his own disintegrated state or lack of self-knowledge. It is emphasized that a high artistic standard is not to be sought. Moreover the aim is for the product to be created within a short space of time so that it forms a basic rather than a contrived product, not one merely expressing consciously thought out representations of a surface conception. And once again the situation is used as a jumping off ground to develop group discussions of the situations created in this way.

Psychodrama is a means of helping the patient to look at problems and significant events in his life by acting them out unrehearsed. The dimension extra to the group discussion is the acting, which may increase confidence and provide the possibility of reliving significant experiences. By putting the participant in another person's place it may render possible first a closer identification with the other person and then an insight into any comparable or related feelings within himself which may need implanting or bringing into recognition

A hypothetical and simplified example may clarify these concepts. If a person has been involved in a fire but has never fully worked through the experience, the scene may be usefully re-enacted for about fifteen minutes by group psychodrama. In the first instance this individual can perhaps only bear to be cast as the fireman and not the victim. Later, however, he may come to see, more clearly than would have been within his power simply on the basis of individual or even group discussion, the essence of the situation. Playing the fireman and not the victim may enable him to recognize and accept that other people would have experienced similar emotions. He can then gain a release from morbid guilt (and escape from the morbid egocentricity of a misconceived need for self-justification), and a feeling for other people's anxieties as well as his own. Thereafter, the value of ordinary group therapy may be made use of during the remainder of the hour. The factors involved are usually much less tangible than this very concrete illustration. But the same principles obtain.

GROUP ACTIVITIES

Sociodrama consists of the acting out, followed by group discussion, of problems of general concern to the group rather than those of a personal nature based on the specific experiences of any particular individual. However there will be occasions on which individual experiences will be involved in the subject-matter as an incidental circumstance, for example in the enactment of a scene in which one member of a family is portrayed as telling the remainder of the family that he is about to enter hospital. This particular situation has clearly been of intimate concern to all the patients in the hospital.

On the other hand the basic principle of sociodrama, which is that it does not primarily involve the individual's past experience but bears mainly on matters of concern to the group as a whole, would be exemplified by a scene representing a job interview.

It will thus be appreciated that sometimes the lines of demarcation between psychodrama and sociodrama can be ill-defined. But one fundamental difference of sociodrama, in contrast to psychodrama, is that since it rests on this general approach it does not involve such deep delving into psychological problems; and in those cases for which it suffices it thereby spares the patient the potential trauma inherent in the more intensive forms of exploration. Careful assessment, having regard to the psychodynamics of each individual and their effects on interrelationships, is therefore an essential prerequisite in the initial decision as to the particular type of these two forms of therapeutic drama which will be the most appropriate. But many other group activities, including those as varied as current affairs discussions or group psychotherapy, can all play their part; while domestic activities, such as cooking, and recreational activities including physical exercises may also be conducted within the context of the group milieu.

GROUP PROJECTS

Ideally the group as a whole decides on the nature of the project. In doing so they should include a consideration of the time element, the project being necessarily of a sort that is capable of completion within the patient's period in the hospital. Another factor involved in the determination of projects must be the form of achievement most needed by the individual patients.

Project work ranges from simple tasks such as painting the inside of a tin and covering it with material for making a wastepaper bin to the more complicated procedures of producing a magazine. And some projects, such as those involving gardening, or assisting families with home decoration, may serve to forge or maintain the links with the community which can so easily become lost or relinquished when patients are largely confined to hospital.

THE INDUSTRIAL UNIT

An Industrial Unit provides a form of rehabilitation in which patients are employed in hospital workshops to carry out jobs for local firms under contract. The activities may include assembling objects, making parts for machinery, packing and wrapping, and a whole range of other procedures relevant to the industrial sphere.

The overall object is to enable patients to regain, or perhaps gain for the first time, the capacity for working to the pattern that characterizes the modern industrial scene; and its aim essentially is to make therapeutic use of its principles rather than to secure a niche in industry after discharge, though in some cases this result may follow as an additional advantage.

The pattern of work undertaken in the industrial unit is thus based on factors such as set time-keeping, the use of machinery, and the concept of production targets. The encouragement of financial rewards and the satisfaction of work achievement combine to form a therapeutically valuable situation for suitably selected cases. In other words, whereas occupational therapy on the whole encourages patients to follow their own spontaneous, creative inclinations with a high degree of freedom from the pressures of direction, in industrial therapy it is the more directed pattern relevant to the industrial world outside the hospital that forms the ethos for improving the level of functioning and raising the self-esteem.

REHABILITATION

The administrative methods for organizing systems of rehabilitation vary from one hospital to another. And the rehabilitation processes themselves differ in the emphasis they receive, different hospitals laying differing stress on different aspects. In one, there may be strong focus on a period of self-catering in a resettlement flat in the hospital as the ultimate stage before discharge to the community resources; another may concentrate more heavily on industrial skills; and so on.

The basis of much rehabilitation, however, is a carefully planned sequence of actions, aimed at re-establishing the social skills by which the patient will eventually recapture the capacity for planning his own life. To acquire mere islets of capacity, such as for cooking or cleaning, is not enough. He must learn to plan his life as a whole, fitting together the isolated activities he has regained into an ongoing and meaningful pattern of events.

Thus a patient afflicted with severe loss of initiative may need to begin with a small series of activities directed towards a limited end—for example those entailed in getting out of bed without being directed by nursing staff. But this limited aim will also be followed by a number of other tasks such as dressing, hairbrushing, and teeth cleaning, designed to lead him through stages of increasingly advanced activities, like attending hospital functions on his own initiative, until he reaches a point at which he can develop the interest and confidence to reach out gradually towards the more distant ambition of leaving the hospital.

This sequence of helping the severely disabled patient first to look after his personal needs and then to bring them together into a coherent theme of progress is carried out essentially as a form of teaching, supplemented by a system of rewards. It therefore has broad affinities with behaviour therapy (chapter 6). These rewards may consist of visible material advantages, of which financial inducements are amongst the most easily dispensed and immediately acceptable. But the development of a sense of achievement, rather than the direct pleasures of material possessions, can be far more potent in furthering the improvement of outlook and activity in a patient receiving rehabilitation.

Not only do the systems of incentives vary, but the environments in which the rehabilitation is conducted also differ according to facilities and circumstances. It may be carried out on particular wards set aside for the purpose containing staff specializing in this work, or on those long-stay wards in which some of the patients have so deteriorated or are so lacking in social support outside the hospital that little hope of discharge can be realistically entertained, but where an improved level of awareness and activity within permanent hospital life remains a worthwhile aim, or on convalescent wards for patients whose illnesses have reached a stage of improvement at which, while treatment on the admission ward is no longer indicated, recovery is not yet sufficient to permit recommendation for discharge. And in some hospitals there is a system of special resettlement flats in which suitable patients may be helped in small groups.

The principle of rehabilitation underlying a hospital resettlement flat is to encourage suitable patients in the final phase of their hospital life towards outside independence. This system, when available, is particularly useful for those with suitable potential who have been in hospital for a prolonged period or who, because of an illness that has lowered their level of vitality or put them at serious risk of relapse either spontaneously or in response to stress, are in need of conditioning into social self-reliance.

Self-catering, shopping, use of money, use of launderettes, the procedures for claiming social security, etc., can sometimes only be learnt by these patients if they themselves carry them out. The period of living in the flat is designed to provide such opportunities.

Changes of social circumstances may also necessitate those adaptations most suitably learned through participation in this type of sheltered setting. These changes are exemplified by a man who, having lost his wife, is then prevented by his illness from learning to cook or use a launderette; or by an incompletely recovered woman whose mental condition renders her incapable of coping intelligently with the changes in the costs of domestic commodities that have occurred during her illness.

Sometimes learning to live in a small community may be valuable as a prelude to a similar life in the flat of a hostel or group home (chapter 12), either of which may be the next link in the rehabilitation chain. On other occasions the patient will proceed directly to live in the community, buttressed when indicated or practicable by relevant community resources.

The rehabilitation of many patients however begins, as we

have seen, at a much earlier stage on a less sophisticated and more highly supervised basis. The object of starting with a maximum degree of supervision, which is gradually diminished until the patient is able to live outside the hospital, is one that ultimately links with community care. Early involvement of relatives and any community worker who will be concerned with the patient's subsequent management should therefore whenever possible form an integral part of the process during the hospital period. Great advantages may accrue from explanations to relatives about the rehabilitation programme. In addition, both the relatives and the community social worker should actively contribute as closely as possible, partly to act as symbolic links of general continuity with the outside world and partly as participants whose specific continuity of relationship will later form the patient's emotional mainstay in the environment.

The history given by relatives may furnish useful data about areas of disability that merit particular remedial effort. Loss of capacity for specific functions may be revealed from these sources. One patient may be reported to have lost confidence over relationships and will now fear meeting people outside the hospital; another may have lost interest in personal appearance; a third may have developed severe anxiety about traffic; yet another may have retained the ability to talk and relate on specific tasks in hand, but with a loss of capacity for other forms of social intercourse such as smiling or making the ordinary comments of conversational interchange.

For many of these patients the planning can be less elementary than for those whose loss of initiative is more general—although in the areas for which it is indicated these patients too may require an equal or even greater intensity of therapeutic effort.

The social worker may be particularly well placed to give assistance in rehabilitation, since she does not have to exercise any degree of custodial or authoritarian regimentation. Unlike those who have the daily responsibility of the wards, she is left comparatively free to relate smoothly, and this will often be seen by the patient as an indication that she understands his inner needs. Also, in her position of witnessing the contrasting circumstances of those patients living in the community and those cared for in hospital, she will become more acutely aware of what it means to patients to lose their privacy and be deprived of the fullest opportunity for creating their own personal world around themselves.

Her role will especially come to the fore when the very improvement in the patient's state highlights the limitations on his further progress imposed by the lack of available objectives for going out. There may be nobody to meet him; or he may have no clear needs that are not already being satisfied by the hospital, with its facilities for walks in the grounds, expeditions to hospital entertainments, use of the shop, and so on. When these facilities have served their purpose and the patient has become well enough to bypass them, the social worker in her close connections with the outside world may help him to do so, and thereby restart the progress of rehabilitation that had temporarily ground to a halt.

It may well be that as time passes it will increasingly come to the notice of community social workers that certain patients have reached the stage of a fair capacity to look after themselves but still have difficulties in passing outwards through the hospital gates. And the patient who has arrived at this point and acquired an ambition to progress further—even if it be ambivalent—may thus be given the chance of a relationship that he will welcome as one in which he can present a new self to a person whose opinions and expectations may in a sense be more encouraging than those of the people who he knows have seen him at his worst. Voluntary workers in this category, acting under the supervision of professional social workers and nursing staff, may thus form very useful members of the wider rehabilitation team.

The material dealt with in the simpler type of group discussions depends on the standard of initiative reached by its members, the factors in their histories, and the experience of the staff. The broad principles of this procedure are that once the most basic skills have been acquired the patients will be brought together, told that the ward or flat must be kept clean, asked to name the jobs that will need to be done, and encouraged to think out and discuss together the problems likely to arise and the details of how they should be met. As they begin to explore possibilities and gain in concentration, ideas are gradually fed into the discussions.

The influence of the staff working alongside the patients can make or mar the prospects of success. During the first phase the staff may give help in planning timetables, exercising intervention or restraint based on the psychological progress of the group as a whole, that of its individual members and the staff members' own experience of other patients' reactions under similar circumstances in the past. But as progress occurs, the patients may begin to make their own unaided plans for the activities of the day, and later for the whole week. At a propitious stage the staff may start to withdraw, leaving them to make their own mistakes and perhaps suffer for them to some extent. If they have not budgeted well enough to obtain a Sunday dinner the situation at least provides material for discussion and improvement of competence.

The principle of encouraging them to look responsibly at what they are doing, rectify their errors when necessary, and discuss possible modifications both in terms of their present needs and future circumstances, thus becomes introduced into the scheme of progress. As at the beginning, it still remains necessary to ensure that they have enough success to carry them forward to the next stage. But by now the scene should have changed from the embryonic one in which group discussions were required for the planning of payment for milk and food, to a situation bearing many of the characteristics of a life of fuller material independence.

While all this attention has been given to the acquisition of practical skills, the patient's loss of social capacity will have been receiving its own emphasis. The loss of ability to communicate in socially acceptable ways has already been mentioned; and it can deprive him of much of the value that would otherwise crown his success in regaining his capacity for dealing with his material needs. Ineptitude in the art of interpersonal relationships can easily render these practical accomplishments hollow and sterile.

The simple basic response of smiling, and the conventional reactions of spoken greetings, may need at first to be re-established through direct methods of retraining. But if the illness has left the potential for communication open to gradual improvement through situations fostering social interaction, and if the patient has redeveloped enough inclination for self-responsibility, he may sometimes become accessible to the more advanced areas of insight provided by formal group therapy.

This situation, like the previous areas of awakening, may be slow in developing its first steps. After his entry into this new dimension of relationships, in which there are discussions of factors on an emotional level such as his problems with relatives, he may quickly revert to a preoccupation with related but less threatening matters of a more practical character, such as concern about why a certain patient may repeatedly get up in the night to make tea and how immediate problems of this sort should be coped with by the group as a whole.

This very development can lead to an improved sense of responsibility and control throughout the group; and dealing with practical matters as a corporate responsibility may itself diminish tensions within the group and pave the way for easier explorations and deeper understanding of individual emotions. Characteristic behaviour patterns of certain other patients and their motivations—recurrent quarrelling for example—may then bring the dawning of insights into the defence mechanisms involved.

The aims sought by individual casework, in modified form and using the forces of the group to enable the patient to see what happens, can be usefully exploited in the rehabilitation of mentally ill people. Often these patients lose a realistic understanding of their behaviour when the illness is at its height; and when its activity has subsided they may need to see more clearly, in the protective setting provided by the circumstances of group therapy, the areas in which their difficulties lie, together with their effects on themselves and others and the alterations required of them. As an adjunct to the drug treatment that has diminished their turbulence and rendered them more emotionally tractable, even though areas of diminished insight remain, it is sometimes within the scope of group therapy to contribute substantial benefit to psychotic patients whose condition has already derived the maximum benefit that can be conferred by drugs alone.

ART THERAPY

Another of the communal treatments about which the social worker should have some understanding is art therapy—a field possessing a number of affinities with group therapy which are fundamental both in their origin and their effects.

The common factor in their origin is that much of the material involved springs from the unconscious; the common factor in their effects is that each offers a milieu in which therapeutic opportunities rest on the opportunity for abreaction, direct 'objectification', and the outward representation in symbolic form of conflict material that would otherwise remain internalized and destructive. Both group and art therapy can serve to facilitate communication between people in whom the capacity for communication is lacking.

In what form, then, and for what reasons may people previously wrapped up in themselves become enabled to communicate more readily with one another through the medium of painting? The answer is that immediate or even rapid success is not necessarily to be anticipated. The proponents of art therapy would be the last people to make such unrealistic assumptions or extravagant claims. Nevertheless, if one is able to accept that some of mankind's most fundamental feelings are derived from the unconscious, and if one is also prepared to recognize that an individual may become severely inhibited as a resistance against their emergence while at the same time standing in need of expressing them, then it is reasonable to postulate that by projecting his inner conflicts in visual forms, in which they receive their expression in acceptable images rather than with the more threatening immediacy of the verbal medium, he may then become more articulate and able to discuss his art. And it is indeed found that in patients suffering from severe inhibitions, images rather than words may at first come to the surface more readily.

This achievement is not always easy; but it is an integral

part of the tenets of art therapy that any temptation to force the pace or exert moral pressures for performance must be resisted. Patients already under pressures from within are hardly likely to respond favourably to additional pressures from outside sources. It is therefore essential for the patient to be helped to feel at ease.

It may be necessary for patients to attend for three or four sessions before they can start to express themselves in painting, and a considerably larger number may be required to pave the way for the hoped-for expansion of their communicative capacities into other channels of expression. All patients, even those who are mute or discouragingly unproductive, should whenever possible be persuaded to attend for several sessions weekly, unless to do so would be running too seriously counter to their inclinations.

The possibility of achieving much improvement in severely apathetic patients may sometimes need to be viewed more as an ideal than as a reality; but as a general approach it is preferable for the art therapist to err on the side of hopeful effort rather than develop reactions of reciprocal apathy. A persistent if restrained hope of success is liable to be rewarded quite unexpectedly by the occurrence of relationships which in turn lead to therapeutic progress that was equally unexpected.

So far we have been thinking mainly about the fundamental principles on which art therapy is based. Now we should proceed to look at its actual practice as illustrated by a typical session. As soon as the patient enters the room the art therapist may try to put him at his ease by talking to him about any matters, whether of general interest or related to his personal affairs, that may be pressed into the service of good rapport. If a relaxed environment already exists in the group—and if the patient himself does not discourage communication by withdrawal or by an attitude of rejection or any other manifestation of undue aversion—then it often happens that other patients will come to greet him spontaneously. On the other hand the art therapist, who will already be aware of his illness, personality and difficulties, may judge that he requires to be actively introduced by her. Yet again, she may take the view that this stage is unpropitious for making formal introductions, in which case she will postpone doing so until a more suitable occasion presents itself. Stilted formality of introduction may be more deleterious than lack of immediate communication.

Next the patient is introduced to the art of painting itself. According to the individual's particular needs he will either be encouraged to start immediately or he will be left to roam around the room, usually unaccompanied so that he can be as free as possible from any sense of constraint. For one or two sessions he may spend his time looking at the work of other patients, making their acquaintance or talking with the art therapist. If he has had no experience of painting it is often necessary for him first to be shown the cupboard containing the various materials—paints, crayons, charcoal, etc. The method of mixing paints is demonstrated to him and if he is too inhibited to make any attempt to paint he may then be invited to paint something he knows about. If he is totally unable to do so it may be useful for him to be given a small paint roller by means of which encouraging marks can be put on to the paper and a start thus be made. Frequently starting is the most difficult part of the procedure. He may well find himself encouraged by being told so.

In addition to such information as may have already been garnered from the patient's general attitude and demeanour during the course of these preliminaries, the size of the paper he chooses may furnish some further data. It may be desirable, therefore, to allow him to make his own choice. Often it is found that a huge piece of paper is overwhelming and is associated with a failure to perform, whereas a smaller piece elicits a more ready response. The inhibited patient therefore often elects to use a piece of smaller size.

When he is about to begin it is naturally very common for the question to be posed, often apprehensively, 'What shall I paint?' He is told to paint anything he wishes but may then protest he is completely untalented and in any case cannot think of anything. If he remains too inhibited, the suggestion of painting simple patterns 'and just see what happens' may provide an effective starting-point. Many patients are emboldened if after about half an hour or so the art therapist holds up their paintings so they can see them from a distance. True visual perspective is unlikely to be achieved at close quarters except perhaps in those instances in which the patient possesses special artistic merit; but the wider purview of his work which he thereby obtains, in contrast to his previous focusing on the individual sectors that mainly engaged his attention while he was bending over them, provides him with a recognition of its total appearance which often he finds unexpectedly pleasing.

It is sometimes necessary for the art therapist to exercise suitable restraint when expressing her praises. A patient too lavishly congratulated on a piece of work may then have some difficulty in emancipating himself from the urge to repeat it endlessly, wishing to retain the approval of the art therapist and preserve the support to his self-regard. A desire to make progress and a readiness to venture into the unknown, both of which are healthy attitudes to be aimed at therapeutically, may become stifled rather than promoted by too heavy an emphasis on the merit of artistic technique. More sagacious and less addictive forms of encouragement are usually preferable. By allowing himself a readiness to advance to work that may seem to him less praiseworthy he may to some extent forfeit his immediate self-regard, but he will not forfeit the approval of the art therapist; and in recompense he stands to gain more than he loses.

If a patient is reluctant to participate in art therapy because of a general attitude of resentment, this aspect will need help in its own right. Similarly, if he has overwhelming inhibitions against self-revelation, these too will need to be recognized, respected and assisted by the avoidance of all semblances of pressure. But if his main difficulty is the lack of confidence he feels in his own artistic ability, the problem can be surmounted much more easily.

However important it may seem to him in the first instance, the presence or absence of artistic talent is largely irrelevant in art therapy. It is in fact the least significant element involved. And when once a start has been made, inhibitions from this source are often swept into insignificance before the greater force of his inner need to proceed. They soon cease to act as a

limiting break, and he ceases to compare his work unfavourably with that of other patients.

If a patient is well enough to walk to the department it is
seldom that he cannot produce some sort of painting, however
untalented. And often the crudest of products reveal information that is far more telling than the pointers that emerge from
those of better artistic standard. Even match-stick men may
portray material that is highly significant. In the simplest of
artistry unmistakable problems may receive expression.

Art therapy contains abreactive possibilities. Abreaction is
the process by which unconscious material, if close enough to
the surface and comparatively ready for acceptance into
consciousness—painful though this process may be—can
sometimes reach representation fairly easily in direct form.
The development that occurs within patients' art activities
may catch them off their guard. They may even be upset by
the sudden emergence. But they may thus be enabled to engage in direct representation of psychological problems, which
although they were clearly near the surface would not have
come about in other circumstances. Though caught off their
guard, at the same time they may basically wish and need
them to emerge, and through the medium of art may succeed
in this end.

Sometimes the representation of problems is direct. But in
many instances it is disguised and symbolic. Patients producing
the latter type of painting usually have greater difficulty in
putting their problems into words, even after they have expressed them in visual form, partly because the origins of their
problems are more distressing and therefore correspondingly
resistant to emergence, and partly because sometimes they are
unaccustomed to giving expression to their feelings even
though they may possess a high degree of fluency for expression of matters of a more emotionally neutral nature.

An example of this indirect type of portrayal—but one that
even so was found capable of giving rise to more direct insight
—was seen in a painting containing clouds, the sun and a
rainbow. During the course of this painting the patient began
to weep without knowing why she did so. She later realized
spontaneously that in painting clouds she had been portraying

her own predicament of emotional detachment and blindness, that the sun represented the hope of warmth and light and strength, and that the rainbow was a symbol of joy whose existence was for her nevertheless at present an illusion rather than a situation immediately open to true attainment.

This process in which material existing in symbolic state becomes manifest in concrete and tangible form may be described by the rather inelegant term 'objectification'. No other examples will be cited; the important point to be appreciated is that one of its values comprises a pinpointing process. It extracts one area of guilt, anxiety or anger from the mass of more obscure and diffuse emotions within which it has its being. This area may then at least be perceived more rationally.

Art therapy is a form of treatment which, while often enjoyable in itself, goes beyond the sphere of merely diversionary amusement. The art therapist must talk with the patient at some stage in his course; and as part of her work and as a member of the hospital team she will need to familiarize herself with those aspects of his history and illness that are considered relevant. As with music therapists, art therapists must have had some training in treatment procedures as well as being artists and musicians.

The art therapist, however, is careful to avoid two pitfalls. First she knows that as a tool of diagnosis the content of paintings must not become the subject of an intemperate enthusiasm for interpretation of symbolism, and even less so for the irresponsibility of wild speculation. Diagnostic assumptions can be made only in relation to the general clinical features and the wider psychological setting within which they occur; and only in consultation with the psychiatrist. He will test the validity of their potential contribution against the criteria of his own knowledge of the case. On the whole they must be tentative rather than dogmatic if their value is not to be jeopardized by the risk of excursions into by-paths of irrelevancy.

Secondly, she knows that she must always exercise stringent economy in her interpretive comments to the patient himself. Indeed she will probably avoid them entirely. She knows that it is not her function to tell patients the meaning of their symbols. Frequently they recognize them for themselves, though often they are unable to do so. There would be many risks attendant on presenting gratuitous or even solicited information to patients. The information might be incorrect and merely a sterile echo of the manipulative patient's efforts to gain attention by producing material deliberately contrived to be of striking impact rather than being of fundamentally causal significance—or it might simply be the art therapist's reading into the situation ideas of her own. Even when interpreted correctly the patient might be unable, as will be seen in other contexts in this book, to face its exposure. And the information imparted to patients might lead them to engage repeatedly in the same material, in the belief that the ultimate value of their artistic activity had already been reached. If left unmolested by inexpedient explanations, however, they will always have expressed something of themselves, and they will always have been creative.

It is for these reasons that the art therapist is trained to avoid interpreting paintings. In so far as she exercises any interpretive function it is that of an essentially passive role in which she acts merely as a sounding board, so that in talking about his art and the problems it reveals the patient is in effect talking about himself. It has already been seen (chapter 3) that this is a cardinal principle common to many areas of psychotherapy. Art therapy is no exception in this respect.

Art therapy need not, and indeed should not, be simply encapsulated within the precincts of the hospital. When we consider the subject of community care we shall see that the concept of social clubs for psychiatric patients living in the community, or for those who have recovered but continue in need of this type of support, has taken firm root over the years in the principles of preventive psychiatry. By taking part in the organization and activities of these clubs the social worker can play an invaluable part (chapter 12). And if her inclinations are sympathetic towards artistic activity, there will be ample scope for her involvement in this sphere.

In some respects the same principle again applies as that which obtains in relation to the patients themselves, namely that it is not necessary for the social worker conducting the sessions to have much artistic ability. But there is one associated disadvantage. If she herself feels diffident and regretful about her relatively low capacity in the artistic sphere, she may set undue store on good artistic standards.

People with striving but self-critical tendencies are sometimes prone to be over-impressed by skills which they themselves do not possess to the extent that they would wish, whereas areas of activity in which such an individual can succeed effortlessly or with comparatively little thought will often be held by him in less awe. Hence an artistically untalented social worker may strive almost automatically to obtain from the patient specimens of work suitable for display, while an art therapist will be free from any inclination to press for successful painting or work that is meaningful by conventional criteria. She should always remember this principle in any work which she may undertake under the supervision of a visiting art therapist with patients taking part in therapeutic club activities in the community.

MUSIC THERAPY

An important application for this field of therapy is with psychoneurotic patients who have shown hopeful signs of potentiality for self-expression and self-evaluation if given suitable help. It can be carried out in various ways—one being as a projective technique by making music, or as subject-matter for discussion by those whose psychological isolation or lack of interests preclude easy communication. It exploits a medium which may draw heavily on the emotions, often those of a particularly deep quality. Therefore it holds the potential power of making individuals more acutely aware on a feeling level of their deeper emotions in need of release, and sometimes brings them into conscious prominence in a form far sharper than can be obtained through less fundamental methods of approach.

In one technique the occupational therapist or music therapist plays music which is relatively unfamiliar, so that the patients will not be able to associate it with previous circumstances of little relevance but will draw on their deeper feelings. Nevertheless it should not be so unfamiliar—such as music from a distant country in another hemisphere—as to be devoid of any material suitable to stimulate the imaginative processes. The object is for the music to conjure up feelings, and for patients to discuss them in relation to their past and present reactions. The therapist tells them to concentrate on the music and talk about what it means to them—the feelings it evokes and any experiences it may remind them of—not confining their responses merely to whether or not they like the music. In other words the music is used as a portal of entry, facilitating a group discussion which then embodies the principles and practice of group dynamics in general.

The other main technique exploring the musical dimension —though one that does not involve the projective approach— lies in encouraging patients to make their own music (perhaps through simple percussion bands), and indeed even to make their own instruments as a related project, for instance with pieces of wood or metal placed in a box to produce a rattle. Long-term patients such as geriatrics and the mentally sub-normal, including children, are sometimes the most suitable subjects for this. A record is played or a pianist performs, and each patient is given an instrument with instructions to use it in time to the music under the guidance of the therapist. It is important for nurses and other workers concerned with these patients to participate as far as possible, so that they have the chance of seeing their patients in this facilitating situation and are available to cope if necessary with any restlessness in the more disturbed members, the therapist being more concerned with organizing the activity. This situation may help to produce an improved level of vitality in those whose illnesses have reduced their interest in activities and in relating; and to those who have previously wished for relationships but have lacked circumstances suitable to dissolve their inhibitions it may give a much needed opportunity to achieve this ambition, putting into abeyance the more threatening aspects of conventional communication and substituting in their place a reassuring situation of agreeable activities easily shared and providing a beneficial sense of unity and achievement.

The assessment opportunities can be multiple. The unexpected emergence of a leader adopting a form of 'authority', in beating the drum for instance, may be illuminating; 'activists' and 'passivists' may reveal themselves in this light for the first time; some patients may be found incapable of withstanding noise and thus recognized as unlikely to be suitable for certain forms of employment; others may show themselves intractably withdrawn, unduly prone to retreat, or unexpectedly possessing a potentiality for 'coming out of themselves' and a certain amount of hidden capacity for mixing and coping which justifies an attempt at placement in suitable social clubs. Finally, any significant capacity for rhythmical activity or appreciation of music may be utilized in appropriate music groups after their discharge from hospital.

Part Three

Psychoneuroses

8

The psychoneurotic client: some theories

Within the whole range of the responsibilities and intricacies of social work, some of the heaviest and most perplexing burdens are to be found amongst the demands on time, thought and emotional resilience imposed by clients with psychoneurotic problems.

These problems are inescapable in every social worker's daily practice. And they are made all the more worrying because often they seem so intractable, and the sufferers so frankly uncooperative or clingingly unwilling to relinquish a therapeutic relationship when it seems to have outlasted its purpose. Sometimes the clients appear perversely determined to create problems for themselves, even in the face of their strongly expressed wishes to be relieved of them and despite all the social worker's efforts to help. At other times they deny the very existence of problems that are clearly present and highly significant to themselves and their dependants.

After a brief period of experience most social workers will have become involved in situations of this sort. Reactions of discouragement, and perhaps aversion, can occur. The lack of an immediately tangible technique for helping these clients can lead to a distressing sense of inadequacy. Appearances of ingratitude can generate resentment.

Only by acquiring some insight into the meanings of psychoneuroses—meanings that go beyond the interpretations of ordinary common sense—can the social worker hope to provide these clients with the sort of acceptance they basically need. Only, for example, by understanding the origins and the effects of possessing an emotionally immature personality can the extent of this particular handicap be really comprehended. The disadvantages of subnormality of intelligence are plain to see, and hence any antisocial effects they may produce usually arouse no more than passing resentment, even though they may be very serious. On the other hand, the difficulties of moving in a world of emotionally mature people, when possessed of only the emotional makeup of a young child, may be much less apparent. But they can be equally disastrous to the powers of adjustment of the sufferer, and are far less likely to receive the understanding to which they are entitled. If only for this last reason the reader should also become as well acquainted as possible with the material discussed in chapter 2.

Again, the implacable rigidity of a severely obsessional personality superficially seems often to justify the designation of wilful stubbornness. But if on the basis of clinical knowledge it is realized that in reality he is the victim of an inflexibility which he himself would much prefer not to possess, and which he often recognizes as seriously conflicting with his own best interests, then a more accepting therapeutic relationship can be established and a more convincing presentation of his difficulties be given to his family when indicated.

In this chapter, therefore, we shall look at some of the theoretical factors lying behind psychoneurotic attitudes.

THE UNCONSCIOUS MIND

For an understanding of psychoneurosis an understanding of the unconscious mind is essential. Three important pioneers of the work in this sphere were Freud, Jung and Adler. But other workers, including in particular the famous physiologist Pavlov, have provided contributions to an appreciation of psychoneurosis of outstanding and fundamental significance.

The writings of Freud and Jung, concerned as they are with unconscious rather than conscious mental processes, not only introduced unique insights into the development and nature of neurosis itself but also made some illuminating commentaries on human activities in general, within which can be included many of the minor aberrations of a homespun quality to which we are all prone. In addition, widespread and searching penetrations were made by these two original thinkers into a great deal of the material found in art, literature and religion. And Pavlov, in his work on conditioning, made discoveries in the field of physiology that have practical as well as theoretical application to psychiatry, psychology, sociology and related areas of knowledge, in particular extending our understanding of the principles of psychoneurosis and forming the foundation of the treatment known as behaviour therapy (chapter 6).

To consider the work of Freud or Jung in anything beyond a brief and very incomplete outline would carry us into details too far removed from the practical approaches often required by the social worker. But this is not to say that a fuller understanding of unconscious material motivating feeling and conduct is without relevance. And although the present context does not lend itself to any very close consideration of these concepts nevertheless any further enlightenment the social worker may choose to acquire in this field will add usefully to her understanding of the motivation of her clients, and may provide her with a means of assessing situations that cannot always be comprehended in any other terms with much coherent logic or practical value.

FREUD

In outline Freud likened the mind to an iceberg, with only the tip being visible above the surface while the bulk is submerged from view. The latter area of the mind he termed the unconscious, or in its less deep levels the subconscious. In it are contained ideas and emotions that are so disturbing to peace of mind that they cannot be permitted to exist in conscious awareness. Insight into the nature of this material, the means by which it has been relegated into the unconscious mind, the means by which it is maintained there—with whatever degree of success or failure—and the effects on conscious life of its re-emergence, in whatever form it then takes, comprise the essential tenets within Freud's tremendous contribution to psychological understanding.

Without for the moment concerning ourselves with any particular material that he postulated as being involved in conflict situations, we must first look at his broad conception. When two contradictory impulses are present in consciousness, the emotions generated by the resulting conflict may reach the point of intensity beyond which their continued presence in consciousness becomes so intolerable as to necessitate exclusion. And when these painful emotions are relegated from the realm of awareness to that of the unconscious mind, the process—termed repression—is automatic. In adults removal of undesired material may on occasions be associated with the more sophisticated procedure of consciously intended deliberation; but 'repression' occurs without conscious intention. Essentially the process of removal from consciousness of the material whose presence there would be too disturbing is one in which the shutters come down automatically, without the conscious intention, and indeed without the knowledge, of the individual engaging in it.

The material removed from awareness thus comes to exist in the unconscious mind as a repressed system of ideas that are charged with painful emotion. Such a system, outside awareness, is termed a complex. Unfortunately the complex does not automatically undergo resolution or become transmuted into a static entity. On the contrary it continues as a dynamic force exercising itself against consciousness, which then remains at risk of falling victim to its readmission—with all the disturbances implied in that possibility.

Freud postulated that to maintain the state of repression the individual develops a mechanism termed the superego, which functions as a custodian of the unconscious—a sort of policeman guarding against the entry of undesirable intruders.

The reader will now appreciate the difference between the term repression—at least in its use in psychiatric nomenclature—and suppression. Suppression is a conscious process adopted by the individual towards others or towards himself. Repression, as we have seen, is a process of whose existence he is unaware. A similar principle obtains in the case of the superego or censor mechanism. Its function of maintaining the painful complexes in a due state of repression is also unknown to the individual engaging in it. It has sometimes been termed, though the analogy is a loose one, the unconscious conscience.

The work of the superego is not continuously and wholly successful. For example it may be too 'thorough', bottling up the individual's emotions with a resulting unhealthy rigidity of feeling and outlook that is sometimes accompanied by a censoriousness of attitude picked up intuitively by others even when the individual tries, with laborious and somewhat guilt-laden attempts, to soften its expression. If too much repression is required, too much energy can be taken up by maintaining the repression. Moreover such a personality, however meritorious and however much he attempts tolerance, is clearly unfulfilled in the quality of his feeling and communication. In spite of all its potentially disruptive effects the unconscious cannot be excessively blocked off with impunity. The human being can only move too far away from his instinctual needs at his peril—hence part of the value of art and symbolism and the need for opportunities for reflective relaxation which the material and psychological enslavements of modern life do not always allow.

But there are also problems that arise from underfunctioning of the superego. In minor degrees these episodes are so common as to be part of the normal human scene. Indeed they were regarded by Freud as protective, in that if they were not to occur the individual could be too rigid and inhibited. According to Freud they may be manifested by ordinary acts of inexplicable folly that are clearly at variance with the individual's conscious wishes and his best interests, but which still bubble up into action or feeling. 'What on earth made me do that?' is a commonly heard phrase that may sometimes contain a wealth of significance in these terms. Irrational actions carried out in a state of lucidity and without organic pathology of the cerebral cortex are apt to have true reasons on a second level of meaning and motivation. Freud believed that even a *lapsus linguae* may be a tell-tale extrusion of underlying truth emerging through a crack in the momentarily lifted curtain of repression.

Situations so common can hardly be called pathological.

But all gradations occur along the scale of control of unconscious material; and it is a matter of everyday experience
that some individuals are frequently assailed by eruptions of
the unconscious—for example of an aggressive or self-punitive
kind—which while not carrying them into frank illness can
nevertheless cause them repeated unhappiness and failures,
especially in the field of human relationships. Freudian ideas
can go a long way towards explaining the unhappy paradoxes
of those who are their own worst enemies, or are at the mercy
of their own intermittent and seemingly gratuitous hostility
towards others whom essentially they hold dear.

In spite of these ordinary aberrations most people cope fairly
satisfactorily at most times because the superego is functioning
adequately enough. But in some cases, as a result of constitutional predisposition, physical factors or psychological stresses,
its efficiency may diminish. Then the individual needs to
muster his psychological defence mechanisms.

PSYCHOLOGICAL DEFENCE MECHANISMS

So far in this brief sketch of the ideas postulated by Freud we
have confined our attention to the general concept of repression.
The actual nature of the repressed material thought to be contained within the unconscious mind will be discussed later.
Nor have we as yet discussed the various defence mechanisms
evoked against the re-emergence of this material into consciousness.

Before looking at these mechanisms individually, four
factors believed to be common to them all must be noted.
Firstly, they take place automatically, without involving intention by the individual in the ordinary sense. Secondly, they
occur unconsciously, the individual being unaware of their
operation. Thirdly, their basic function consists of investing
the emerging underlying material with a disguise that safeguards consciousness against the disturbing effects which its
admission in direct and undisguised form would entail.
Fourthly, although they are defensive in their purpose, they are
nevertheless only partially successful. Hence while to a greater
or lesser extent they safeguard consciousness against the direct
impact of material from the unconscious, at the same time they

raise their own problems in consciousness itself—sometimes clinical in degree—since even in its disguised forms this emergent material, though rendered less traumatic and painful, still often has a markedly disturbing character.

Having understood these general properties, the social worker can now usefully familiarize herself with the names and definitions of at least some of these mechanisms. Among the most important are reaction formation, dissociation and projection.

Since difficulties within the family setting form the largest part of the inter-personal problems for which the social worker's aid will be sought, she will frequently see instances of the interactions of these mechanisms between the members within a family—between parents and children for instance.

Let us look at the first of these mechanisms—reaction formation—and consider a simple illustrative situation in which it could take place between an adult and a child.

Reaction formation is a defence mechanism in which underlying feelings are kept out of conscious awareness by an exaggeration of the tendency opposite to that which has undergone repression. For our illustration of this mechanism, we may consider a child's insecure feelings that are presenting themselves in a disguised form which is unrecognized as such, and which is therefore failing to bring him the reassurance he needs from his parents. Suppose, for example, that a mother is trying to help to dress a child who has been disturbed by a previous admission to hospital at an early and crucial stage of his development and in circumstances under which the separation was maximally traumatic and led to continuing insecurity. Such a child may well refuse to accept her help, pushing her away and rejecting her further advances.

The mother may at first react by accusing the child of never having needed her, of always wanting to do everything for himself, of not even having recognized her when she came back from hospital or missing her while she was away. Eventually she feels little interest in the child's feelings and needs in relation to herself, wishing to avoid involvement with him. This mother's approach having been rejected by the child, her unfulfilled wish to believe that he accepts her has become abandoned as unattainable and too painful to persist in.

This exaggeration of the tendency opposite to that which has been removed from awareness for self-protection brings its own problems, being a falsification rather than a resolution of the basic situation. And it is worth remembering that it is not uncommon for a child to fail to make much acknowledgement of the mother's return from hospital, this being his own defensive response to the combined separation and sibling jealousy. This false front of independence adopted by the child is of course an example of reaction formation within the child himself.

Another mechanism that can be usefully thought about is dissociation. This defence mechanism consists of a splitting of consciousness—not the type of splitting that characterizes schizophrenia, but a state in which groups of ideas remain more or less in their own compartments unaffected by the logic in the others. Some examples will make it clear. First we may look at dissociation in an adult, again operating within the family setting. A young child may be playing with a toy which then breaks, perhaps the head falling off a doll. The mother may fail to comply with the requests to mend it, and a tantrum may result. It is perfectly natural that at this age the child wants his own way and cannot tolerate much frustration.

It is obviously natural and healthy for adults also to have their limits and become angry under the ordinary stresses of life. On the other hand if, for example, a child falls over, hurting his knee and making his clothes dirty, and if the mother herself is severely immature emotionally—commonly as a sequel to her own emotionally disturbed early background—then she may react by hitting the child, shrieking at him, stripping off his clothes, sending him to bed, and neglecting the knee. The mechanism of dissociation may be present. She fails to console the child, taking no notice of his feelings, from which she is dissociated, or of the disproportionate nature of her own reactions. This dissociative defence reaction arises from her own basic lack of maturation, or from a current stage of regression that may be remediable by suitable help.

With increasing experience of family histories and situations the reader will come to recognize this mechanism in relation to some of the cases of florid adult hysteria; and on being told by these adult clients about their own childhoods or by witnessing the present developmental problems in childhood situations themselves, the caseworker may recognize the basis of the difficulties that afflict some of these clients who have remained unable to make deep or sustained relationships.

Another example of this mechanism may be exemplified by the case of a child subjected to erosion of his loyalty to one parent by the other, or when he is constantly assaulted by a parent's criticism against him which is of the neurotic quality destined to cut too deeply into his sense of acceptance and security. Thus an overwrought mother may be seen by a young and impressionable child to be criticizing her husband, telling her neighbour or the social worker that she will leave home and saying in the child's presence that the child constantly whines, fails to occupy himself, and incessantly hangs around her feet. The child, on the other hand, may hardly notice, continuing to hum to himself nonchalantly.

Here by the mechanism of dissociation the child is disregarding the situation. If he were really to take it in, the pain would be too great. He shows little concern, since he has needed to defend himself against emotionally threatening situations of this sort so often in the past. He cannot allow emotions to penetrate, and so he grows up emotionally shallow. Although in these circumstances feelings in later life are often intense on the surface, he develops little depth into which he can anchor his reactions in a stable and secure way.

Again, a child may be incontinent as a result of regression (chapter 3), wetting his pants but clearly unconcerned. The mother will be angry, accusing him of being lazy, messy, dirty and indifferent. This too may be a defence reaction of dissociation in the child. He is denying to himself that anything is amiss, though realizing that she is angry.

After a time this child may come up to his mother with the object, for example, of receiving a sweet from a tin out of which she has taken one for herself. In asking ingenuously for a sweet he reveals that he has not been able to register his mother's anger in a normal way. He had dissociated himself from it. He denies to himself the fact of her punitiveness. This makes her even more angry, because she assumes that in the ordinary sense he simply does not care.

One last example of dissociation may be useful. It is one sometimes seen in connection with sibling rivalry. The mother may be paying an excess of attention to a child's sibling, comparing this sibling too unfavourably with the child. She may say that the sibling is quite different and does not whine all the time etc. The child may then kiss the sibling so hard that it hurts. This is another example of dissociation. The child is partially denying to himself the aggression aroused in him by the pangs of sibling jealousy. In one sense he is being kind and loving, but in another it is an act of aggression towards the favoured sibling and possibly a manipulation to gain praise.

The sort of conflict between the aggressive feelings which a child who has been pathologically mishandled has accumulated towards his parents, and the love or anxiety which prevents his giving expression to them, is sometimes dealt with by the mechanism of projection. Being afraid to recognize his own aggressive feelings he projects them on to people and situations that are essentially inappropriate. Fighting with other children, perhaps stealing from school coats, or similarly 'unprovoked' and 'unreasonable' behaviour are frequent outcomes of this mechanism.

Projection is the mechanism whereby the individual assuages his sense of guilt, however caused, by ascribing it irrationally to other people rather than to himself. For example, a mother with an hysterical personality may implant into a child an unjustified sense of guilt by adopting a morbidly martyred attitude, retiring to bed with a headache and accusing the child of having made her ill with the noise and the worry he causes her. He in turn may then blame his sibling, saying that it was not his fault but the fault of his brother.

Over the years, in severe cases an increasing sense of guilt may become so unbearable that he almost constantly disencumbers himself of it by repeated use of this mechanism. But it is only partially successful and does not lead to self-acceptance of a healthy variety. Moreover when this pattern of reaction becomes established and spreads widely over the environment of his life it brings, naturally and inevitably, counter-criticisms and counter-pressures from the environment as a whole.

These counter-reactions reinforce his insecurity and contribute their own part to the vicious circle in which he is caught up. On reaching adult life he continues to project, perhaps putting his own child off his school work by forcing homework help on to him—while blaming the school for incompetence. Or the mechanism of dissociation may be brought into play. Thereby he may practice double standards and fail to see any connection, for example chain smoking while reprimanding others for lighting cigarettes.

There are other defence mechanisms. Thus rationalization refers to the making of a judgement on emotional grounds by an individual who believes it to have been arrived at by logic; and sublimation is a mechansim whereby unacceptable instinctual energy is deflected into socially acceptable channels of expression. But whether the child develops unhealthily by direct absorption of morbid attitudes, or whether by these defence reactions against them, the long-term result can clearly become an established state, crippling and lifelong, if the causal factors in childhood are severe and continue unrelieved.

FREUDIAN CONCEPTS OF DEVELOPMENT

Freud's concepts of the contents of the unconscious mind relate closely to his belief in the crucial part played by sex in the development of neurosis—and indeed its part in influencing attitudes over a whole range of thinking and feeling which at first sight would not appear to have any connection with this aspect of life.

Amongst his extensive commentaries on psychological matters, it is his theory of early childhood sexuality that is the one perhaps the most alien to the areas of understanding ordinarily held by those unfamiliar with his work. Partly for this reason it is also the one which at the time of its inception generated the most widespread and heated controversy. Nevertheless many of the insights to which it gave birth have been found increasingly convincing with the passage of time, and much of the resistance evoked by the initial aversion and clinical conservatism has now subsided, even though a few workers still elect to sidestep as far as possible the unacceptable implications they assume it to carry. But most people, whatever their primary fields of interest, recognize that each of the major analytical schools propounding psychological motivations has its place in our total scheme of understanding, and that no school of thought, even one emanating from such a genius of original thinking as Freud, can validly claim a monopoly of psychological insight. That the unconscious mind can exert a profound influence, however, is beyond dispute.

Freud derived his theory of development from the studies on neurosis which he carried out by a technique known as 'free association', in which thoughts were traced backwards, if possible to their origins, by the patient trying to allow them to flow freely and without hindrance, adopting as relaxed an attitude as could be achieved and taking all steps to avoid withholding information about himself through anxiety, shame or indeed any motive that might impede their free expression. These are still the criteria aimed at for patients undergoing Freudian psychoanalysis.

The details of Freudian theory are extensive and complex, and we would not be justified in pursuing them in much depth in the present description. Only a very brief thumbnail sketch will therefore be given. First, his theory of infantile sexuality.

Infantile sexuality

The essence of Freud's theory of infantile sexuality is that the child inherently passes through certain developmental stages during the course of early life which leave effects that linger into adult life and lurk unrecognized behind many adult attitudes seemingly unrelated to them. He conceived these developmental stages as consisting of three main phases termed the infantile stage, the latency period and puberty.

The social workers should be aware of the existence of these phases, and should have some knowledge of the contents postulated as part of each one, since the seeds of neurosis that lie within them may be in process of implantation into the children of any of the families with whom she is dealing. Moreover the adult members of these families may themselves have acquired neurotic difficulties, about which she should have some understanding, tied up with prior happenings in these same phases in their own early development.

The first phase, the infantile phase, is also termed the auto-erotic stage. Within this phase Freud conceived the infant as passing through three consecutive sub-divisions of developmental progress which he terms the oral, anal and genital phases. Each of these phases he regarded as being associated with the experiencing of a particular type of sensory pleasure by the infant. The oral phase in his view involves sensory pleasure through the mucous membranes of the mouth; the anal phase involves the deriving of satisfaction associated with the processes of excretion; and the genital phase contains a source of physical enjoyment derived from this bodily area.

Unless fixation occurs at any of these stages, according to the Freudian theory, the child normally passes through each stage of emotional development satisfactorily. But if he fails to do so and becomes 'fixated' at a particular phase, he will carry into adult life emotions and relationship urges relevant to the infantile state concerned. And although not present in consciousness, they will influence his feelings, the nature of his relationships, and his capacity for adjustment.

We must now turn to a particular situation believed by Freud to occur in these early years which, though embodying a concept that was first described by him in detail in the nineteenth century, had broadly been foreshadowed in mythological terms in ancient Greece. It is the widely known, but less widely understood, Oedipus complex.

The Oedipal complex

In ancient Greek literature Oedipus was a tragic figure who slew his father and later married his own mother. Freud postulated an important parallel between this fictional theme and certain conflicts that are liable to sow the seeds of neurosis in the early stages of a boy's normal development within the realm of observable non-fictional reality, holding that a strong emotional attachment by the boy to the mother occurs as a universal phase of early development, from which he normally becomes healthily emancipated but in which, if unhealthy circumstances so decree, he may become 'fixated', and predisposed to later difficulties in sexual relationships.

Attention having been focused on to it, the essence of the concept is easy to recognize. What is more natural than that a young boy—dependent since birth on the love of his mother, which he continues to need and grows to reciprocate—should jealously resent the intrusion of his father's rivalry in the triangular relationship? And what is more understandable than that his resentment will also be mixed with conflicting feelings about the intruding male parent, from whom retaliation is to be feared but towards whom he has also developed feelings of warmth and on whom it is in any case his developing nature to model himself? The corollary that inner emotions of guilt and anxiety will characterize this early stage of his development, and colour his future attitudes if unresolved, need hardly be a matter of surprise.

The social worker, keen on achieving an understanding of her client in practical terms, may be apt to think of the Oedipal complex as being merely an esoteric and somewhat unreal concept, unrelated to the reality with which she herself is concerned. Such is not thought to be the case, however, by those who believe in its significance; and it will be worth our briefly relating this concept to some of the everyday circumstances that she encounters.

The ultimate significance of the Oedipal situation depends on how well it is resolved—a highly practical matter in which her own understanding and efforts may go far towards ensuring success instead of the far-reaching consequences that are postulated, probably correctly, as being sometimes the price of failure. Supposedly the happy resolution is that normally the boy subsequently attaches himself emotionally in a healthy manner to his father, with whom he identifies, and thereby eventually becomes a healthy man. If, however, the Oedipal attachment is not resolved, then the boy vies for his mother's attention, being at risk of becoming a 'mummy's boy' who grows up over-dependent, lacking in essential masculinity and prone to make an unhappy marriage because he still has an unduly strong primary need for a mother-figure relationship.

It is not only on the domestic front that difficulties may arise. A far wider spectrum of life—including the working situation—is sometimes thought liable to receive reverberations from these early circumstances. Fear of the rivalry of other males, as a legacy of unresolved feelings concerning his father, is thought apt to ensue, because in effect he remains pursuing the mother relationship and unconsciously feels in peril of other males standing for father. This fear of rivalry may then produce irrational envies and emotions, including anxieties about the possibility of his rivals' greater competence. Any hint of competition may evoke intolerable anxiety so that he shrivels into incompetence, perhaps reacting with petty resentments that render him a disagreeable colleague with equals, or becomes prone to surround himself with nonentities whose competition he need not fear. Ordinary anxieties, healthy restraint and the modesty of fulfilment are part of the mature individual's characteristics. But the timidity and its defensive consequences postulated as Oedipal in origin are thought to be of a different quality.

It is believed that the healthy cessation of the Oedipal situation depends on the existence of ordinarily favourable circumstances of family life. Anything that seriously disrupts the closeness of a marital relationship may conspire to the unhealthy perpetuation of the Oedipal state. Sometimes, for example, difficulties may be introduced by a father's repeated long absences from home through the needs of work as a result of which, unless steps are taken to avoid it, he and his son may grow apart. Moreover on his return home he may be heavily drained by his work, with little vitality for relating to the child. The normal closeness between the mother and son may thus become abnormally intense or prolonged.

Some of the factors other than physical absence that may

cause emotional isolation of marital partners are discussed elsewhere, and many others may reveal themselves to social workers over the course of years. These circumstances may leave the mother feeling starved of affection. Nature abhors a vacuum, and if she fails to receive it from her marital partner she may well turn to her young son to fill the emotional void. The boy, having acquired a taste for the situation, may then himself proceed to set the pace, and an unwitting state of collusion between mother and son may become a self-perpetuating system, though without intention by either to cause family distress or neurotic disturbance.

Although lack of stable marital affection may be the sad reality—frequently as a legacy of the partners' early life experiences—nevertheless a genuine marital affection may be present which, because the man is undemonstrative to his wife, passes unrecognized and therefore fails to forestall the Oedipal problem. But, whatever the reason for the prolongation of the infantile closeness of relationship between mother and son, even if the divisive circumstances eventually subside and the father reasserts his emotional claims on his wife the boy may then become further disturbed by the resulting shift in the balance of emotional relationships.

The Electra complex

Comparable difficulties may arise in relation to the situation known as the Electra complex.

The Electra complex—a term also derived from Greek legend—postulates a phase of developmental attachment between the girl and her father in early life. Apt, like the Oedipal situation, to become perpetuated on an unintentionally collusive basis it too can constitute a situation redolent with psychoneurotic potentialities.

According to these psychoanalytical teachings, if for any reason a girl fails to identify with her mother but over-identifies with her father she is unconsciously liable to retain the fantasy-image of an ideal male based on a little girl's concept of her father as a God-like figure. When her marital partner in later life is unable to measure up to this fantasy-concept and idealized notion, marital resentments and discord may develop. Moreover this ambivalent aversion to ordinary mundane males—her reaction to her father was itself an ambivalent attachment—though unrecognized by herself, may communicate itself to her daughters, who absorb it during their own childhoods and later suffer corresponding difficulties in adjusting to their own marital relationships. Sexual frigidity, thought in some circumstances to be the sexual expression of a marital resentment arising from this attachment or even the outward manifestation of an unconscious incest taboo, may add its own marital difficulties.

While it is always important to avoid the pitfall of forcing an interpretation of individual situations into preconceived abstract moulds, the social worker will nevertheless encounter cases in which this sequence of events can be recognized as likely in the light of the observed facts. Clear expression of love for a child is an essential requisite from both parents from the outset of the child's life. But the excessive doting over a girl by her father to an extent that interferes with the mother's position may contain the seeds of many later difficulties in the child. Not only may the mother's basic emotional relationship with her daughter and her husband become impaired, but her practical authority may be undermined. For various reasons, therefore, she may become classed in the eyes of the daughter as a less attractive proposition for self identification, and the child's healthy developmental identification with her mother may thus become impeded.

If the parents then begin to pull together early enough and healthily enough to rectify the girl's insidiously distorted developmental needs, the factors are unlikely to lead to significant consequences. But if parental jealousies due to their own immaturity prevent this possiblity, her normal milestones of emotional development may remain unpassed. And ultimately the father too will be unhappy in the reaping of what he has sown. The girl may well grow into a resentful and manipulative 'little madam'. When she reaches the teenage phase, if the emotional attachment has persisted unhealthily he may become embarrassed by her boy-friends, possibly adopting a volte-face of sharp withdrawal from the girl, which will be emotionally disturbing to her at a time when her need for security is paramount. And if she has become strongly conditioned into the art of male/female manipulation, she may exercise her newly found powers by importing boy-friends as rivals into the situation. Some of the more subtle effects believed to flow sometimes from her attitude towards her father in relation to her later long-term ambivalence towards males have already been mentioned.

The latency period

After these early years in which the phases of infantile sexuality have been developing and in which the seeds of later-life sexual adjustment or maladjustment have been sown, there comes the sexually quiescent period of the 'latency phase'.

The latency period starts at around the fourth year and continues until puberty. It is the phase of childhood during which there takes place a consolidation of the repressions initiated in the previous stages—with the residual memories of these earlier emotions retreating from awareness—and in which there occurs a new means of preventing their re-emergence. This last mechanism is referred to as sublimation.

Sublimation is the process through which unacceptable instinctual tendencies become deflected by the individual into channels of expression that are socially approved and desirable. This mechanism, which exists as part of the process of acquiring healthy patterns of behaviour and outlook, is unknown to the individual practising it. But these years of the latency period, in which the earlier repressions are consolidated and the necessary sublimations brought into being, play a vital part in the shaping and fashioning of the individual's future. Any effort the social worker may make towards modifying any morbid factors impeding the healthy progress of this phase of development will therefore prove amply worthwhile if they are well-directed.

Aspects of dream life

In the minor revelations of repressed material that constitute the features of neurosis the material is disguised, though in waking life it often shows some relationship to the reality that characterizes the world of ordinary life. In sleep, however, the situation is very different. Rational meaning often seems virtually non-existent and, according to the Freudian explanation of dreams, it is here that the unconscious material often asserts itself in its most intensely irrational form.

Many factors are involved in dream life, and the following is only a resumé of this one school of thought. During sleep the superego and its associated defence mechanisms, like many other processes in the organism, function at a lower level of activity. Hence in sleep the underlying material has comparatively unbridled opportunities to exert a more direct influence on mental activity. And this material, being unchanged by the logic of conscious thought processes, commonly reveals itself to the dreamer in forms far more bizarre than those which obtain when it intrudes into the waking state.

But even in sleep, it is believed, modifying mechanisms operate. Here too the symbolic representations that we have already seen to be a potent source of irrational feelings in conscious life appear to play their part in determining content. From the basis of his emphasis on sexual drives as the determinants of mental development and unconscious influences, it was a logical concept that Freud regarded these sexual influences as the attributes that receive the symbolic representation in dreams. Freudian symbolism in both sleeping and waking life is the aspect of his teaching that is perhaps the best known. But it is not always the more subtle pressures, arising from the deeper levels of the unconscious mind in its clamourings for emergence, that receive their expression in dreams. Sometimes material that is quite directly and obviously in the nature of wish fulfilment is experienced.

The analysis of dreams can of course only be carried out by a skilled psychoanalyst. Incomprehensibly bizarre fragments of thoughts may be strung together in broken sequences whose meanings may for a long time or even permanently elude confident interpretation. Defence mechanisms may operate whereby emphasis becomes displaced in the dream from crucially important material on to that which in point of fact is much less significant. And the dream content may become overlaid with secondary material imposed on it by the dreamer after waking.

The fact that the material of dreams is usually forgotten so rapidly, even when it has been vividly unpleasant, lends its own confirmation to the basic concept of repression. A process of active repression, rather than the mere forgetting of such vivid material—which otherwise would hardly fade over such a short period—is clearly the operative mechanism. On resumption of its normal level of functioning on waking, the mechanism of repression becomes reactivated.

A knowledge of all these theoretical points, apart from its general interest, is of value to the social worker because it highlights with further clarity—for her awareness in relation to the more direct aspects of her work—the existence and importance of unconscious material and processes in the sphere of the irrational. The reverberations amongst a client's family and associates that occur when underlying material remains unrecognized form the substance of many of the difficulties the social worker meets in practice.

JUNG

Another great analytical psychologist whose ideas are particularly worth attention by the social worker is the Swiss psychiatrist Carl Jung. As a young man Jung was a pupil of Freud and it is therefore natural that throughout his life his views bore the imprint of his teacher in that he accepted, at least in their broad form, some of the fundamental tenets which Freud himself evolved. Like Freud, for example, he accepted the existence of the unconscious mind, and with Freud he shared the recognition that its workings are of fundamental importance both in health and illness. Another broad basis of similarity was their common belief in the immature and indeed infantile quality of the symptoms of psycho-neurosis, which both men considered to be related to the patient's emotional ties within the family relationships. And the corollary to these beliefs, which again reflects a fundamental agreement in broad conceptions, was that the techniques of treatment of psychoneurotic symptoms were to be viewed, both in their theoretical basis and their practical implementation, in terms of the value of following symptoms backwards into the realms of infantile reality.

In many other aspects however—and these too were very fundamental—Jung's evaluation of psychological processes differed widely from those of Freud. In much of its content this divergence of outlook from that of his teacher was of a radical nature. After absorbing his basic influences, he broke away from Freud and formulated his own elaborations and modifications, which made for a gulf between their work that was to prove unbridgeable.

One of the most basic areas of his disagreement concerned his conception of libido and its part in normal and abnormal mental life. Whereas Freud ascribed to the libido a heavily sexual role in which disturbed emotional attachments lead to the sort of fixations already described, Jung viewed it as a broader force of life having a nature far less sexually-toned than that envisaged by Freud. As we have seen, Freud taught that neurosis is essentially a state of fixation, and lies in a morbid continuation of, rather than a healthy emancipation from, infantile emotional attachments—with forms of un-conscious psychologically incestuous situations thus remaining in later life. Jung, on the other hand, emphasized that failures in the present, rather than in the past, comprise the basic in-gredient of psychoneurotic illness. Regression from the present —where he conceived the essence of the illness to lie—back into the past, rather than a primary morbid attachment that arose in previous developmental phases, was one of the con-trasting keystones embodied in his own thinking.

There are two areas of psychology in which the ideas advanced by Jung are particularly well known. One is his classification of personalities into introverts and extroverts. The other is his concept of the 'collective unconscious'.

The terms introvert and extrovert are so widely used that they have become part of everyday conversation. It is less well known that Jung also subdivided each of these types into four further categories. This reluctance to endow people with crudely generalized and oversimplified labels seems in keeping with his religiously-oriented outlook concerning the uniqueness of the individual. The four additional qualities with which he concerned himself were those of thinking, feeling, sensation and intuition. Thus he postulated eight categories, still broad but determined by whichever of these four qualities is predominantly contained within the particular introvert or extrovert of his basically twofold classification. These further subdivisions brought a more finely calibrated system of perception.

These types are found to accord closely with many individuals met with in daily practice. But Jung carried his postulates to a still deeper level, advancing the concept that introverts and extroverts each unconsciously exert an internal force towards redressing the balance of the predominant attribute of extroversion or introversion. This notion too is in line with the daily observation that at least some people, recognizing their own imbalance, make quite conscious attempts to exert a pull in the opposite direction. It seems likely that those without conscious recognition of this process may also carry it out at a deeper level.

Jung's concept of the collective unconscious arose from his investigations into the customs and modes of thought and feeling found amongst primitive peoples. On the basis of detailed studies, he concluded that a great deal of common material is contained in religious beliefs, in dreams, and in myths and legends; and he discovered that much of this material was widespread and often existed within isolated communities which at the time of his studies had received no communication from outside sources to account for its presence. He therefore deduced that these tendencies in thinking and feeling, which he termed archetypes, were ingrained into the unconscious mind as archaic material on a collective basis of racial heredity and racial evolution, rather than being primarily implanted by the individual's personal life-experience. His belief in the significance of symbolism therefore went beyond that of Freud. In Jung's view unconscious life has both personal and also archaic contents, the origins of the latter being essentially collective and independent of the circumstances of the individual's life history.

ADLER

The predominant theme in the psychology propounded by Adler was an emphasis on a striving to obtain masterful dominance over the environment and thus compensate for a sense of inferiority. The concepts of 'inferiority complex' and 'overcompensation' were basic in his teachings. In his explanation of the content of the sense of inferiority, with the resulting ineptitudes in outlook and relationships to which the overcompensation against it may give rise, Adler stressed particularly heavily the notion of 'organ inferiority' as the stimulus prompting the overcompensation. These concepts often have an obvious application to many of the cases of maladjustment that lead to problems in which the social worker may become implicated. But they may also have their relevance in states of maladjustment in which this origin and mode of operation is less apparent. With increasing experience however, they will be found to provide the social worker with a structure of explanation within which the keys to a large number of misunderstandings, both suffered and generated by psychoneurotic clients, may be recognized.

An application of the Adlerian principle of overcompensation, for example, may be found in many clients in whom the sense of inferiority, and the consequent drive to overcome it, is reflected in their overcompensated attitudes towards the social worker as an authority figure. Since the social worker is so open to be 'type cast' as an authority figure—at least in the client's fantasy—the client is automatically liable to feel inferior and dependent. Unless the social worker has successfully safeguarded the client's self-esteem, problems become added from this source also. But even on a more general basis it is not always easy for people to feel that they are being helped, and social workers do not always appreciate the full extent to which a client who is genuinely relieved and grateful for her help may also feel disadvantages, and then overcompensate by hostility and morbid self-assertiveness.

Other important methods of psychotherapy have developed from those of the pioneers discussed. Melanie Klein, for instance, elaborated on the concepts of Freud by focusing in detail on the processes involved in the earliest levels of human emotional development. This work has led to techniques of psychoanalytically orientated play therapy for disturbed children. The reader will have recognized that a number of schools of psychological teaching may thus have simultaneous applications in the explanation and management of any problem confronting her. The last situation, involving Adlerian concepts, exemplifies this principle. In the particular instance we have considered, namely hostile feelings towards a social worker, explanations in terms of the early fantasies concerning family figures, and the long-term consequences that may flow from the symbolic representations involved, are presented by Freudian concepts of unconscious motivations. But at the same time this situation may be explained by the Adlerian principle of overcompensation, which may coexist with these Freudian mechanisms. And examples of Pavlovian mechanisms, in which associations with previous traumatic experiences can provoke conditioned responses, will simultaneously be found to lie behind many of the problems encountered in psychoneurotic situations.

PAVLOV

Psychoanalysts, as we have seen, concern themselves with the unconscious. Another great worker, however, the physiologist Pavlov, by contrast approached the study of mental processes exclusively in terms of studies of the conscious mind, regarding mental processes as the expression of an area of purely physiological functioning. He did not regard the unconscious mind as a valid concept.

The most widely known physiological experiment of Pavlov consisted of placing suitable food in front of a dog, which would then salivate. If the food was placed in front of the same dog on a number of occasions and a bell was rung in association with its arrival, the dog would eventually salivate in the absence of food in response to the sound of the bell alone. This salivation in response to the bell sound is known as a conditioned reflex—a reflex modified by experience, the original stimulus being replaced by another but the response remaining unchanged. Thus if a neutral stimulus, i.e. one that does not produce an inborn or unconditioned reflex response (in this case the bell), is given repeatedly immediately before an unconditioned stimulus, i.e. a stimulus that produces an unconditioned response (in this experiment the food), then the animal learns to associate the neutral stimulus with the unconditioned stimulus and responds to the neutral stimulus in the absence of the unconditioned stimulus. The fundamental concepts in Pavlovian theory thus relate to learning and association.

The material discussed in this chapter is based on guiding principles rather than rules of the sort that characterize the physical sciences. Many of these explanations about relationships rest on hypotheses that arose in the first place from clinical observations on patients—amongst the most notable being those carried out by Freud. Apart from Pavlovian principles their validity rests on reasoning of a clinical character rather than procedures of a scientific nature.

These concepts, particularly on their deeper levels, do not in general lend themselves easily to the methods of scientific research that can be applied with such value in other fields of psychiatry. But inaccessibility to scientific approach does not invalidate assumptions based on the daily experience of many psychiatrists in clinical practice. With increasing experience the social worker too will meet more and more cases in which she will see that many of the factors laid before her in this chapter will have a strong claim to relevance to the current problems with which she is coping. The awareness of the possibility that they may be present should help towards a better understanding of many of those situations which at first sight seem inexplicable, inaccessible and even on occasions alarming.

9

The psychoneurotic client: some illnesses

Psychological maladjustment, using the term in its widest sense, occurs throughout the population as a continuum that ranges from the minor difficulties arising from being unduly 'defended', at one end of the scale, to the clear-cut syndromes of the overtly psychoneurotic illnesses at the other.

If the social worker tries to look along the length of this scale, starting at the end containing the minor aberrations, she will now be in a better position to recognize the fuller significance of some of these commoner psychological problems. For an understanding of the more formal psychoneurotic illnesses, however, she will need a knowledge of the particular symptoms of each individual illness. The collection of symptoms comprising an illness is known as its syndrome. The three conditions whose syndromes will be most worth some understanding are anxiety states, hysteria and obsessional neurosis.

SYNDROMES

ANXIETY STATES

Normal anxiety, being a biological endowment necessary for efficiency and even survival, naturally is experienced universally amongst normal people. It can be regarded to a greater or lesser extent as morbid, on the other hand, when aroused by irrelevant factors, is unduly intense, or continues beyond the point at which subsidence would normally occur. There are also conditions of pathological lack of anxiety—not to be confused with courage—as for example in hysterical dissociation, schizophrenic apathy (chapter 11) or organic dementia (chapter 13).

The manifestations of anxiety may be subjective or objective. Subjectively, anxiety consists of a feeling of marked apprehension, either free floating or focused more narrowly on to individual fears, or occurring as a mixture of the two. Objectively, it receives its expression in mental states, and often forms of behaviour, coloured with this emotion—either expressed directly or to be inferred indirectly if disguised through recognizable defence mechanisms. It may also take the form of physical symptoms. The discharge of the tension through physical channels may even give rise to suspicions of organic disease that require physical investigation. Sweating, tremor, palpitations, diarrhoea, abdominal pain, shortness of breath and innumerable other bodily responses may then be found to have a purely psychogenic basis.

Diagnostic mistakes may occur in three directions. The mental outcome of a physical disease that affects brain function may dominate the picture, dangerously deflecting attention away from the need for treatment of the physical condition itself. Such a mistake, liable to occur for example in certain forms of thyroid disease (chapter 13), may prove serious. Secondly, through ignorance, or reluctance to accept the supposed stigma of even a temporary psychological infirmity, a primarily physical label may be wrongly appended to features that are in fact psychogenic in basic origin. Instances are found in families in which one of the members is regarded as physically 'delicate'. A woman with a pain under the left breast known as *angina innocens*—a condition which is nervous in origin—may throughout the whole of her life be thought by herself and her family to have a 'bad heart' when in reality the heart is perfectly sound.

Thirdly, anxiety may merely be a component of another psychiatric condition. Thus in an agitated depression, which basically needs anti-depressive treatment, the anxiety may be so prominent that the depressive features are overshadowed and overlooked. Similarly an obsessional neurosis may present itself as a problem of anxiety; and only on close enquiry will it then be found that the anxiety features are an integral part of a primary obsessional neurosis. In some cases of schizophrenia the general perplexity and failure of mental functioning,

however hard the sufferer tries to resist the inexorable progress
of the illness, may lead to anxiety of a still different origin.
Again, the process of learning by association, already mentioned in connection with the work of Pavlov, provides an
important explanation of many cases of anxiety. Anxiety
reactions can clearly be learnt processes—learnt not through
formal education but through the many experiences of living
that modify.

There are various kinds of normal learning. Processes of
classical conditioning may provide an explanation of certain
forms of pathological anxiety on the principle that such states
are the end-points of maladaptive learning. Association can
clearly be highly significant in these cases. The person who in
wartime has come to associate the sound of aeroplanes with
the dropping of bombs, and then continues in peacetime to
palpitate at the sound of an aeroplane, furnishes a well known
example that is obvious enough. Here an association with
previously disturbing experiences is provoking a conditioned
response of anxiety in the absence of the original stimulus,
comparable with the experimental findings with Pavlov's dogs
(chapter 8). But anxiety states having a more subtle initial
stimulus and more complex chains of association—chains in
which many associative factors become successively involved
and obscured over a period of years—may form pathological
conditions whose basis is less easily recognized. In these cases
the original trauma may be unknown; but the associations
provoke responses through a mechanism that is fundamentally
similar though less readily discernible.

HYSTERIA

Hysteria is a condition about whose nature there is widespread
misunderstanding. To the layman it often signifies an 'attack
of the screams', with a douche of cold water as the time-
honoured remedy richly deserved and most likely to be
effective. But while it is true that screaming and occasionally
convulsions may arise—and sometimes require to be distinguished from other conditions—episodes of this type are
comparatively unusual. A far wider range of manifestations
forms the commoner substance of this condition.

These manifestations fall into two main categories—the personality and the neurosis. There is a certain type of personality, met with commonly and varying in degree, which is termed the hysterical personality. And there is a group of symptoms, occurring occasionally in everybody and frequently or even almost constantly in some, that constitutes the illness of hysterical neurosis.

For ordinary purposes the hysterical personality and the neurosis may be thought of as separate entities. This personality, while rendering the individual less well adjusted to life as a whole, does not necessarily lead to frank symptoms of neurosis. Similarly, under sufficient stress hysterical symptoms can arise even in a well-integrated individual devoid of these personality characteristics. Hence there is no obligatory relationship between the two. Nevertheless such a relationship frequently exists. The social worker will often find that under the influence of stress the attributes of an hysterical personality become accentuated to a level producing emotional problems or manifest symptoms which in their more severe instances may point to the need for formal psychiatric help, social support, or assistance through casework.

The attributes of this over-reactive and sometimes frothy personality reflect to a greater or lesser extent a state of emotional immaturity. They often include rapid changes of mood, a love of naïve enthusiasms, a tendency to think and talk in superlatives, volatile emotions having far more surface intensity than depth, a strong inclination to histrionic scenes often created to compensate for inner emptiness or to divert self-awareness away from the disturbances of underlying insecurities, and a capacity for selective observation and forgetting based on the need for self-protection and wish fulfilment. The intensity of the distress sometimes displayed by the hysterical personality would, if occurring in another type of personality, signify an ominous degree of reactive depression: in the hysterical personality it is liable to pass quite quickly, leaving the individual remarkably unruffled.

Descriptions of conditions containing attributes that are found in lesser degree in many well adjusted people can be misleading. Unless this fact is kept fully in mind many personalities that are sound, well adjusted and even of superior and valuable capacity for subjective understanding will inevitably fall under misplaced suspicion of being pathological. A sense of perspective is always a diagnostic *sine qua non* in assessing the presence or absence of psychoneurosis.

The symptoms of hysterical illness, as distinct from those of the hysterical personality with which they nevertheless often overlap, are very numerous. Often they mimic those which the sufferer believes to be associated with organic illnesses. And they can intrude into the sphere of both mental and physical functioning. Their essence is that they are unknowingly adopted for gain.

In the mental sphere, an intensification of the normal features of this personality may take on a severity which then merges into the clearly pathological. For example, its basic tendency to selective lack of concentration or retrospective disregard may in gross cases reach a state of fugue, where the repression from awareness extends into large areas of life, leaving the sufferer in extreme instances even unaware of his own identity and present circumstances; or there may be a memory block for long periods of life containing only patchy islets of recall.

A vulnerable immaturity of outlook and a tendency to flight into self-deception are key factors in hysteria; and any of the defence mechanisms already described may become involved (chapter 8). Dissociation is particularly common. The extreme examples of this mechanism, leading to multiple personality development in which each personality is unaware of the existence of the others, are very rare. But minor degrees of dissociation enabling the individual ingenuously to reconcile in his outlook disparate factors whose irreconcilability is obvious to other people, are seen fairly commonly. Double standards of outlook and behaviour may sometimes contain this mechanism. Yet another example of dissociation is seen in hysterical *belle indifférence*, in which the sufferer displays distressing symptoms with a bland manner of resigned acceptance, sometimes ignorantly or charitably misinterpreted as a shining example of ordinary fortitude and very apt to be exercised at the expense of other people.

Alternatively the symptoms may be displayed with florid ostentation.

Hysterical depression is a condition that often causes considerable concern to onlookers, and not infrequently results in admissions to hospital because of the anxieties provoked by expressions of suicidal intention or the occurrence of supposedly suicidal behaviour. Usually these episodes embody attention-seeking techniques staged under circumstances in which almost immediate detection and treatment is to be anticipated. But occasionally a client's errors of judgement about this course of events, or ignorance of the effects of the drugs ingested or the wound self-inflicted, may produce serious consequences.

These attacks of depression are real; but they differ from the type of depression described in chapter 11 in all but the most superficial of appearances. To the experienced eye even the depressed demeanour itself carries the stamp of its hysterical quality. The genuine but often petulant and self-pitying feeling of misery when seen in its more extreme form is frequently unmistakable. Typically also these depressions are sudden—sometimes almost instantaneous—both in their onset and cessation, and often they are highly reactive to current happenings or thoughts. Commonly they last as little as an hour or two, having been precipitated by an unpleasant occurrence, and they are as rapidly dispelled by a pleasing one. Many such mood swings may take place within a single day.

A distinction between hysterical and endogenous depression frequently needs to be made as a basis for clinical action. For this purpose a number of contrasts should be looked for—between the erratic mood swings of one, and the regular diurnal variation of the other; the self pity, in contrast to the self reproach; between the often sullen and blatant taciturnity of hysterical attacks, and the slowed-up and laborious efforts at conscientious response found in endogenous depression; the sudden onset and brief duration and sometimes flagrant display of the hysterical attacks, compared with the insidious development and protracted course of the other type of depression (see chapter 11).

Hysterical stupor comprising a state of extreme withdrawal

to a point of gross inability to comprehend the surroundings is rare; but minor examples of hysterical 'confusion'—a state of bemused and 'stunned' psychological disintegration not amounting to a state of fugue—are seen fairly commonly.

In the sphere of physical symptoms, the fundamental attributes of the features of hysteria are again that they are motivated for a purpose but that this fact is unknown to the individual producing them. These two criteria, it will be recalled, apply equally to the mental symptoms. The symptoms, however crude or histrionically presented, are not in the nature of pretence. Features paraded for gain when there is dishonesty known to the perpetrator constitute malingering. Hysteria is an illness in which the motivations lying beneath its symptoms —escape from difficult problems, seeking of attention, exaltation of self regard, or exercise of aggression—are unknown to the sufferer.

These physical symptoms may include loss of powers of movement, or increase of muscular movement as in hysterical vomiting; or they may consist of changes in bodily sensations such as tingling, patches of insensitivity of the skin to pain, or other sensory disorders like impairment of vision and hearing. Gross examples of paralysis, loss of speech due to spasm of the vocal chords, spasms or flagrant tremors of muscles may all occur. More commonly, however, the symptoms are less striking, consisting of 'lightheaded' and 'woolly' feelings, a feeling of a tight band around the forehead, or a sense of pressure on the scalp, etc.

But not all psychosomatic symptoms are hysterical. Only if they are purposively-motivated can an hysterical quality be validly ascribed to them. Anxiety, without any intention for gain, can often provoke the initial psychosomatic reaction. Perpetuation on a purposively-motivated hysterical basis may or may not supervene. It should also be realized that all these physical symptoms are true experiences. The patient indeed cannot move muscles paralysed by hysteria or loosen those in hysterical spasm; it is objectively found possible to insert needles into areas of hysterical anaesthesia without any sensation of pain occurring; and in the light of these sorts of observable verifications it is quite legitimate to conclude that expressions of pain without any organic origin are an equal reality. Clearly the sufferer feels pain irrespective of the absence of physical disease. The origin is hysterical, but he is not shamming.

OBSESSIONAL STATES

The term obsessional shares with hysteria the principle that within the general designation a distinction can be drawn between the personality and the neurosis—again with overlapping on occasions. The obsessional personality does not in itself form a pathological entity. It varies widely in degree; and in moderation it contains many features of great value both to the individual and to the community. But when its features exist in an excess that leads to severe impairment of internal or external adjustment, then it is abnormal.

Its characteristics (chapter 11) may include a love of order and tidiness, meticulous exactitude, a need for unnecessarily ponderous hesitation before embarking on action coupled with a somewhat crippling reluctance—or in severe cases almost an inability—to change any attitude or course of action once set in motion, the seeking of clearcut and predictable patterns of procedure, and often a hankering after perfection in various fields of work or social relationships with a difficulty in tolerating its lack in others, even though specific efforts to acquire a sense of tolerance may be dutifully made. As we shall see, if people possessing this type of personality happen to develop mental illness—and they are no more likely to do so than those who possess other forms of personality makeup —the resulting disability is usually an endogenous depression. Rather strangely, an obsessional neurosis is not the most common pathological development arising from this personality, although features of obsessional neurosis sometimes become mixed into those of the endogenous depressive syndrome. In a full-blown obsessional neurosis, however, any depressive component is more usually a development secondary to the distress of the neurosis itself.

Clinical obsessions, as distinct from the features of the basic personality, may occur in the form of ruminations, acts or fears. The features of the ruminations or acts are that they are compulsive, intrusive, repetitive or continuous, and are associated with a state of mental tension which is partially relieved if the sufferer complies with the tendencies but increased by his resisting them.

This last component, the dilemma of the tension factor, forms a central predicament. If the sufferer indulges in the compulsions in order to relieve the tension, he is deflected from constructive thought and activity by his untrammelled performance of the obsessions. If on the other hand he resists the intrusions, the tension becomes increased possibly to a point that is unendurable. He is caught in a cleft stick. The intrusions are not in the ordinary sense enjoyable to him, as in this form of illness he would wish to be disencumbered of them.

The compulsive thoughts are liable to involve intrusive ruminations about 'philosophical' or 'religious' matters; but other sorts of material may form their content, sometimes floridly nonsensical. It is the insight possessed by the sufferer into the irrational and unconstructive nature of the ruminations and ritualistic acts—such as repeated irrational hand-washing or repetitive thoughts of no relevant value—that distinguishes this neurosis from a psychotic state.

The sine qua non of insight also exists in relation to the various compulsive fears termed phobias. The person who is afraid of entering a telephone box or passing close to a telegraph pole through the fear that rays will emanate from the mechanism and affect his body lacks insight. He has a psychosis. But the claustrophobic person, intensely anxious about these situations because of obsessively compulsive tension, while aware of the unreasonableness of his aversion, has an obsessional neurosis.

Minor obsessions, such as mild discomforts on heights or in crowds, are so common as to be of negligible significance. But serious obsessions may benefit by treatment, though they are usually difficult to treat. There is, however, another value to be drawn from a knowledge of obsessional neurosis, namely that the psychoanalytical explanation of some of its symptoms gives a still further illustration of a number of defence mechanisms whose significance stretches over a vastly wider area of application than this particular condition. For example, according to the Freudian concept the origin of this neurosis lies in the stage of infantile development at which the young child has an intense interest in excreta—a fact of normal development to which every mother can testify. A fairly common symptom in marked obsessional neurosis is repetitive hand washing. In severe cases these repetitions may be so frequent that the skin becomes affected.

According to this explanation, the mechanism involved is reaction formation, or inversion, i.e. an exaggeration of the tendency opposite to the one that has undergone repression. The young child's need to express an interest in dirt, having been repressed by him from his own awareness—and therefore retained unconsciously in an unresolved state, is kept in a state of continued repression by the use of this mechanism of inversion. In other words the unresolved desire for dirt becomes defensively transmuted into a similarly intense hatred of it— with resulting fears of germs and contamination to a degree that is flagrantly pathological but clearly does not occur without reason.

Another general mechanism exemplified in the psychoanalytical explanation of obsessional illness is displacement. Phobic anxieties are thought to arise through displacement of the repressed emotions on to entities in the environment which may be emotionally neutral but which then come to form focal points for the underlying material that is essentially irrelevant to themselves. Under these circumstances these intrinsically neutral entities become invested with the pathological anxiety relevant to the underlying emotion, for which they have unknowingly become the symbols and substitutes. They themselves then become sources of symptom-production, sometimes severe. A person with a severe phobia of telegraph poles may choose to walk miles in order to avoid passing within their proximity.

Here again there is illustrated a situation with far wider applications. If the focal point is manifestly neutral, such as an inanimate object or situation, at least an insight into the irrationality of the reactions is preserved. But if the inappropriate and merely symbolic nature of the situation is not

perceived so clearly, as when the emotions become directed
on to a marital partner or child, then the consequent inter-
personal reactions may contain counter-responses and misunderstandings which lead to endless problems and unhappiness.

Finally, Freud regarded obsessional acts as rituals for pro-
pitiation and expiation—invocations of the powers of magic.
They can indeed be often observed to be highly ritualistic, in
that the compulsive behaviour may be carried out with a rigid
enslavement to a system dominated by the treadmill of an
inescapable craving for numerical exactitude, compelling the
sufferers to engage in their acts in groups of sharply specified
numbers sometimes even followed by exact multiples of the
original figure. If the premise is accepted that the motivating
material is guilt-laden and unconsciously thought to be
deserving of punishment—which was the child's reaction at
the time of its repression—then the fact that the acts may be
carried out for expiation of guilt and appeasement of a potentially punishing source is not an illogical explanation. The
observable facts that the obsessional personality is heavily
preoccupied by considerations of 'right and wrong', and that
the obsessional acts bring relief of the tension, which is
assumed by this explanation to be associated with anxiety and
guilt, lend clinical credence to these psychoanalytical explanations. And if they are related to a wider setting, it will be
realized that the invoking of 'magic' by 'touching wood' etc.
is an ordinary practice which, though normal and even engaged in with humour, may well be akin to these factors in
its basic origin.

ANOREXIA NERVOSA

Anorexia nervosa is a psychoneurotic illness sufficiently serious
to require separate mention. This term refers to a loss of
appetite, not associated with endogenous depression or psychosis, mainly found in adolescent girls or young women but
seldom occurring in the third or subsequent decades. It is a
condition whose potentialities are so serious that it can never
be disregarded. Indeed if left untreated a significant risk of
death may arise. It is therefore important for the social worker

to be aware of its most obvious features and when necessary to be ready to use all possible influence, not only with the sufferer but also the family, to ensure that medical advice is sought and the recommendations followed.

Often there is a history of food consciousness and weight preoccupation, with the rigours of a slimming diet having passed into an almost total lack of interest in food and even an intractable revulsion against food of any type. Physical changes, such as cessation of the monthly periods, naturally exist. In its more advanced stages the illness may be obvious from the loss of weight itself, perhaps of several stones, with an accompanying loss of elasticity of the skin shown by its dry, loose quality. An impoverishment of circulation may occur in the hands and feet, which can become strikingly cold and blue. Moreover all manner of deceit may be practised in resisting efforts to be helped, food sometimes being hidden and thrown away with a skill that can easily mislead those unfamiliar with the severity of the revulsion felt against it.

Treatment is often less difficult in the earlier than in the later stages. It necessitates admission to hospital for supervision of feeding and perhaps treatment with medication. But to whatever extent any speculative constitutional or self-perpetuating physical factors may have seemed relevant, the illness has commonly developed within the context of previous psychological difficulties. Attention to the psychiatric state is therefore of paramount importance. Not infrequently parents appear to have been over-anxious and emotionally disturbing, and their difficulties too need consideration and help as part of the total system of management. This principle, however, is common to all the syndromes described in this chapter—a point that should never be lost sight of even though the social worker's main focus of attention will commonly be needed by the sufferers themselves.

THE PSYCHOPATHIC PERSONALITY
Before leaving these brief descriptions of psychoneurotic syndromes, mention should be made of the state termed the psychopathic personality. In itself it is not classified as a psychoneurosis. But it commonly becomes associated with

psychoneurotic attributes, partly because the early-life experiences of these individuals has frequently also led to their possessing ingrained psychoneurotic proclivities and partly because the conflicts with society brought about by the behaviour of the psychopathic personality readily provoke reactions of anxiety, hysteria etc.

The problem of the diagnosis of psychopathy has always tended to be very difficult, if only because of the uncertainty of the diagnosis which frequently exists in the light of the existence of other individuals whose personality deviations have features in common with this state but whose capacity for adjustment is much less seriously diminished.

The undesirability of designating such individuals as psychopaths, with the seriously antisocial and prognostic connotations associated with this diagnosis, has led to an increasing use of the term personality disorder. A more useful clarification of the nomenclature may possibly be arrived at when the present Mental Health Act is amended (chapter 6), but it is equally clear that, from the very nature of these various disabilities, considerable diagnostic difficulties will inevitably continue in relation to many sufferers whose problems are the outcome of poor powers of adjustment rather than mental illness itself.

Since social workers are liable to become drawn into these situations they should be as clearly aware as possible of the typical patterns of behaviour and attitudes traditionally described as psychopathic. The Mental Health Act (chapter 6) will in due course be the subject of further parliamentary debate, and the laws it embodies will no doubt undergo a certain amount of revision. At present, however, psychopathic disorder is defined legally as 'a persistent disorder or disability of mind (whether or not including subnormality of intelligence) which results in abnormally aggressive or seriously irresponsible conduct on the part of the patient, and requires or is susceptible to treatment'. In practice, unless this condition is recognized by the social worker as a likely harbinger of repeated failures of any efforts she may make to produce a sustained adjustment, a great deal of supportive time may be spent to little purpose.

It is not always easy for the inexperienced social worker, nor even for the most shrewdly perspicacious, to refrain from attempts to answer the calls for help made by these unfortunate clients. The reality of their difficulties, coupled with a convincing plausibility, sometimes a charm of manner and a touching appearance of gratitude for any sign of intention to help, will readily induce a social worker to make laborious efforts to do so, but these efforts will be followed by painful disillusionments destined to recur time after time in relation to a never-ending series of crises. One of these clients alone, whose prospects of acquiring stability are so woefully slim, may consume so much energy and disorganize a social worker's timetable so radically that she becomes unable to help a whole series of other clients fortunate enough to be capable of deriving more lasting benefit.

Whatever the current problem experienced by the psychopathic personality, the nature of this long-term prognosis needs to be borne fully in mind when his position on the scale of priorities for attention is being assessed. Nevertheless psychopathy exists in degrees; and while unhappily it is a condition whose features are present in such heavy loading that only a pessimistic outlook can be reasonably held, there is also a substantial fringe area of individuals in which supportive help seems at least to reduce the frequency of their irresponsible or antisocial episodes. And it is always important to avoid making an overpessimistic assessment without full cause.

Typically the psychopathic personality is compounded of a pattern of ineradicable irresponsibility and frequently an incorrigible though plausible untruthfulness, together with a generally antisocial attitude that represents a fundamental if concealed inability to identify with the needs and feelings of others. The maladjustment, often reflected either in a state of self-isolation or a gregarious existence amongst personalities similarly dedicated to antisocial pursuits, may result in sudden and unexpected departures by suicide from a world in which the capacity for adaptation is too seriously lacking. These suicidal episodes are rather apt to be carried out by violent techniques, such as self-wounding, which accord with the aggressive inclinations. In these circumstances the aggressive attitude is turned by the individual against himself. Other features include a lack of foresight, a lack of ability to learn from experience, an employment background often containing a very large number of jobs, not uncommonly severe alcoholic tendencies and sometimes abuse of drugs and sexual perversions, though not all these indicate psychopathic personality.

Viciously or sometimes dangerously aggressive outbursts may occur; but not all psychopathic personalities are aggressively explosive. In many the irresponsible behaviour is docile and passive. Nevertheless in a significant proportion aggressive explosions form an integral part. These episodes are characterized by a low flashpoint, in which the explosion is often provoked unexpectedly by trivial slights or acts of opposition. They are often instantaneous in their occurrence and acute enough to inflict severe physical injury on the person towards whom they are directed. They pass rapidly, and are typically replaced by an attitude of detached unconcern. Any disturbance felt by the perpetrator relates only to the problems which the episode may bring to himself. These personalities, who sometimes appear remarkably ingenuous, will usually state quite frankly that they are 'all right until somebody say something out of line'. Unfortunately, to place them in circumstances appropriate to the needs of this last attribute is too often a hope inevitably foredoomed to prolonged failure, though with the onset of middle age they gradually tend towards detonating less readily and intensely.

The explanations put forward to account for their ominous inability to identify with others vary. A nebulous form of brain abnormality in the physical sense is sometimes postulated, perhaps at times on grounds that are valid though intangible. The brain damage caused by the virus of *encephalitis lethargica* or sleepy sickness, for example (chapter 4), is known to lead to loss of capacity for sympathy and moral feeling; and this fact, amongst others, has given rise to the speculation that vague antenatal, constitutional or birth factors may produce a state of 'minimal brain damage' and a resulting psychopathic attitude. Certainly a correlation sometimes exists between the explosive behaviour and the psychopath's electro-encephalographic brain rhythms, their electrical rhythms on occasions being demonstrably of an immature variety. However, the direction of any causal relationship between the immaturely uncontrolled behaviour and any detectable physiological substrata cannot be confidently asserted. Again, the explosive nature of the psychopathic outbursts, and the amnesia apt to be associated with it, imply to some observers that an epileptic type of basis may exist. This reasoning is often equally speculative.

Most frequently a history of serious deprivation of love in the early formative stages of life is present—in particular there have often been multiple changes of substitute parents likely to have led to an irreversible sense of rejection and an inability for constructive relationships (chapters 2 and 5). It can then be reasonably argued that what was not received at this early stage may not be present to be given in later life; while associated experiences that were plainly destined to engender an ingrained sense of hatred can often be seen to have existed.

In these circumstances the ability to sympathize and identify with the needs of others, not having been built in during the most crucial stages for its later application, may be seriously lacking; and sympathy may be as meaningless to some psychopathic personalities as is the significance of musical sound to the tone deaf or colour to the colour blind. It is believed that they can only understand the feelings of others indirectly and not essentially, through what is basically a limited or even fruitless process of mere deductive reasoning. In spite of normal or even superior intelligence, the essential psychological machinery for this purpose does not appear to be present. Hence however serious their offences they cannot on this logic be held fully accountable for their failure to exercise a quality they do not possess.

DRUG DEPENDENCE

A group of clients that contains a high proportion of people with primary psychoneurotic difficulties is formed by those caught on the treadmill of drug dependence or addiction.

There are, however, many reasons why individuals may take drugs as an artificial means of obtaining satisfaction. A wish to achieve membership of a particular group, the urge for experimentation in the era of adolescent emergence, a need for stimulation to counteract psychoneurotic emptiness or psychotic inertia, the seeking of relief from anxiety when personal vulnerability or life circumstances have led to states of intolerable stress, or the restless searching for new and more satisfying experiences in an improvident and ill-adjusted psychopathic personality may all form the basis from which drug experimentation, abuse, dependence and even addiction may spring.

The broad facts of this problem are well known. Some drugs such as heroin and cocaine can lead to a physiologically-based pattern of craving for them and a 'tolerance' which necessitates an ever-increasing dose and renders the situation unbearable unless a commensurate increase in the supply is obtained. 'Withdrawal symptoms' may occur involving mental prostration, diarrhoea, abdominal cramps etc. if the drug is discontinued or sharply reduced. These withdrawal features may be so distressing as to lead to a further dose being taken as a forestalling measure, sometimes by intravenous injection.

Of the other drugs—the 'soft drugs' such as Amphetamine, LSD, or marihuana, also known as cannabis—many do not appear to produce physiological dependence. But the individual taking this group may experience states of euphoria, welcome though sometimes antisocial disinhibition and excitability, hallucinations, changes in perception of time, place and colour, or other psychological aberrations according to the particular drug, which even if not associated with physiological dependence nevertheless play into any psychological need impelling an inclination for substitute experiences. This need can then lead to dependence on the drug if the individual remains in need of, or develops a preference for, its artificial solace.

Any individual case of drug abuse can only be assessed in its own terms and managed by reference to the particular factors involved. The field is complex, understanding is still far from complete, and a full assessment clearly cannot rest with the social worker. Her own form of help lies in attempts to eliminate or modify any difficulties, material and psychological, that may have led to the situation, together with support for the family in the burden of their distress. These principles apply equally to those cases of chronic alcoholism that have defied clinical attempts at reversal. Indeed support for the family may itself diminish stress which would otherwise lead to continuation of the habits perhaps even forestalling the passage from abuse to dependence.

SOME POSSIBLE EFFECTS ON THE SOCIAL WORKER

Each of the personalities described in this chapter tends to produce its own responses in social workers. The anxious personality, certainly if severe, commonly induces an automatic reaction of sympathy. The psychopathic personality is apt to generate, at least in the inexperienced social worker, conflicting impulses to help a needy client and to refrain from allowing the intelligence of the head to be dominated by unrealistic hopes of the heart.

The hysterical personality and the obsessional personality are liable to provoke less clear-cut though often more disturbing feelings. A few words about these last two reactions may therefore be helpful. It is obvious as a general principle, though not always as easy to adjust to in living instances, that insecure personalities tend to 'put on the style', whether by display of social position, good looks, intelligence, erudition or any other attributes that may appear to lend themselves conveniently to the purpose. Hysterical personalities are a prime example in which this tendency is frequently seen. Often the possessors of these personalities also have a knack of discovering the most sensitive spots in those with whom they are involved and of prodding at them painfully, either directly or by innuendo. But the flauntings presented by these sufferers need cause no anxiety in those trying to help them. Even if an hysteric is a duchess or a member of MENSA, no emotional reactions except the appropriate form of sympathy can be justifiably felt. Such sufferers are not to be feared for their airs and graces, even when based on one level of reality. They would be far better off with different gifts of fortune, for example with less intelligence but less areas of the crippling blindness or painful jealousies which mere intelligence or financial possessions, however high, cannot reach. The social worker need never be overawed by these clients; and certainly she cannot help them satisfactorily if she too becomes emotionally toppled.

Markedly obsessional personalities are also liable to evoke reciprocal emotional difficulties, sometimes giving rise to painful inhibitions amongst those in contact with them. Even in everyday working relationships many people are unreasonably inclined to compare themselves disparagingly with the perfectionist, even though no criticism has been expressed or intended against them. Feeling themselves unable to contribute with sufficient success by comparison, they sag into a sense of inhibiting inadequacy and from there freeze into a state of painful incompetence. And in a professional relationship involving casework, comparable reactions can occur. Fears of failure to measure up to the obsessional client's standards of slavery to duty or capacity for reliability and exactitude may obscure from the social worker that it is compulsive characteristics themselves that have been responsible for the client's downfall.

These attributes need not therefore be enviously emulated, nor guiltily construed by the social worker as indices of incompetence in herself. Here again, to exercise the art of conscientious but realistic self orientation will be an essential part of the social worker's skill; and it can only be achieved with benefit to the client if the necessary objectivity is reached and sustained.

Finally, it should always be remembered that while a tremendous number of people stand in need of the social worker's active help, in other cases too active an involvement will not serve the best psychological interests of the client. Clients and their relatives are not necessarily the best judges of their own needs, however volubly expressed, aggressively demanded or importunately sought. Feeding by an unwise compliance into the manipulative tendencies of an hysterical client, or intensifying the excessive dependence of inadequate personalities by responding too automatically and 'supportively' to their pleas for help, are reactions which in practice may be the antithesis of good psychological management. There are times when a judicious economy of involvement may be the best form of therapy. Adopting this attitude may itself be distressing to a conscientious social worker; and when in doubt an inexperienced or emotionally-involved social worker may be helped in this dilemma by discussing the situation with other workers more suitably placed to make an objective assessment.

PROGNOSTIC CRITERIA

This difficulty in assessing the amount of time that should either be devoted to or withheld from those suffering from psychoneurosis demands a certain amount of understanding of the prognostic factors that can bear on psychiatric states in general. It is important for social workers to be aware of at least some of the guiding criteria for determining whether or not to enter professionally into certain types of problem situation. Often these situations simultaneously invite and discourage; and how far she should go in any particular instance, in the event of her deciding to do so, in her efforts to produce some sort of modification is a question that can pose anxieties needing appraisal on the basis of the most realistic evidence that can be mustered. A number of concrete facts as well as intuitive assessments must be brought into this process of decision.

We should therefore look at some broad prognostic factors. In order to evaluate the patient's accessibility to any efforts that she may have in mind—and thus to gain a reasoned impression about whether or not she should embark on a course of action that may prove very time-consuming—the social worker should look as closely as possible at the frequency of any previous breakdowns. She should also try to note the discrepancy, or alternatively the degree of correspondence, that existed between the severity of any precipitating stresses and the intensity of the responses they evoked. This relationship may point broadly to the individual's susceptibility or resistance to stress.

In addition, the nature of these stresses and their duration, the duration of the breakdowns, and the responses to any methods of help that may have been applied will all need to be looked at as closely as possible. Attempts should also be made to determine whether the client's susceptibility appears to relate to problems that are predominantly specific, or whether the susceptibility is of a more broadly based type. If the former, her efforts may be most usefully directed towards removing or reducing the offending circumstances and safeguarding against their recurrence in specific ways. If the latter, a more general form of psychological support may be called for.

There are two prognostic errors that need particular emphasis, namely the failures to distinguish between coincidence and cause, and between cause and effect. For example, in a truly reactive depression the ruminations are understandable in the light of the circumstances that preceded their onset, the depressive content maintains a close connection with the precipitating circumstances, and the condition subsides if and when they are accepted or rectified. In an endogenous depression, on the other hand (chapter 11), the factors preceding it are either causally irrelevant—mere fortuitous accompaniments—or simply final precipitants whose presence becomes swallowed up in other elements in the depressive ruminations and whose removal, by contrast, does not produce the hoped for recovery or ensure against recurrences of the depressive illness.

It will be useful to look at some of the practical correlates of these principles. To organize a holiday for instance in the erroneous belief that the lack of a diverting environment is responsible for an illness may simply be to impose on the client a disturbing need to adapt to a change of surroundings which merely exacerbates the depressive condition, since basically this cause was in fact more apparent than real. Both the circumstances that may have fortuitously surrounded the onset of an illness and also the symptoms themselves—such as the poor sleeping or loss of appetite—are apt to be misleadingly regarded as primary causes.

Another practical error is to arrange for a change of work on the erroneous assumption that anxieties about this particular work are the primary source of a psychotic depression rather than its effects, for here again this measure may merely add the additional strains of attempting to readjust to new requirements. As in the case of the supposedly therapeutic holiday, the depressed person may find himself still more distressed by his inability to benefit from the working concessions given, which in any case he is apt to regard himself as unworthy to receive. Even suicide may thus be unwittingly encouraged.

Other types of psychosis, such as schizophrenia (chapter 11), may similarly give rise to prognostic assumptions leading to measures more deleterious than beneficial. An error easily committed by the inexperienced in schizophrenia is to accept without regard to the essence of the illness the relatives' sincere belief that a client's bad relationship with neighbours warrants a move to another area. Such a move does not in itself necessarily solve the problems of a person with a paranoid illness. The illness may be only transferred from one domicile to another. If a move is in fact to be undertaken, usually it should be made only after treatment has been given and preferably after a period of observation in the improved or recovered state, so as to confirm or eliminate any doubt about the need for the requested action. But in reactive depressions, and in some hysterical depressions in which the general liability to recurrence is not too high, great value may be conferred by modification of social precipitants or by provision of psychological support.

10

The psychoneurotic client: some aspects of management

GENERAL CONSIDERATIONS

Although a proportion of psychoneurotic people will always appear to be defeating all attempts to help them, it is also a matter of frequent experience that in other cases their regressive phases may become largely resolved as the relevant stresses are mitigated and as the client's self-regard and self-sufficiency are supported; effects arising from primary abnormal fixations may recede with suitable help; and the more clear-cut clinical illnesses may improve under the more specific clinical treatments.

But in general the management of psychoneurosis cannot be confined to narrowly specific remedies. Since constitutional, physical and environmental elements all have their relevance in causation, a comparably multiple approach in the management too is often required. Referral for medical assessment may lead to the administration of helpful medication, or even to discovery of vitally important physical conditions, as in thyrotoxicosis (chapter 13), or to useful psychotherapy, occasionally psychoanalysis, behaviour therapy, or very rarely one of the modern forms of brain operation. It is important that the social worker should know of the existence of these possible measures, so that in potentially suitable cases the client may be encouraged to seek medical opinion. Alternatively, or in addition, casework carried out by the social worker with the individual, or arrangements for alleviations of family difficulties through attendance at special groups for family psychotherapy, may be the primary or supplementary needs.

MEDICATION

Medication with sedatives or tranquillizers may prove helpful; but as the sole method of management drugs may be a poor substitute both for deep psychotherapy or the less technical and more general forms of psychological support. Nevertheless new drug preparations appear on the market almost continuously, and pharmacological 'breakthroughs' for helping psychoneurosis are an ever-present possibility. For example, certain forms of medication in current use now sometimes seem to be proving more effective in obsessional neurosis than those used for this condition in former times.

PSYCHOTHERAPEUTIC SUPPORT

Psychological exploration is usually conducted with the patient in a state of clear consciousness; and in this area the social worker may, as part of her psychologically supportive role, have a certain part to play (chapter 3). But occasionally it is felt desirable for the process to be facilitated by the use of an intravenous injection of a barbiturate drug to 'loosen' the patient, putting inhibitions into abeyance and creating conditions for 'breakthroughs' into consciousness of psychological material that would otherwise remain imprisoned within the unconscious. Benefit may then accrue from the recognition of this material; but the possibility of adverse consequences flowing from unacceptable insight always needs to be weighed in the balance when the procedure is contemplated.

Not only does the use of intravenous drugs in psychological exploration sometimes facilitate the release of psychological material. It may also suspend the individual's functions of critical evaluation. The result can be an increase in his suggestibility, and this state may be utilized for clinical improvement, as for example in 'suggesting away' disabling symptoms in cases of hysteria. Nevertheless if the underlying conflict is left unresolved, the superficiality of this form of approach may limit its efficacy, with the removal of one symptom being

followed by substitute symptoms differing in form but emanating from the same underlying source.

Another release mechanism in which the use of drugs may
be exploited, though nowadays very rarely, is the excitatory
form of abreaction brought about by a stimulant drug, rather
than the release of underlying material within the setting of a
calming state created by sedative drugs. One such technique
consists of therapeutically-controlled inhalation of ether, so
that in passing through the stages of excitability associated
with the loss of orientation for time and place induced by this
drug the patient relives the distressing past experiences in the
temporary belief that they exist as a present objective reality.
The associated release of emotional tension has brought a high
degree of relief in suitable cases.

This particular process had its main application in this
country in the treatment of war neuroses in the 1940s and
1950s. Its main field of value was with patients with sound
basic personalities who had broken down in response to intense and clear-cut stresses such as those imposed by insupportable battle experiences. It has little function, however, in
the neuroses of peacetime, which are more deep seated in their
childhood or constitutional origins and not relevant for this
relatively superficial approach.

The social worker's own role in psychotherapy will be either
to try to help the client herself (chapter 3) or to persuade him
to seek an opinion on the need for specialized methods.
These specialized methods, group or individual, may be required in relation to the age of the client or the nature of the
problem. Suitable adolescent groups, groups for mothers of
disturbed children (chapter 3), and even groups for toddlers
may be necessary according to circumstances.

In many areas helpful facilities can be made available—on
the basis of prior discussion with the family doctor—through
the local child guidance clinic, day hospital or club for
psychiatric patients. Social workers should make a point of
familiarizing themselves with all such relevant facilities for
psychiatric help in their areas. Their psychotherapeutic efforts,
determined by the client's needs and their own understanding
and experience, may range from the most basic and general

befriending, such as that which is provided by the very helpful and widespread work of the Samaritan movement, to the more complex involvement of psychodynamic concepts, which arise from psychoanalytical concepts themselves.

On the superficial level, listening to a problem, even when essentially irremedial, may prove of great help if only on the basis that troubles shared are troubles halved. Practical explanations relating to material problems, or simple guidance concerning psychological predicaments, may also be of considerable value, well conceived discussions on such matters often alleviating a client's traumatic sense of powerlessness. Reassurances may resolve distressing doubts. Strong persuasion when indicated may form a therapeutic antidote to a client's sterile vacillations, bringing the relief and self-respect associated with a definite line of action.

When engaging in the deeper levels of psychotherapeutic help, however, the social worker will particularly need to bear in mind the concepts involved in listening (chapter 3), immaturity (chapter 2), and the significance of childhood experiences on later-life attitudes towards members—children and adults—within their own families and towards others in general.

The concepts involved in these functions will not be reiterated; but from the emphasis already placed on emotional immaturity it will be clear that a relationship between the adult client and those concepts pertaining to child psychiatry will often be highly relevant. The reader is therefore recommended to study again the first three chapters of this book, and in general to acquire as much understanding as possible of the modes of reaction in normal and disturbed childhood and the factors lying behind them.

Nevertheless, not all psychoneurosis consists of immaturity. Many patients with anxiety states or obsessional neurosis, for example, show none of the features especially associated with childhood feelings and behaviour. On the contrary, such patients often have a marked maturity of outlook and are characterized by behaviour and attitudes that are highly responsible and reliable. Moreover, even in the case of a basically immature or manifestly regressed psychoneurotic person it would be an unwarrantable denigration, and indeed an unrealistic error, to equate these attributes in this adult patient—whether permanent or temporary—with the totality of the outlook and behaviour of the child. In states of psychoneurotic regression, or even fixation, people usually embody mixtures of maturity and immaturity in juxtaposition. Every child himself is obviously a mixture of attributes, the most tangible often being in respect of intellectual skills, which vary from one area of aptitude to another—good at some subjects, bad at others. And it will often be one of the functions of the social worker, when she is attempting to support the immature adult, to find and build upon his positive attributes, nurturing self-esteem and tactfully fostering the will to grow up in those particular areas of immaturity that have their relevance to the difficulties concerned.

An important area in which an understanding of childhood attributes sometimes facilitates an understanding of adult psychoneurosis is the recognition of the long-term significance of the child's propensity to play off one adult against another. The adult client who plays off the health visitor, the school, and the clinic staff against one another, for instance, replicates the mode of behaviour of earlier immaturity. If she has this facet of insight into the particular adult reactions, the social worker can receive them impersonally and without rancour or misunderstanding. The jealous child in heavy need of emotional attention is apt to attempt to split his parents, such children sometimes literally inserting themselves between the parents in bed. Hence criticisms against the social worker made to her colleagues by an adult in the throes of regression need not necessarily be taken at their face value. Residual needs of early life to monopolize relationships may sometimes be highly relevant to current attitudes in this sort of way. Uncooperative attitudes may have many symbolic origins. An easily recognizable example is that in the same way as a child who has had a strict paternal upbringing may then stand in dread of his headmaster, so also in adult life the fact that the social worker is a fantasied parent-figure may introduce residual distortions into the relationship that will cause corresponding difficulties if she fails to recognize them. But they may be utilized to the advantage of the client if she understands and accepts their presence.

The 'testing out techniques' and sibling rivalries in connection with children explained in chapter 2 may have their counterparts in the problems of adult psychoneurosis. A psychoneurotic person's early type testing out behaviour can too easily sour the relationship between a social worker and her client if its significance is not recognized and allowed for. A client's need for reassurance of his acceptability however bad his behaviour, comparable with the mechanism described in relation to disturbed children, may sometimes activate the tiresome behaviour of those adults unfortunate enough to be in the grip of psychoneurotic regression. And sometimes it will only be after the client has gone through potentially vexatious and wearisome stages of experimentation that the social worker will be able to perceive the real unhappiness and cry for help that lay beneath their occurrence.

When they are in process she may need to exercise a great deal of strength, patience and acceptance; and she will only be able to do so if her tolerance is born of an insight into her client's unresolved needs. Only then can the client's testing out behaviour succeed in its necessary purpose of securing the reassurance for which it is designed, rather than confirming the suspicion of unacceptability that led to its adoption. She need not, and indeed should not, be manipulated. But to respond by an attitude inadvertently implying rejection or withdrawal would not only be to portray a lack of psychological perceptiveness. It would often reinforce the very difficulties that she hopes to eliminate.

The opposite reaction may also be seen. Instead of the repetitiously 'testing out' forms of behaviour presented by the immature or regressed personality—in which are exhibited the various features designed to displease and thus to test the level of acceptance that may be present in spite of the unattractive qualities displayed—there may on the contrary be an attitude in which attempts to please the social worker are made with such an abnormal degree of effort that this situation too can be reasonably construed as pointing to probable insecurity in need of help. Again a parallel can be seen between this mode of feeling and that of an insecure child who, uncertain and haunted with fears of rejection, is morbidly incapable of allowing the parent to see the envy, spite and greed which he feels would threaten his acceptability and jeopardize his emotional needs.

The social worker's chronologically adult but emotionally immature clients may sometimes present her with a deceptive appearance of excessive competence, docility or kindness, adopted through an inability to believe that she could accept them unreservedly if their actual qualities were to become known to her. Until they realize that she can in fact accept them in spite of their inadequacies—such as their feelings of hatred towards a child or marital partner—little real progress will be made. After the eventual disclosure of these feelings they may hate the social worker for having found them out; but this situation, if well handled, will be likely to hold out more hope of eventual adjustment than will the essentially static situation that will otherwise obtain.

Sibling jealousies of childhood too may sometimes seem to be recapitulated in adult life, the marital partner appearing to represent the sibling rather than the parent towards whom the ambivalent resentment was felt. This problem may become highlighted when a couple are first interviewed together but later seen separately, one partner then revealing signs of anxiety that go beyond the mere lack of confidence due to loss of support by the spouse in the interview situation. The latter may be an element in the anxiety; but a reactivation of the tensions of early difficulties of parent/sibling relationships may be a significant factor. These fears by one partner that unwelcome disclosures will become possible in his or her absence may well have affinities with the severe anxieties experienced in childhood over a sibling's 'tale telling' to the parent. Sometimes such a possibility may be felt by the client to carry the risk of revealing the falsity of any pose of excessive confidence, etc., that has constituted the type of defence previously adopted.

PSYCHOANALYSIS

The techniques of formal psychoanalysis vary with the school to which the analyst belongs. Sometimes for example it is carried out by 'free association', sometimes by the patient 'associating' on a list of key words presented to him for the purpose (chapter 8). In some forms, the release of emotional tension, termed abreaction or catharsis, and the achievement of insight are considered the essential needs; in others, a further system of rebuilding is regarded as an indispensable key in the healing process.

In general, psychoanalysis is a method requiring the individual to be intelligent enough for the necessary degree of understanding of the psychological material revealed, and young enough to be still free from such a profusion of accumulated experience that the essence of the problem remains inextricable and its effect too hardened. In addition, the deeper psychoanalytical work undertaken on a basis of private practice, being a long and highly specialized process requiring frequent sessions, is often heavily expensive. For one reason or another, therefore, the deeper forms of psychoanalysis are recommended comparatively rarely in relation to the number of people with psychoneurotic difficulties. Behaviour therapy, also a highly specialized treatment for closely selected forms of psychoneurotic illness, may similarly be of help to only a relatively small percentage of sufferers (chapter 6).

Part Four

Care in the community

11

The psychotic client

THE CONCEPT OF COMMUNITY CARE

The concept of community care—a belief that patients who are chronically ill mentally should be looked after by their own families, or at least within the community rather than, as formerly, almost exclusively in mental hospitals—is one that is well established in the ethos of today and deeply entrenched in current ways of thought. It has given rise to a complex structure of administrative effort still lurching uncertainly in its relatively early stages, cumbersome, inadequate and fragmented. Its synthesis continues to present a heavy challenge to organizational enterprise. Its ultimate nature cannot be clearly foreseen.

The causes of this concept of community care were multiple, and reactions to its development diverse. It followed partly as a logical extension on the tidal wave of enthusiasm for the hospital as a therapeutic community, in which the breakdown of the traditionally rigid boundaries between the patient and the various professional groups within the hospital and within the groups themselves—or at least the blunting of their sharp edges of demarcation—was found to lead to clinical improvement in many longstay patients. Freedom within the hospital, though with suitable preservation of order, was found to pay good clinical dividends.

Therefore, so ran the argument, a similar benefit should follow the adoption of a more liberalizing acceptance of the human status of the patient within the general community itself. The hospital was seen as the microcosm and miniature reflection of the outside world, and comparable principles were anticipated as being potentially operative there too.

These speculations had been germinating within the soil of the spectacular advances in the clinical field, and this fortunate fact catalysed the course of their history. Advances in physical treatments in psychiatry had been taking place throughout the previous few decades with meteoric rapidity, and had transformed (chapter 6) the prognosis in some of the most devastating forms of mental illness. Patients helplessly and hopelessly crippled with anti-social behaviour, or with states of withdrawal and inertia so severe as to necessitate lifelong detention in hospital, often become calm, tractable and even appreciative—though still with less than average sensitivity—of the quality of their surroundings.

Furthermore, these illnesses had been so anxiety-provoking to the relatives that the tendency shown by some—though by no means all—to withdraw in horror, leaving the patient unwanted, unvisited and often abandoned without any form of communication to the staff or even to the patient himself, could hardly be wondered at. To see these patients sedated with drugs to the point of stupefaction, reducing their dignity to levels bordering on a vegetative and seemingly subhuman existence, overtaxed too heavily the emotions of many kindly and basically well-intentioned relatives.

Within the space of a few years, however, the change in the clinical picture and prognosis had lighted up embryonic ideas amongst the staff of involving the relatives. Speculations about 'halfway houses' between hospital and the outside world began to take shape. Within the confines of the hospital walls the dawn of community care was breaking.

The fact that it was not entirely an innovation was recognized with satisfaction. In Geel, in Belgium, mentally disabled people had from early times been living amongst the citizens of the town; they had been employed, smoothly integrated into their community and contentedly assisting in work such as dairy produce and manufacture of woollen goods, lace, and tobacco. Their acceptance by the people of Geel had long been held up as a testimony to the higher qualities of mankind and a splendid example of the effects of humane extramural management; but, although it has endured to the present day, the Geel community had been apt to be thought of as a special and rather picturesque way of life, far removed from the mainstream of life and hardly embodying an aspect of practical living. Now, however, it came into focus as the potential prototype of a widespread principle in the twentieth century.

Nevertheless, reactions to the concept of community care varied. By some it was greeted with suspicion. A few cynics attributed to it the machinations of politicians anxious to avoid financial expenditure on massive rebuilding programmes of large hospitals, most of which had been built in the last century. Others pointed fingers of scorn at those of their colleagues in high places called upon to advise on government policy, regarding them as either toeing the party line to curry favour, or as falling victims to their own self-persuasiveness. Still others were less sweepingly censorious, but overemphasized the obvious—and in itself very important—fact that a small nucleus of patients inevitably remain irrevocably undischargeable and therefore in need of permanent hospital care.

But in spite of these individual reactions and reservations, people of goodwill were quick to recognize the humane qualities and prospects of change for the better inherent in the new and imaginative thinking. Cooperation, albeit at first as much on a level of tacit approval as of active assistance, was from the outset forthcoming from psychiatrists as a whole. And it has grown. Community care is permanently with us; and it is for us to ensure that it produces the maximum benefit with the minimum damage.

THE SOCIAL WORKER'S INITIAL INVOLVEMENT

One of the ways in which the social worker may equip herself for this task will be first to consider some of the thoughts that can usefully pass through her mind when a patient with a psychotic illness is referred for her help.

Often her opening step should be to address further detailed enquiries—after careful reflection on the data already provided—to the referral source, since sometimes the information given by the person by whom she was first approached will have been of such limited scope or of such indeterminate character as to be of little value or perhaps even misleading. But having obtained this clarification she may still need to direct her

attention to sources of possible data from people other than
the one who first approached her. Ethical considerations may
then impose on her the obligation to obtain the client's permission to extend enquiries into these other areas.

The sources from which the original approach may have
come to the community social worker vary widely. General
practitioners, local authority community agencies, voluntary
societies of various sorts, the mental hospital medical or social
worker staff, or the patient himself or his relatives may all
bring her into the picture. At times her appearance on the
scene may be in response to a call from a general practitioner,
police surgeon or doctor in a general hospital to take part in a
compulsory admission to a mental hospital.

The community social worker's involvement with the
hospital may arise before her client's admission, during the
course of his stay in hospital, or after his discharge. But from
whatever source the call may have come, her first task will be
to define and articulate the problem as clearly and accurately
as possible. What has not been clearly defined and expressed
cannot be clearly understood, or dealt with as rationally as
necessary.

Any assessment of psychiatric features should be made as
soon as the necessary material is to hand. But not only should
a provisional assessment be attempted merely in clinical terms,
so that the presence or absence of psychiatric indications for
referral for further help can be evaluated. In the process of this
aspect of the assessment it is also important to guard against
being deflected from looking closely enough at the more
general situation within the home itself, where factors such as
the presence of a disturbed child or a geriatric problem, or
indeed many less concrete forms of family difficulty, may
bear closely on the management required.

All these environmental possibilities reflect the social
worker's fundamental role—concern with the family as a
whole. But to exercise this broad function in relation to a
psychotic client she needs to possess a certain amount of
specialized understanding of the clinical manifestations of
several of the major psychoses.

SOME PSYCHOTIC SYNDROMES

It is not the object in this book to present an elaborate picture of the psychotic illnesses in their wide variety of detail and colouring. But presented with the bare outlines of these syndromes, the reader can first acquire—if adequate opportunity for personal experience is available—a working ability to recognize and interpret the fuller details and then achieve a more sophisticated skill in sensing the subtler changes of behaviour and feeling they contain. The treatments too will not be described in anything more than empirical terms, even in those instances in which their modes of action have to some extent become understood. The aim is merely to provide enough broad knowledge to enable social workers to support their psychotic clients in the community as effectively as possible, and to initiate medical referrals when indicated.

Only three conditions will be described—depression, mania and schizophrenia.

DEPRESSION

Clinical features

Depression, like schizophrenia, may take many forms. The hysterical and reactive types, for instance (chapter 9), manifest themselves differently from the type of illness we are considering in the present chapter, which is the psychotic variety, characterized by ideas that are not necessarily merely strong reactions to circumstances in quantitative terms but are essentially delusional in their quality.

Broadly, psychotic depression arises on the basis of two different types of personality. One is the obsessional personality (chapter 9), the main features of which, it may be recalled, are an extreme love of tidiness, order, exactitude, predictable patterns of procedure, and perfection. Such personalities tend to be rigid, are inclined to be self-contained in expression of feeling, are prone to engage in excessive reflection before action can be embarked on, and experience no difficulties in adapting to changed circumstances when once a course of action has been set in train. Many patients subject to psychotic depression without any history of attacks of mania possess this sort of basic personality.

The other type of personality from which psychotic depression may spring is that of the ebullient, warm, unselfconscious, unworrying, easily coping individual—not infrequently associated with a thick-set, robust, strong and well-covered bodily physique. This is the sort of individual whose attack of depression often causes great astonishment amongst friends and relatives, since he has always ridden the storms of life with such buoyant ease and unflagging strength. Understandably in their way of thinking, his depressive lack of confidence could never have been reasonably predicted. The anomaly, however, is that this depression is one side of the two-sided coin known as manic-depressive psychosis. Such patients are also liable to be afflicted by attacks of mania; and the high confidence shown during the latter phases is, though pathological, usually a matter causing relatives far less surprise.

What are the features of these psychotic depressions? The first point to remember is that they come from within. Failure to recognize this principle can lead to fundamental mismanagement. A second misleading aspect is that, partly because of the rather self-contained and stoic personality which tends to characterize the sufferer's attitude if the illness occurs on the basis of an obsessional personality, the client may fail to volunteer information about his difficulties. This can obscure from bystanders the fact that any illness is present. Subjectively the sufferer himself feels painfully different; but the difference will not necessarily be apparent objectively.

Often therefore it may be essential to ask him leading questions, to which he usually replies revealingly and truthfully though slowly. Important depressive features, such as a decline in his interests, his initiative and his capacity for decision-making, will usually need to be enquired about specifically, both from himself and other relevant sources. Frequently it will be found that work and domestic duties have been tailing off, though people will tend to have covered up for him because of the admiration and protective inclinations engendered by his previously high standards of service.

Bound up with these features is the state known as psycho-motor retardation. Psychomotor retardation, as the name implies, is a slowing up of psychological processes and bodily movements. The extreme of this condition, seldom seen today, is termed depressive stupor, in which there is to a large extent a suppression of all visible mental and bodily movements, the patient in extreme instances being frozen into an almost statue-like state. In the vastly commoner and much less severe cases the posture is merely droopy, the speech slow and perhaps scarcely audible, and the facial expression set into a lack of movement. Also a general lack of movement throughout the whole body may be detected, which has given rise to the simile of a film in slow motion. But even when these features are not to be seen, the patient will agree on questioning that his concentration has diminished and that he must constantly steel himself to make conscious efforts to drag out thoughts or carry out simple activities, all of which would previously have been quite effortless and spontaneous.

In addition to the slowing of the thinking processes in depression their content also is disordered—in severe cases to the point of blatant delusions. It is therefore important for the social worker to be familiar with the various types of delusions that can point to depressive illness. In psychotic or endogenous depression, delusions of unworthiness and its associated self-reproach, of futility, of hypochondriasis and of poverty are the most characteristic. And it must be recognized that delusions, in whatever illness they may occur, are false beliefs, out of keeping with the patient's cultural background, which cannot be removed by appealing to his sense of logic. They are not founded in logic and they cannot be dispelled by discussions based on logic.

Clients with even mild endogenous depressions may blame themselves for inadequacies of various sorts, which in these circumstances must be recognized as springing from primary depression. Superficially some of these self-accusations, partially brought about by the depression itself, may contain an element of reason; but basically they are rooted in illness. Kindness is indicated; reassurance is virtually useless.

Clients' depressive feelings of futility, similarly delusional, may vary in their intensity from a comparatively mild though unmistakable distress associated with the conviction that recovery is very unlikely to occur, to a more heavily tormented sense of everything being irrevocably lost and black, without hope for the future or salvation for themselves. Very occasionally these ideas may become seriously projected on to their nearest and dearest, this delusion perhaps lying behind those rare acts of infanticide in which a psychotically depressed mother kills her baby to spare him the ordeal of an existence of supposed futility.

Delusions of hypochondriasis and poverty do not necessarily occur. However, psychotic preoccupations with the bodily state tend to be found in depressions of middle age—particularly in women with menopausal psychotic depressive illnesses and in the aged. In these illnesses the hypochondriacal ideas may be weird and flagrant, for example a belief that the gullet stops abruptly short or that the stomach does not exist. Delusions of poverty are commonest in the elderly or senile; and clients whom the social worker finds on investigation to be financially solvent may intractably believe themselves financially ruined.

A few final points need memorizing. Loss of appetite, loss of sexual enjoyment, and a pattern of insomnia in which the person wakes during the night or early hours of the morning, distressed perhaps to the point of suicide by an unceasing and delusionally-coloured round of unconstructive ruminations, are all characteristic. Another typical feature is diurnal variation—a term describing a pattern of maximal depression in the mornings, a gradual lifting with perhaps some improvement in the diminished powers of decision and concentration later in the day, and a return of the full depressive features again at the outset of the following morning. And the possibility of suicide, apt to be fatal and undertaken without prior statement of the intention or even any indication, must be constantly remembered.

Treatment

Electric treatment

The most potent treatment for this type of depression, at least in the sense of the quickest acting though not the most convenient, is electrical treatment. For its use in hospital readers should refer back to chapter 6. But the community social worker's main concern is often related to its administration on an outpatient basis.

The same medical techniques are adopted in these circumstances as those within the hospital, and she can reassure her client that on an outpatient basis it is equally painless. But on waking he may feel a little 'fuzzy' and therefore should not drive or undertake responsible work on the same day. And a tendency to amnesia may sometimes occur—a side effect seldom of much significance though while present it may impair working capacity—which usually lasts only for the duration of the treatment and for a short period afterwards.

Transport problems sometimes deter clients. But hospitals where this treatment is given on an outpatient basis commonly arrange transport if necessary, collecting the patient, returning him home, and perhaps providing a mid-day meal. Another deterring anxiety sometimes expressed by clients is that they have known other patients who have received this treatment without benefit. This observation may sometimes be correct; but these failures were often due to an admixture of other psychiatric elements present within the syndrome, so that although the clinical depression was dispelled the coexisting symptoms, not being of the sort amenable to electric treatment, naturally remained unchanged. For a client to deprive himself of this highly beneficial treatment on the basis of an imperfect understanding of it—which may also predispose him to react to it by developing symptoms originating from this very anxiety and to which on rare occasions he may then cling tenaciously—is a regrettable and sometimes far-reaching act of unwarrantable equation with other and irrelevant cases. A social worker in possession of reassuring facts which have been rejected by her client at their first telling may herself be able to secure his agreement subsequently.

Drugs

Other medical treatments for depression, though mainly indicated for less severe cases, exist in the form of tablets. A few points relating to one or two of the drugs used in other psychoses will also be worth presenting as each illness is dealt with in turn. Only a few of the preparations at present available will be mentioned; and still others will come into use as research progresses.

Clearly it is not the function of a social worker to remain in contact with a client simply for surveillance of the drug aspects. She is not a clinician. But in the course of her general involvement she may be able to ensure, for example, that a forgetful or reluctant client attends for any necessary blood estimations. And if familiar with potential side-effects of the drugs prescribed she may be able to recognize the need to arrange for medical appointment to be sought for their interpretation at an early stage if suggestive features occur. It may then be found that any such effects, perhaps unless they subsequently increase, are to be regarded as acceptable and inevitable; or further observations or immediate alterations may be required.

For depression various drugs may be prescribed. The main tricyclic drugs, so called because of their chemical composition, are Tofranil or Imipramine and Tryptizol or Amitriptyline. These tablets, when effective, may produce relief of depression within a few days; but this effect may not occur until they have been taken for as long as a month.

The social worker should be aware of this fact, so that logical encouragement to help the patient to persist with the treatment can when necessary be given at the time of his and his relatives' greatest despair about its value. If she knows about this possibility of delayed action, her attempts to induce her client to put faith in the medication and persist in taking it will be likely to contain a more confident and therefore more effective note than would exist in the absence of an understanding of this element in its mode of action. Other medications some-times prescribed in depression, such as sedatives to blunt the edge of any associated tension, may sometimes produce im-provement in this particular feature, albeit restricted in its depth of therapeutic penetration, within a few days—an effect sometimes also produced by tricyclic drugs themselves before their antidepressive action becomes apparent.

A knowledge of some of the possible side-effects of tricyclic drugs can also be helpful. They may include dryness of the mouth, constipation, sweating, blurring of vision, dizziness, palpitations, increased rapidity of the heartbeats, and skin rashes. Unless they are involving the patient in situations of physical danger, such as may arise from dizziness or disturb-ance of vision, the only action required may be reassurance that these features are usually merely annoying side-effects. This reassurance may be necessary to alleviate a depressed person's unspoken fears that their development signifies an ominous disease.

These effects are the commonest. But, just as there are many important drugs in medicine as a whole which may produce potentially serious side-effects as a remote possibility, any slight risk attendant on the use of anti-depressive drugs too has to be balanced against the usually much more important factor of the need to achieve an improvement in the condition for which they are prescribed. Nevertheless if any physical development arises during the course of drug treatment for depression or any other psychiatric illness it is prudent to obtain medical opinion about its nature, if only because en-tirely independent illnesses, as well as occasional serious drug effects, may intervene.

There are also certain circumstances under which it may be desirable for tricyclic drugs to be withheld; and since mentally ill patients may fail to grasp or remember instructions given by the doctor it may be useful on occasions for a social worker to be aware of the following points. Patients not infrequently retain a supply of tablets given in previous attacks. Mixtures of these tricyclic drugs with other antidepressive drugs or with one another—and particularly with the monoamine-oxidase inhibitors which will be mentioned later—may all be unsafe. Clients whose illnesses render them incompetent, or who are desperate or improvident, may endanger themselves by taking such mixtures.

For the social worker to remind them of the need to avoid mixing any incompatible treatments can thus be a worthwhile service. Another piece of medical advice which clients may overlook is the necessity to leave a gap of fourteen days after taking the last tablet of any of the monoamineoxidase inhibitor drugs, about to be discussed, before starting to take Tofranil or Tryptizol. Also, patients known to be suffering from heart or thyroid diseases or who have had any attacks of retention of urine should obtain medical advice before taking any tricyclic drugs already in their possession, since in these circumstances also dangerous effects may ensue. Finally, if a client under treatment with any of these drugs begins to develop features suggestive of hypomania, which may imply a tendency to suffer from attacks of this illness in addition to the tendency to depressive attacks, then the drug should be discontinued until medical review has been carried out.

In addition to the tricyclic compounds there is the group of antidepressive drugs, already referred to, known as the monoamineoxidase inhibitors. This group includes Nardil, Parnate, Parstelin, Marplan and Marsilid. Here again a number of side-effects may occur—dizziness, drowsiness, weakness, puffiness, dryness of the mouth, gastric and intestinal reactions, headache, blurred vision, and other symptoms. However, they are usually minor and commonly subside during the treatment.

A more significant point is that the use of each of these monoamineoxidase inhibitor drugs requires precautions because of its liability to react unfavourably with certain other drugs and foodstuffs. Some of the drugs used for pain relief and anaethesia, for instance, such as morphine and its related preparations, may constitute a dangerous combination with monoamineoxidase inhibitors, and Amphetamines, too, sometimes taken illicitly for mental stimulation, should not be combined with monoamineoxidase inhibitors. Nose drops should be withheld. Indeed with any medicines a doctor's opinion will be needed about their safety if combined with a

member of this group of antidepressives. The social worker
may usefully remind clients of this fact if she knows for
example that they intend to take cough or cold cures, laxatives,
tonics, or pain relievers including those that may be ad-
ministered for dental operations.

Among the foodstuffs from which people must refrain while
taking these drugs are cheese—plain or cooked—pickled
herring or broad bean pods, Bovril, Oxo, Marmite, or any
similar meat or yeast extracts, and alcohol except in moderation. Chianti wine should never be taken. If these foods are
inadvertently taken the resulting reaction may consist of a
serious rise in blood pressure accompanied by intense headache and acute incapacity.

Help over its effects

Some knowledge of electric treatment and the use of drugs,
though having its relevance to the role of the social worker, is
not her primary concern. Her central therapeutic function is
that of mitigating the inter-personal and social effects of this
illness. These effects are therefore worth memorizing. For
example, the marital partner may misconstrue the depressive
loss of warmth—conversational or sexual—as a basic loss of
affection even justifying retaliatory infidelity; the repeated
loss of sleep occasioned in the marital partner by the depressed
person's restless insomnia may deplete energy and eventually
erode capacity for tolerance and acceptance; depressive in-
decisiveness may at first be merely vexatious, but eventually
may prove destructive of the respect previously felt; depressive
failure to attend to ordinary domestic affairs may give rise in
the marital partner to an unjustified suspicion of hitherto unrecognized egocentricity, leading to a feeling of distressing and
isolating disenchantment; the incompetence created by recognized depressive illness may worry or even antagonize employers, threatening the sufferer's job security or bringing an
unwarrantable reputation for dangerous unreliability that can
never be lived down.

Hence to the misfortune of the illness there can become
added the misfortune of undeserved recriminations arising
from uninformed misinterpretations of many of its features.

These misunderstandings may be eliminated by a good social worker's explanations to the family; and, if conducted in parallel with the clinical measures, such explanations may prove of inestimable value in the general management of the situation.

In spite of the value which her participation may provide in this way, the limitations of the social worker's functions must also be remembered. This illness essentially comes from within. An important practical corollary therefore is to take steps to ensure that the client is promptly referred for medical help. Casework and alterations of the social environment are not the major methods for tackling the condition, at least not until the symptoms have been dispelled by medical treatment. Not being due to external factors—contrary to what may too easily be assumed—psychotic depression cannot be primarily dealt with by reference to external factors. Attempts to change the environment will merely leave the condition itself unchanged; or may impose on to the sufferer the kindly-meant but burdensome and sometimes insupportable strains of the need to adjust to the altered circumstances. In severe cases an over-zealous attempt to deal with a supposed cause that is in fact more apparent than real may itself tip the client into suicide, perhaps through increasing his sense of inadequacy by unwittingly demonstrating his inability to respond to the very efforts—albeit ill-founded—made to help him.

Thus, as with many other mental illnesses, all too commonly symptoms are regarded as causes. For instance, the patient's failures are often the result of the illness rather than the cause of it—and even in those cases in which the illness has been genuinely brought about by a fairly obvious causal factor, this factor has been the precipitant but not the essence of the condition. A related pitfall awaiting inexperienced social workers is their potential failure to recognize as delusional those psychotic ideas that are only minimal in the intensity of their expression. But any delusion is by definition a false belief not amenable to reason. If therefore a social worker attempts to dissuade a client of the false nature of a belief of this sort, no good will be achieved. The client may appear to acquiesce for the sake of peace; but he will feel misunderstood. And in relation to this matter he will be correct. The true quality of his belief will indeed not have been appreciated.

A flagrant depressive delusion can be recognized; minor degrees are less easily appreciated. But they are governed by the same natural laws relating to the ineradicability of delusional convictions by this means. The difference is merely in degree of intensity; minor degrees of delusions, such as mild depressive self reproach, are equally impervious to modification by reassurance. It is of great practical importance to recognize this principle which is so commonly overlooked.

Finally, a special point about the assessment of suicidal risk must be borne in mind. Every patient suffering from this form of depression is a potential suicide throughout the illness. But there are certain phases during which he may be most likely to make the attempt. Paradoxically, and sometimes to the surprise of inexperienced nursing staff impressed by these patients' improvement after a few electric treatments or during a course of antidepressive medication, the patient may attempt suicide at the stage when he has become less depressed. The psychomotor retardation may have become diminished, and while still deluded and wretched he may then have the initiative to commit suicide. The ability to kill himself has been restored; but the inclination to do so has not at that stage become sufficiently diminished. The situation may thus be seriously deceptive. For a social worker to be forewarned of this principle may lead to a closer watch on the situation, with lifesaving results. Suicide may be at its most dangerous level when the client is passing into, or emerging from, the deeper levels of his depressive misery.

MANIA

Clinical features

It was mentioned earlier that often the form of depression just discussed comprises only one side of the two-sided coin known as manic-depressive psychosis; or, putting the position in another way, the total psychosis has as its essential nature the characteristic of bipolarity—it has two poles, one of which is the depressive state, and at the opposite pole is the state of mania. Each of these states typically runs a phasic course of substantial duration, often for weeks or months, in contrast to the short-lived reactions found in hysterical depression or elation. And each may be followed either by a period of normality (which indeed may remain as a permanent condition uninterrupted by further attacks), or by a recurrence of the same condition, or by an attack of the opposite type of illness. Sometimes one phase merges directly into the other, the state during this transitory period on occasions partaking of features of both illnesses. The latter condition, known as a mixed affective syndrome, tends to be difficult to diagnose and in any case is uncommon.

The social worker can most easily remember the features of a typical attack of mania by recalling in succession each individual feature of the depressive illness and then thinking of the opposite condition. These features will comprise the characteristic syndrome of mania, classified in the mind in a form suitable for practical application.

The miserable and self-reproachful sense of inadequacy, for example, found in depression has its mood counterpart in mania as an abnormality taking the form there of a display of extreme confidence—sometimes overweening and arrogant but frequently at the same time warm and jovial—which is as much a reflection of delusional belief as is the depressive's opposite conviction of his unworthiness. Again, the depressive's withdrawal from the environment contrasts with the manic patient's extraverted entry into affairs outside himself, which often takes the form of a bouncing interference in other people's concerns and antagonizes its recipients in spite of its associated warmth and bonhomie. The counterpart of the depressive's lack of responsiveness to approach may be seen in the manic's highly responsive reactions of irritation and momentary hostility (in severe cases sometimes leading to physical as well as verbal violence)—particularly if the approach contains any semblance of opposition—though soon the warmth of manner returns and euphoria again exudes.

A feature common to both mania and depression is the fact that each, when severe, intrudes inevitably into the functioning of both mind and body. But here again a contrast exists. In place of the mental and physical slowing of depressive psycho-motor retardation, in mania there is an elevation of the mood, the speed of thinking and the level of physical activity. The union of expansiveness of mood, increased speed of thought and general loss of inhibition results in gratuitous and garrulous communication and a restless physical overactivity in which the flamboyant and uninhibited gestures (classically the manic patient is said to shake hands from the shoulder) are the complete antithesis of the shrinking and silent immobility of the patient in the grip of clinical depression.

In talking to a patient suspected of suffering from a develop-ing manic state, two points in particular should be looked for. One is termed flight of ideas; the other is known as distracta-bility.

Flight of ideas is an outcome of the person's increased pressure of thought and speed of association; and it expresses itself as one idea leading to another with undue rapidity, thoughts being increased in number but diminished in depth. In spite of this superficiality, in the early stages of a first attack, before it has reached manifestly pathological intensity, the picture may be mistaken for cleverness—'such a quick brain, he's three jumps ahead of everybody'. But if the condition progresses the thinking becomes so fragmented that it is recognizably abnormal; and in severe cases it may eventually lead to extreme incoherence.

The second point, distractability, is a manic phenomenon related to the external environment. By this term is meant that the sufferer's attention is repeatedly diverted by chance stimuli in the environment which in normal health would remain largely unheeded. A noise outside the room, an object on the table, an insect on the window, may catch the patient's atten-tion, evoke his cheerful comments, and break still further the already tenuous thread of consistency in his garrulous and ever-changing topics of conversation.

This feature of distractability—again diametrically opposed to the depressive's lack of interest in his environment—has an obvious affinity with another attribute of manic illness, namely the tendency to embark on more and more activities. His sense of superior personal ability and status—be it concerned with ideas about his mental powers, physical strength or financial position—is often bound up with this phenomenon. It is the other side of the coin to the depressive's feelings of futility.

The manic's certainty of his superiority may communicate itself so convincingly to the simple or unwary that employers and others may be misled into espousing similar assumptions. The result may be that he is commissioned to undertake responsible ventures in which his heightened energies may indeed bring outstanding successes in the early stages. But with the increasing internal pressure and loss of inhibition, one task after another is left restlessly uncompleted. This pattern of having undertaken an increasing number of activities, none of which reached its completion, is often recognized after recovery by the sufferer himself as having been pathological. But at the time of its occurrence he is incapable of comprehending or controlling it.

An equally pathological form of overactivity frequently found in manic patients is a tendency to overspend. A combination of delusions of wealth or grandeur, overactivity, and his powers of confident persuasiveness born of psychotic conviction, can result in regrettable or even disastrous financial transactions. This financial prodigality and confident persuasiveness may constitute an urgent indication for compulsory admission to hospital. But it is a step for which the patient sees absolutely no need, protesting with complete honesty that he has never felt better or more capable throughout the whole of his life.

This constellation of increasing expansiveness, inordinate warmth and euphoria, gesticulating garrulousness, ill-conceived intrusions into the affairs of others, pathological mental agility leading to ultimate incoherence, and increased pressure of libido sometimes leading to promiscuity and marital discord, may bring in the social worker from many sources—doctors, relatives, employers, clergymen, samaritans, marriage guidance counsellors. Even if such a condition is only of subclinical intensity it must be taken seriously and careful enquiries made about any history of phases of depression—perhaps subacute and unrecognized at the time.

Treatment

Although many cases of even mild mania (termed hypomania), and certainly of mania, require treatment in hospital, mild hypomanic illness amounting to little more than a slight persistent elevation of mood and heightening of physical and mental activities may subside entirely within the general community, treated or untreated. Indeed when an attack of mania occurs for the first time, there may be reports of mild symptoms of this condition in the past whose significance was slight and passed entirely unrecognized. In addition a history of attacks of features only retrospectively recognizable as mild depressive illnesses may be found in patients developing a manic attack. Knowledge of these facts may enable a social worker to perceive the potential significance of—and therefore recommend that early medical advice be sought for—behaviour that would otherwise pass without the necessary attention until reaching a point at which treatment would be more difficult or even refused.

Of the drugs used for mania the commonest at present are Haloperidol and Lithium. Haloperidol, or Serenace, a drug whose tranquillizing effect can be exploited in the relief both of manic and schizophrenic excitability, may, like the phenothiazines, produce the side-effect of Parkinsonism (described later), though usually it is only at the higher doses that this development arises. Antiparkinsonian drugs must then be simultaneously taken, such as Artane, Benzhexol or Cogentin.

The effect of Haloperidol in reducing the overactivity of a patient suffering from mania is often very striking both in its rapidity and degree. Nevertheless it is unwise to acquiesce in a patient's belief that improvement while taking drugs necessarily renders him suitable for discharge from hospital. Sometimes when this request is first made the symptoms are merely held in pharmacological abeyance. The patient's imperceptive euphoria can then be both a disadvantage and a safeguard. The disadvantage lies in the likelihood of a cheerful neglect of taking the medication after discharge, and a consequent relapse. The safeguard is the amiable nature of the euphoria that fortunately often leads him to agree to the recommendation to remain in hospital. If, however, he leaves against advice, the social worker's knowledge that the illness may still be in a state of underlying activity will alert her to the possible need for further help, and may give her conviction in her own efforts at persuading him to accept any medical advice for readmission.

Lithium is a drug which, though commonly efficacious for its own purposes to a greater or lesser degree, is without many of the disadvantages of the antidepressives. Unlike the tricyclic compounds, it can be mixed with other drugs without danger. Unlike the monoamineoxidase inhibitors, no steps to avoid unsuitable foodstuffs are required. It is also believed by many psychiatrists to provide the possibility not only of dispelling illness, but of forestalling its recurrence, and is therefore often prescribed as a 'mood normalizer' to be taken over the years, even after recovery, on the assumption that in the manic-depressive patient it may stave off future attacks of depression as well as mania.

But it brings its problems of observation and organization. Observation is needed, apart from the ordinary assessment of psychiatric progress, to detect any developing toxic effects. Organization is required, so that the level of the drug in the blood stream can be seen. The dose can then be reduced if the toxic level is drawing too close, or increased when necessary if it is found that a suitable margin of reserve is available for this purpose. A little blood is removed from a vein for the initial estimation and thereafter at intervals which are determined by factors such as the current dosage, the clinical progress—for instance an anticipated deterioration of the psychiatric state may presage the need for higher doses—and the length of time during which the patient has been receiving the drug.

It may happen—for example if a person receiving the medication has inadvertently taken an excessive quantity and failed to attend for observation—that toxic manifestations occur. They may include loss of appetite, diarrhoea, vomiting, and various effects on the central nervous system such as drowsiness, dizziness, unsteadiness in walking, tremors, noises in the ears, blurring of vision and muscular twitching. If any of these features are known to have developed, no further tablets should be taken, but an immediate medical examination arranged.

A variant of this drug, Priadel, has the same essential therapeutic action but carries the advantage of 'controlled release', which enables a once-daily dose to cover the patient's therapeutic needs continuously, providing a constant level of availability to the brain. Again the possibility of toxic effects similar to those of Lithium, will necessitate review of dosage and point to the need for estimation of the level of the drug in the blood stream by chemical analysis, similarly undertaken at the particular frequency evaluated by the medical adviser. The blood specimens for this purpose must be taken before the daily dose – a point which the social worker may help to ensure. Another point worth her knowing is that the first blood estimation should be taken within four or five days, and at the most a week, after the treatment has been started.

SCHIZOPHRENIA

Clinical features

Schizophrenia tends to be a recurring or chronic illness. It is therefore self-evident that the relatives of people who suffer, or in the past have suffered, from schizophrenia need some practical knowledge of the illness. And this need continues to increase yearly as those patients who in a former era would have been custodially retained for long periods in hospital— or would at least have been readmitted at frequent intervals— now spend all or most of their lives at home, living in a state of mental health that has been greatly improved by their treatment but which nevertheless still depends in large measure on an enlightened understanding amongst those by whom they are surrounded. Similarly, the relatives' own well-being, and sometimes even their own health, depend on the patient's improvement being adequately maintained.

This illness has many facets about which relatives therefore need to be suitably informed. They include its manifestations, its management, and the legal machinery relating to the admission of sufferers to hospital. One approach to the manifestations of schizophrenia is to consider them in terms of the condition's four main types, namely its simple, hebephrenic, catatonic and paranoid varieties. These types are not sharply divided from one another, and each may contain features of each of the others.

However, the present approach will be to consider the illness from a somewhat different angle, not distinguishing between the different types of illnesses but considering the aggregate features of a typical composite case.

The system of classification of the symptoms of such a case can be usefully presented by a division into two categories of features: firstly those arising from disorders of thinking, and secondly those arising from disorders of the emotions. This twofold classification forms a simplified aid to memory. Before embarking on a description of each of these categories, two further points will be mentioned. One should bring confidence and consolation to relatives. The other sounds a warning note. Each point may need to be conveyed to them.

The consoling point is that although in order to present a sufficiently comprehensive picture of the possibilities of the illness this description will include features which at first sight may appear distressingly ominous, nevertheless very many cases are instrinsically much less destructive to the personality than is suggested by the inclusion in this description of those features that exist at the severe end of the scale. In addition, the effects of treatment can often reduce the severity of these conditions to a state at which a good level of adjustment is achieved and excellently maintained. Happily this is a common finding, though better community facilities for buttressing the welfare of the less well-recovered cases are badly needed.

The warning, on the other hand, is that the changes in the person which herald the development of the illness—or of a relapse into a further attack—may at first be misleadingly unobtrusive, except perhaps to those who know the individual very well and are tuned in to the slight nuances of change in manner which may be the only features by which the illness declares itself, at least in its early stages. The development of slight but persisting withdrawal from social contacts, a certain loss of warmth of feeling, a strangeness of manner or an increasing oddness of outlook may sometimes signify more to the sensitive and discerning eye of a near relative than to a doctor who has less familiarity with the patient's day-to-day demeanour and psychological makeup. Relaxed and confident vigilance by close acquaintances is important if relapses are to be averted.

Of course we all have slight temporary mood changes. But while keeping this fact in mind, and trying to avoid over-anxiety, relatives should not discount the possible significance of subtle changes when seen taking place in a previously improved or recovered patient if they persist over a period of a week or two. It is true that in some cases schizophrenia is an illness with manifestations that are concrete to the point of being unmistakable—bizarre delusions for instance. But in others it takes forms which at first sight seem so minor that explanations for the failing powers may be put forward which are far removed from the true reality and may easily obscure detection of the illness. This last situation is most apt to arise when the brunt of the condition falls into the sphere of the emotions, causing a loss of emotional warmth and drive which leads the patient to withdraw from social and family activities but makes insufficient impression to arouse suspicions of serious illness in the minds of those comparatively unfamiliar with this condition.

Disorders of thinking

In the first category of symptoms that we shall consider—the disorders of thinking—the production of ideas by the patient goes seriously awry, so that they become changed in quantity or quality or both. Quantitatively, a smaller number of ideas appear to pass through his mind. His intellectual functioning is reduced both in its vitality and in the number of normal thoughts, while at the same time he indulges in excursions of imagination into areas of thought that are often frankly delusional. His constructive thinking may be reduced to such a low level that he becomes incapable of sustained employment, of attending to domestic duties, or in extreme cases even of carrying out the needs of ordinary personal hygiene.

The schizophrenic diminution of the amount of ideas and interests is very characteristic to the experienced observer.

As to the qualitative changes, the most difficult to recognize is often a minor degree of what is sometimes termed tangential thinking. His ideas may become irrelevant, causing the process of thinking to go off at a tangent and lead to nowhere in particular. When this tangential thinking is severe it is quite apparent. But when it is of minor degree it may be very difficult to detect. Indeed if a schizophrenic patient's answers are only minimally 'off the target' on each occasion, the resulting discussion may have led nowhere; but it may be impossible to pinpoint any particular example of irrelevancy at any stage of the conversation when it is subsequently reviewed. The observer's feeling that his own mind is losing its grip is a well known and sometimes disquieting reaction that may nevertheless play its own part in diagnosing schizophrenic disorder in those cases in which tangential thinking is only subacute in its manifestations.

Other qualitative disturbances of thinking are usually easier to recognize. A resultingly remote and detached manner, a facial expression of inert perplexity, sudden interruptions in the stream of thinking with the result that the patient goes abruptly blank and fails to return to the previous theme, woolly thought processes with loss of former precision and incisiveness, metaphor ineptly and nebulously used, the shading of thinking into delusional material liable to embody spurious philosophical and metaphysical ruminations, and even the introduction into speech of invented words unknown in ordinary language, may all reflect a schizophrenic process. Some of these features too when undramatic may pass unrecognized by the inexperienced or untaught.

Gross thought disorder can hardly be overlooked. Bizarre and even macabre ideas may abound. Their nature is endless. Sometimes they involve weird hypochondriacal beliefs, sometimes patients express an ability to hear their own thinking as hallucinatory experience, sometimes they have the conviction that thoughts are put into or taken out of their minds, sometimes that their thoughts can be read, that their food is poisoned, and so on.

Two symptoms are especially characteristic, though like all the features of schizophrenia they are not necessarily present in any individual case. Each comprises a particular form of delusional expression of persecution. They are known as passivity feelings and ideas of reference. In passivity feelings the patient believes that he is under the malicious influence of agencies outside himself, such as rays malevolently emanating from the sky, machines directing vibrations on to him that pass through walls and influence his mind or body, or that gases or thought waves from indeterminate sources influence his thoughts, feelings or conduct. Such ideas will be held with total and impervious conviction.

In ideas of reference, on the other hand, inanimate beings do not form the delusional content. Here the patient believes that other human beings are referring to him in various derogatory ways. Newspaper articles, television comments, innocent discussions or exchanges of glances between neighbours may be construed as carrying communications impugning his character or plotting his downfall. These delusions may lead him to engage in violent quarrels with the supposed persecutors, to lodge complaints with the police, or even perpetrate physical assaults.

All the ideas of this sort found in a schizophrenic patient are delusions. But there is another very characteristic feature of thought disorder which, like delusions, may occur in forms of mental illness other than schizophrenia and which, again like delusions, are also completely inaccessible to appeal to reason. They are the experiences referred to as hallucinations.

Hallucinations are false perceptions; or put in another way they are perceptions that have no sensory foundation in the environment. Defined more simply, they are experiences in which the patient hears sounds which exist only in his own mind, sees visions which similarly do not in fact exist outside his own imagination, or experiences smells, bodily sensations or even tastes which again are derived only from his own mental processes. In schizophrenia much the commonest hallucinatory experiences are those in which he hears non-existent voices.

Disorders of emotion

Earlier we saw that the disorders of thinking in schizophrenia comprise only one major dimension of this illness. The other, namely disorders of the emotions, equally need to be appreciated. People with only limited understanding of the illness are apt to consider that the disordered thinking is the essence of the condition, and that the emotional changes are mere subsidiary accompaniments. Such is not the case.

This imbalance in clinical interpretation arises largely because the disorders of thought, such as the bizarre delusions, often impinge more strikingly on the awareness of the observer than do the disorders in the emotional sphere, which can sometimes pass unnoticed. And even where there is loss of emotional vitality so gross as to be unmistakable, if there are no detectable delusions coexisting the condition is liable to be interpreted as a mild case. But in some instances—in teenagers and young adults for example—the destructive effects on the emotions produced by this illness, though potentially reversible, may prove to be much the most sinister aspect.

The emotional effects most often declare themselves in a grave, though sometimes insidious, leaking away of the capacity for emotional response. The resulting state is sometimes termed schizophrenic indifference, or affective loss. The sufferer loses his previous capacity for warmth of feeling—a different situation from the 'dissociative' withdrawal that sometimes occurs as a defence mechanism in psychoneurosis. Those towards whom he had previously felt affection, such as parents, marital partner and children, now cease to generate and receive this response. Not only does he become cool towards his loved ones, but he also loses the emotional drive which formerly prompted his interest in work and in the general affairs of his environment. A withdrawn, flat, and sometimes simpering vacancy, perhaps with a fatuous passivity of manner, may in some cases be the crippling end-point of this destructive process.

On occasions his emotional reactions may be frankly inappropriate, with serious matters evoking a quiet facile giggle, or pleasant considerations leading to a brief reaction of inert tearfulness. It is this split between the thought content and the emotional response—these two spheres of mental life being out of gear—that gives rise to the designation 'the split mind'. The 'splitting' in this illness, contrary to common lay belief, is not the 'Jekyll and Hyde' dual personality. The latter is an expression of hysterical dissociation (chapters 8 and 9).

Sometimes the loss of capacity for sympathy associated with the diminished emotional warmth leaves his basic instinctual drives relatively unopposed by the normal safeguards of warmth and kindness. Callous attitudes or even episodes of impulsive violence, sometimes in response to hallucinatory voices, usually indicate the need for increase in the pheno-thiazine drugs, described later, so that their calming effects on his schizophrenic reactions can bring about the necessary state of inner stability and external adjustment.

The degree of this emotional loss and social withdrawal is liable to be related to the age of the individual. It tends to be greatest in the younger age groups and less marked if the illness first attacks in later life, when the emotional capacity may in fact remain quite well preserved and the emotional responses retain their appropriateness to the thought content. Paradoxically the greater turbulence of, let us say, a paranoid schizophrenic patient towards a neighbour in those circumstances may be of good portent clinically in spite of its distressing nature from the social point of view. Acute cases, with rapid onset and extreme withdrawal or excitability, do not necessarily carry the worst prognosis—often it is better than for those with unobtrusively insidious deterioration or a less strident social impact.

The mental spectacle of a human being degenerated into the extreme of incapacitating indifference and inertia is one that may be chilling to the imaginations of many readers. But it should be re-emphasized that although collectively this group contains a substantial number of the unemployable 'loners', drifters and vagrants, nevertheless within the broad psychotic community the individuals destined for this unfortunate end-point form only a small minority of schizophrenic people. Psychiatrists dealing with the panorama of psychotic referrals are able to keep the scene in its true and happier perspective, finding that only an occasional case reaches this tragic outcome amongst the much larger numbers who go into gratifying reversal, or at least are held in a state of undeteriorating abeyance.

Treatment

Although the management of the clinical aspects of this illness is not the primary role of social workers—on the contrary it is the community nurse, as will be seen later, who mainly bears this responsibility—nevertheless their involvement in these situations, in whatever capacity, requires that they possess sufficient understanding of the drugs in common use to render the client's reactions meaningful and to make for a service that will be as effective as possible.

An historical survey will not be given concerning the efforts undertaken in the past to bring this crippling illness under control, except to mention that some of the major work carried out so energetically in the earlier part of the present century has not stood the test of time in providing therapy that is sufficiently practicable or effective. A famous example of earlier therapeutic endeavour, ephemeral but protracted, which in this country is no longer a live issue is that of deep insulin coma treatment for schizophrenia.

This treatment entailed an immense amount of work for little if any therapeutic return of proven benefit, and was eventually widely abandoned. Nevertheless the strains devolving on doctors and nurses in carrying out such skilled, demanding, potentially dangerous and on occasions lethal treatment—and the careful work required by the research workers concerned to evaluate its effects—were by no means wasted. The climate of outlook induced by the methods of close observation required by insulin coma treatment and the need for the vigorous scientific evaluation of the results, set the tone for an attitude that was the foundation from which subsequent discoveries of immense and long-lasting value have been made. This more scientifically disciplined attitude thus came to be established into the forefront of the approach that is adopted with such value towards psychotic illnesses in the present day.

The most significant pharmacological breakthrough into the modern psychiatric era began with the arrival of the phenothiazine group of drugs, of which the drug Largactil was the first example in the 1950s. Like all drugs it is not without its side-effects, amongst the most striking of which are the state known as Parkinsonism, which will be described later in this chapter, and a tendency to skin reactions that occur particularly under the influence of the summer sun. These two side-effects can be controlled by the use respectively of anti-parkinsonian drugs and a cream applied to the exposed areas of the skin. Very rarely jaundice may occur and require discontinuation of the treatment.

The typical effect of Largactil is that it usually enables the patient to disregard his psychotic ideas to a large extent. One does not anticipate, however, that they will necessarily cease to exist. But at least the delusions and hallucinations often cease to disturb his conduct, and no longer impair his concentration as seriously. In some cases they may indeed peter out while he is receiving the drug, but in these circumstances it is sometimes difficult, until the effects of reducing or omitting the drug have been observed, to decide with confidence whether or not a spontaneous subsidence has simply taken place as part of the natural course of the illness, since this course towards recovery was occasionally observed even before these drugs had come into existence. Because in the majority of cases the delusions and hallucinations do not actually disappear, there often remains a need for the patient to continue to receive long-term 'maintenance' treatment after his discharge back into the community so that their comparatively innocuous nature now achieved can then be maintained.

Obviously an effective drug having the least significant side-effects is usually to be preferred to one in which such complications are known to occur more readily. Many years after the introduction of Largactil another drug, Stelazine, came into being. This drug, though sometimes producing Parkinsonism as a side-effect, fortunately does not possess as many possible side-effects as its otherwise comparable predecessor.

Other drugs, such as Melleril, have similar advantages. They are therefore widely used in the management of this illness. However, Largactil also continues in use as a valuable, if less readily prescribed tool in schizophrenia under appropriate circumstances.

Some cases seem to respond more satisfactorily to one drug, while others respond better to others. Every clinical problem needs assessment on its own merits, and one of the functions of the psychiatrist is to balance the advantages and disadvantages of the various drugs, either alone or in combination, in relation to the individual's own reactions.

The change of scene brought about by the introduction of these drugs into mental hospitals was referred to in chapter 6. And with their continuing use the environment outside the hospital became correspondingly more receptive of the patient's return. It will be recalled that patients hitherto undischargeable became capable of return to the community, no longer impelled by their delusions and hallucinations to offend or alarm others, and no longer preoccupied with psychotic ideas to an extent that precluded their ability to earn their livelihoods—or at least they sometimes became able to make a modified working contribution to the family's welfare. And those cases still unable to work often regained the capacity to make a general adjustment within the home.

Even before the advent of the present supporting services this medical procedure for achieving great improvement had already taken root. But the maintenance of the patient's improvement rested on his continuing to take the drug in the form of tablets or medicines by mouth. Unfortunately, as we shall see when discussing the work of the community nurse, frequently patients fail to continue to take their medication. The result is too often a relapse and re-admission—a factor which in the past has seriously limited the long-term value of these pharmacological advances in the community.

This limitation has become diminished, though not entirely eliminated, by a further advance during the last decade. The development of long-acting phenothiazine drugs available for injection, in contrast to those prepared in forms that could only be taken by mouth, has now made it possible to ensure that an adequate level of the medication is maintained within the patient's system for a substantial period, often for several weeks or a month. Perhaps rather surprisingly, patients unwilling or unable to take multiple tablets regularly will frequently accept this method contentedly and with enormous benefit to themselves and their families. At present the phenothiazine drugs called Moditen and Modecate are used for injection; but future research may well bring other drugs, both for oral and intramuscular use.

There is no easy rule of thumb for establishing the regime of treatment by the method of injection of phenothiazines, beyond the broad generalization that the drug should be administered on a basis leading to an optimal therapeutic benefit with a minimum of side-effects. Weighing practical factors involved in this principle requires experience and care. It is usually necessary for the process to be undertaken and completed with the patient in hospital, so that after his discharge a known and satisfactory system will have been established as a foundation for his long-term management in the community.

In hospital the main variables that need to be brought into a suitably fixed pattern include the frequency of the injections and the dose injected. The eventual interval between injections usually ranges from a month to a week. It may be observed, for instance, that if injections are given once monthly the patient shows signs of relapse after, let us say, three weeks. Either an increase in the dose or a reduction of the interval to perhaps two weeks is then required, followed by continued observation and possibly still more modification of dose, frequency or both, according to the further clinical findings and the social circumstances. At the same time the correct dosage of antiparkinsonian tablets is assessed, again by trial and error, in relation to the modifications.

When these procedures have been completed, and the patient is ready for discharge, the same regime often remains suitable for continuation in the community. But at other times the situation after discharge may revert to one that is less satisfactory. For example, in addition to the patient omitting to attend for his injections after leaving hospital, he may in fact accept them on the prescribed basis but discontinue taking his antiparkinsonian tablets, or lapse into taking them capriciously. Recrudescence of Parkinsonism—sometimes arising as an alarmingly acute reaction necessitating emergency readmission, but usually developing more slowly—then takes place. Furthermore, as a result of a spontaneous change at any time in the level of intensity of the patient's schizophrenic illness, it may become inadequately controlled if no corresponding change in the pattern of medication has been made. If social workers (and members of other caring professions liable to find themselves in close and regular contact with people afflicted with schizophrenia) can be aware of these considerations in broad and general terms they will be better able to forestall relapses. The important side-effect of Parkinsonism is a matter about which they should therefore have some detailed knowledge.

Parkinsonism is a condition liable to arise from the administration of any type of phenothiazine drug, whether taken by mouth or given by intramuscular injection. It is also a condition that may occur under other circumstances, such as following an attack of encephalitis or as a result of senile degenerative changes in certain brain areas; and basically it is due to interference with the normal working of the brain machinery responsible for inhibition of the tone in muscles. The consequence, not unnaturally, is the development of an increased tone in these muscles.

This increased tone—known as spasticity—may produce a degree of paralysis. But in Parkinsonism the most striking feature is usually the tremors that result from this increased muscle tone, observed particularly in the characteristic 'pill-rolling' movements of fingers and thumb, and the clumsy shakiness of hand movements. The increased tone of the muscles of the face often gives rise to a staring, unblinking, mask-like expression, with slurring of speech and a dribbling of saliva resulting from the involvement of the muscles of the mouth and lips. In marked instances the patient's posture resembles a statue, with a tendency to turn *en bloc*. Occasionally, while shuffling along he may move helplessly forward with an increasing momentum, chasing his own centre of gravity.

In order that this Parkinsonism produced by the phenothiazine drugs, whether given by injections or tablets, can be
satisfactorily combated it is necessary for the patient to take
some additional medication such as Artane or Cogentin. Up
to the present stage of pharmacological science such drugs are
mainly available in tablet form. If taken regularly, however,
they relieve—thus lessening any undesirable need for reduction of the phenothiazine dosage—the complicating factors of
Parkinsonian tremors, mask-like facial expression, difficulties
in speech and writing, troublesome salivation, impairment of
swallowing, diminished capacity for walking, and the insomnia liable to be associated with the discomforts of the
muscular rigidity.

Recognition of the side-effects of drugs should not automatically induce the social worker to dissuade the patient from
persisting with the treatment, since serious relapse of the
schizophrenic illness may follow, but the presence of side-
effects may need to be drawn to the attention of the medical
adviser. Commonly a balance is then achieved, acceptable to
patient and family and satisfactory to the clinician. And as
long as the medication is taken punctiliously, a combination
of an optimal psychiatric effect with a freedom from physical
discomfort usually provides these patients with lives that are
much happier and incomparably more productive than the lives
of so many of their unfortunate predecessors in the first half
of the century.

There is a still further element that requires watching. The
process of balancing the medication includes the need to look
for any potential side-effects arising from the antiparkinsonian
drugs themselves. These effects may include dryness of the
mouth, blurred vision, nausea, occasionally vomiting and
nervous tension or drowsiness. In large doses muscular weakness may occur. But such complications, which in practice
seldom form too serious a stumbling block if duly attended
to, can usually be overcome by adjustments in the doses of
these drugs too when necessary.

In other words, the dosage and frequency of administration
of the phenothiazines are pushed high enough to ensure adequate help for the mental illness, but at the same time is pitched

at a low enough level to avoid a degree of Parkinsonism whose control beyond a certain point may bring its own problems. Within fairly wide limits there are variations in the responses, both therapeutic and adverse, amongst the recipients. And in general the greater the experience of the psychiatric and nursing staff in this field, the greater will be their success in tailoring the medication to the mental and physical requirements of the individual.

Another important drug given by intramuscular injection which has come into use more recently is Depixol. This medication has little tendency to produce Parkinsonism. It also has an activating property of value for those schizophrenic sufferers who show inertia, though where excitability is present this attribute may limit its value.

But it is important to underline once again that at the present stage of medical history the only outcome of any anti-schizophrenic medication that can be relied on is that the patient will often be rendered relatively well able to disregard his psychotic ideas. If as an additional advantage the psychotic ideas are abolished as well as being rendered less significant, so much the better. In practice a complete return of insight may in fact take place; and this gratifying outcome is by no means rare.

Nevertheless one cannot assume that the disordered thinking will be entirely abolished. When it has become likely that within the foreseeable future the patient will only reach this first level of improved adjustment, namely the ability to live contentedly and inoffensively, then the treatment must often be accepted as having achieved its object. The immense value of this limited achievement should never be underestimated by social workers or relatives. The extent to which treatment by phenothiazine or other medication, which sometimes needs to be continued in the community over a period of many years, can render a previously unmanageable patient readily containable in the community and acceptable in the domestic setting should never become obscured by any understandable but misconceived forebodings arising from memories of his state before treatment started.

For relatives to withhold their re-acceptance of the patient into the community on the anxious grounds that 'he's still got the same silly ideas and therefore isn't fit to come home' is commonly an unwarrantable attitude based on ignorance. In point of fact, when he has become able to conduct himself satisfactorily apart from expressing the 'silly ideas'—which in any case by that stage are usually expressed much less frequently and forcefully—more often than not it is quite reasonable and indeed proper that he should return to his family or other circumstances in the community, remaining under medical supervision, and take up the threads of his life, if necessary at a modified level.

For those cases deteriorating into a condition in which delusional ideas and hallucinatory experiences nevertheless come to exist within a seriously disabling state of fragmented thinking—especially if accompanied by aggressive attitudes or severe loss of constructive vitality—long-term institutional care rather than hospital care may be necessary and the possibility of hostel or other forms of community accommodation (chapter 12) may then be worth considering. But such cases are in the minority. The majority of sufferers return to live with their families. And within this context the community psychiatric nurse, discussed in the chapter that follows, is commonly a keystone in the system of support.

In the aggregate the psychoses we have discussed in this chapter form a comparatively common group of illnesses. And they remain amongst the major clinical scourges of mankind. Some of their sting has been removed by the various advances in treatment, which more recently have come to be combined with supervision conducted in the community setting. But while these clinical developments in the twentieth century have brought into practical possibility the humane principle that sufferers from psychosis should be spared the additional fate of prolonged or permanent incarceration in institutions, it will only be through the simultaneous provision of a widening range of resources within the community itself that this increased freedom will be suitably achieved and any potentially disturbing effects on the families and community satisfactorily nullified. In the next chapter, therefore, we shall include a survey of some of the further community services that can smooth away these problems.

To the extent that the concept of community care becomes underpinned with suitable supportive services, the outlook for the management of schizophrenia, already greatly improved by the clinical advances, will be still further enhanced. The need for such services should not be underestimated. A very significant proportion of homeless vagrants, devoid of accommodation and incapable of adequate self-care by day or night, have been found to consist of people disabled by this illness. In spite of the improved prognosis of schizophrenia in general, therefore, failures still occur; and they continue to need all the social and clinical efforts that can be mustered.

Some further resources in the community

To embrace principles embodied in theoretical concepts clearly is sometimes less difficult than to launch them into practice with hard cash. The sound administrator will naturally feel some hesitation in authorizing expenditure on early and un-tried schemes at the expense of withholding financial support from other areas of the administrative machine, however loud the exhortations to do so and however lofty the sources from which they emanate.

The Mental Health Act 1959 placed on local authority administrators the responsibility of supplying supportive services for community care. And the early stages of some of the resources that are now buttressing community psychiatry were in fact slow to come into being. Indeed in many of the present fields of need these resources continue to lag woefully behind the basic requirements. Nevertheless, during the 1960s progressive local authorities began to lay the practical founda-tions of the preventive psychiatry that had been implicit in the spirit of the Act.

When one surveys the field of these resources one soon finds that in practice no clear-cut classification exists. This lack of clarity is inevitable. Psychological needs are ubiquitous, and the points at which the needs of normality shade into those of abnormality are apt to be arbitrary in their manifestations. One loose classification of these widely varying resources may be attempted in terms of the administrative bodies responsible for their provision and organization. Another may be made in terms of the various clinical conditions they serve and by reference to some of the normal developmental processes whose very normality it is the function of preventive psychiatry to preserve.

In this chapter therefore we shall simply select at random a few of those resources for which the psychological indications are relatively tangible—facilities for improved social life, hostels for patients discharged from mental hospitals, group homes, the work of the community psychiatric nurse, day hospitals, day centres, domiciliary occupational therapy, industrial units and resources for the elderly.

NON-RESIDENTIAL ACTIVITIES

After a psychotic illness a patient may be left so disabled that not only will his working capacity be impaired but he will be unable to make his own way back into social circles without the most careful introduction. With his initiative lost, this patient will often be ineptly uninterested in the affairs of the community in which he formerly participated with success and enjoyment. Moreover the very anxieties he will feel about his changed state—if his illness has not altogether obliterated the insight and capacity for such feelings—may add their own fuel to this disinclination to participate. If he is then allowed to drift into a state of chronic withdrawal, he may easily pass into an irreversible inertia that restricts his life to a mere shadow of normal existence, setting it at an unwarrantably low level even in relation to the reduced potential produced by the illness itself.

How can the social worker in the community help to avert, or at least minimize, this personal disaster befalling a disabled patient discharged from hospital? How can she direct him along channels through which constructive social relationships can first be established and later made to fructify? Various possibilities are open to her, in consultation with the hospital staff. For instance, useful information about his social tendencies may be elicited from former friends whom with his permission she may approach on his behalf if he himself has lost the initiative to do so. At the same time she can take the opportunity of assessing their own suitability to relate helpfully to his changed mental state. If he agrees she can apprise them of his difficulties and needs, working out jointly with them a system of relationships that may be beneficial to him and acceptable to them. In other words she can smooth over the necessary path of his return to their acquaintance.

Another service she can supply is that of assessing his suitability for whatever range of social clubs for the normal population she finds existing within his area. She will need to familiarize herself with these clubs, talk—again with the patient's agreement—to the warden or leader, and if necessary introduce the patient in person. Because of his impaired capacity to make relationships on a general basis, it will often be preferable to put him in touch with a club having an emphasis on one or more specialized activity, that may have a specific appeal and form a definable common bond, rather than involving him in a club with little more than sitting, talking and dancing as its functions.

It is obvious that the married patient, despite all the difficulties of mutual adjustment to his family when he returns from hospital, often has a great advantage over his unmarried counterpart. Although casework may be needed with the family (chapter 3), frequently its success will be fluctuating. But unless the patient has been excluded from returning home, at least a family environment is present. The single person on the other hand, may have no family, or even no environment at all, to which to return.

Too often when an unmarried patient's initiative has been crippled by a psychotic process from which he has been able to make only partial recovery his welfare is tacitly regarded by his previous acquaintances and employers as being no concern of their own. It seems often to be vaguely assumed to be the responsibility of some nebulous form of officialdom, which though unspecified nevertheless exonerates the tax-paying citizen from any individual obligation. And while more often than not this assumption is likely to arise from a sense of powerlessness and anxiety rather than a callous loss of sympathy, its effects on the patient can be indistinguishable.

Either at the outset of his discharge from hospital, therefore, or after a subsequent period of help from the social worker on a one-to-one basis, such a patient often needs to be introduced not only to individual friendships but also to sources of collective acceptance. Her understanding of the various types of social clubs that exist in her area is an important part of the social worker's knowledge—whether the client be single or married.

The aim in the first instance will often be to provide an opportunity for participation in suitable communal activities which do not involve competitive results or place emphasis on any form of achievement in which his slowness or poverty of concentration might mar his performance and cause him embarrassment. However, placed in a suitable club setting which has a definite activity, he will usually experience less difficulty in adjusting than in an environment in which social relationships can be acquired only by unaided initiative. And if his confidence is overtaxed by even this simplified form of opportunity, it may still prove possible to coax him into gradual relationships through the minimal contact of attending an evening class, rather than a formal club, where a learning situation places him in human proximity that facilitates a more spontaneous approach through the shared interests and ambitions.

Another useful vehicle of communication and bridge to constructive relationships which makes use of a common denominator is the social club consisting exclusively of psychiatric patients, many of whom will themselves have previously been in hospital. These clubs similarly vary in the range of their orientation, spreading widely over a spectrum from the opportunity for patients to talk together, over coffee and bingo, to the facilities for organizing their own jumble sales and outings to theatres or producing their own dramatic works. In some of these clubs there may be group discussion, not necessarily based on formal group therapy but designed to concentrate on the everyday problems of being an ex-patient.

RESIDENTIAL CARE

In the light of her information on the patient's illness, its prognosis and the social situation surrounding it—which includes the degree of support to be anticipated from neighbours and workmates—the social worker may conclude that more is needed than casework combined with introduction to social activities. She can then usefully consider looking for any resources for residential care in her area that may assist the local community to reabsorb the patient. It must be remembered that residential care and community acceptance do not necessarily cancel each other out. Often they operate in unison, the community tolerating more easily those of its disabled members known to be subject to the safeguarding forms of supervision that residential care is seen to provide. Nor are they necessarily interchangeable alternatives. The local community may be prepared to help exclusively, but it may not be in the patient's best interests for it to do so.

The criterion for residential care is a client's inability to live in the community as a result of his psychiatric disability, even when supported by his family and any help available from the social services department or other bodies. The support of living constantly in a suitable group, in order to develop an interest in other people and therefore an improved quality of interest in themselves, will sometimes be a paramount need for this category of clients. The security of the group structure and the impetus to conform that are supplied by the demands of a residential group are provisions which the mental hospital social worker may already have considered for particular patients, especially for those with schizophrenic inertia.

HOSTELS

The indications for, and the possibility of obtaining the services of, a local authority hostel or, in suitable cases, a group home which is self-governing, should always be considered with great care. The patient, if he is to be suitably placed, must find himself amongst other residents with comparable difficulties. The environment must be one in which acceptance, respect, interaction and social reciprocity are generated by encouragement based on judicious restraint of criticism, praise and the maximum demands for routine work from each individual that lie within his limitations and that will benefit the group as a whole. The hope will be that a gradual increase in working and sociability may eventually lead to attendance at social events, first within the hostel itself and ultimately elsewhere.

The social worker will readily appreciate that if a hostel is too custodial in its orientation the system, however benevolent its intentions, will be likely to act against these principles. But even amongst those hostels where the outlook is predominantly non-custodial, i.e. where people are sheltered from full responsibility but are encouraged to be more independent, there will be variations in the amount of independence demanded.

Some ultimately aim at almost total independence; others accept that their patients may never go out to work but try to help them to take responsibility for the hostel as a self-governing group—for example, through carrying out cooking and cleaning and organizing outings and membership of local clubs—though with the warden taking the ultimate responsibility for decision-making. Some hostels largely confine their rehabilitation to these more homespun domestic functions; others, such as some Richmond Fellowship hostels, have as their object the fostering of emotional growth through relatively formal methods of group therapy which are designed to promote in the patient a more insightful awareness into his own attitudes and behaviour and into how these factors relate to other people. But even in the most therapeutically sophisticated environments some patients will inevitably ignore the effects of their group membership, while others will use it for self-understanding and an improvement of their ability to cope.

Hostels, then, vary in their forms of provision for what is therapeutically the most suitable ethos and regime, their systems of help being determined by the particular type of client they are concerned to serve. And while at one end of the scale there may be a regime that fosters the maximum of personal initiative and the most sophisticated forms of insight, and at the other end those hostels whose orientations are more strongly custodial, the philosophy of the latter is no less benevolent than is that of the more 'liberal' establishments. It is merely geared to the type of client in need of this particular system of approach.

The custodially-based hostels are in general run on lines in which comparatively little is left to the initiative of the individual and in which the principle of collective self-government that characterizes some of the other types of hostel is not demanded. Their residents are those who have suffered degrees of mental damage which are more seriously and unremittingly crippling, and of such a nature that little hope for restoration of independent initiative can be reasonably entertained. This group of residents includes many patients who would formerly have been consigned to permanent mental hospital care.

Whatever the nature of the mental disability, and therefore whatever the type of hostel to be sought, once the decision has been made that some form of residential management is required, then a certain amount of casework of appropriate depth and intensity will commonly need to be carried out with members of the family, either to persuade them to accept an immediate recommendation for transfer to the hostel or to render the prospect of any separation sufficiently palatable to form the foundation for their eventual agreement. When the relatives' resistance is too great, postponement without pressure may be needed, perhaps for several years. Otherwise the tension within a family whose members have prematurely acquiesced against their current inclinations can develop into a prolonged or even permanent anxiety or resentment so strong that it acts against the client's own happiness and adjustment, outweighing the advantage which his eventual transfer to the hostel would otherwise bring.

Initial reactions are not necessarily reliable. Parents may rightly ask for an adult psychotic son or daughter to be placed in a hostel, only to withdraw their request if it is acted on, raising strong and sometimes specious arguments in support. The very reasons initially put forward for removal—lack of confidence, for instance—may now be presented as grounds for retaining the patient within the home. Reasons that are indisputably realistic may be advanced. But they may also be complicated by emotions of overpossessiveness, understandable but undesirable, as a result of which the parent or spouse, while having the patient's best interest at heart, still clings desperately to the patient, torn between the desire to be relieved of the burden he imposes on the family and the personal need to maintain the continuity of the relationship in undivided form. At other times these conflicting emotions within the relatives may introduce uncertainties in their minds about the soundness of the advice being proferred.

The family psychodynamics will therefore always need to be looked at carefully from the outset. Another trap into which the inexperienced social worker may fall is the fact that sometimes a hostel placement may on the contrary seem to offer a comparatively easy solution, particularly if it is the one most rapidly obtainable. But the recommendation, however well founded, should not be pressed until the family psychodynamics have been brought to the propitious stage. Otherwise, as we have seen, the situation will be apt to break down. Even in those cases in which the aim has been to secure only a temporary hostel placement, with a view to the client returning to the family after a limited period there, if action has been precipitately taken before the emotional difficulties of the relatives have been adequately resolved they may unwittingly encourage him in overreacting to the sense of dissatisfaction with which many residents will inevitably respond from time to time. And anxious relatives, with their conflicts still insufficiently resolved by casework designed to support them in their sense of loss, and disencumber them of the sense of guilt to which they are so prone, may then feel themselves justified in demanding his return home on a basis which they view as a dutiful intercession on his behalf. Such a premature return may well prove deleterious to his recovery.

A great deal of prior discussion may be needed with the client also, if his best cooperation is to be obtained. He may well need to visit and comment on a number of hostels before his long-term interests can be clarified to him to his best advantage. Excessive or precipitate persuasion, perhaps adopted under the pressure of his illness or his family's need for relief, may produce only a partial and poorly sustained solution, leading him either to accept a hostel on a basis that proves merely transitory or to agree to one where his initial reluctance, having received too little understanding and concession at the outset, will remain an unresolved irritant, robbing him of his capacity for optimal adaptation there and the opportunity of the life of greater fulfilment that would otherwise have been within his power.

GROUP HOMES

There is a category of patients who are so mentally disabled that they need more support than is forthcoming in the family setting, but nevertheless do not need an environment as structured as that of a hostel. In the absence of a group home the only alternative available for this disabled but relatively well-preserved group may be consignment to a bedsitting room—an existence embodying a precarious and psychologically unhealthy situation all too apt to smoulder unhappily or fulminate into frank breakdown, with disturbing effects on the environment and a reinforcement of the patient's sense of insecurity.

For clients in this category a group home may provide the only source of psychological salvation. These homes receive their clients from mental hospitals or psychiatric hostels. Their nature varies, but they rest on common principles. In contrast to the psychiatric hostels, where residential staff are employed, the group homes have no residential staff. Usually they contain between four and eight residents, this number not only being the most satisfactory in terms of material practicalities but also the one most in accord with the principles of group psychodynamics. An ordinary house in the community is used, which provides both single and double bedrooms and shared living rooms, kitchen and bathroom. Frequently a social worker is attached for regular visits.

Amongst the most important principles of group homes is the concept that each client must be capable of using social relationships to the therapeutic advantage of himself and the other residents. In the place of those group pressures which in the past have contributed to his maladaptive behaviour, the group home now brings its own remedial group influences as a form of resocialization, the constant proximity of those with shared difficulties supplying a continuously supportive—if intermittently traumatic—framework for readjustment. Some form of group support, ordinarily available as a family unit, is a basic human need. The group home constitutes a substitute situation for psychologically disabled people who are deprived of such support by separation, divorce, death or lack of accommodation—or who cannot avail themselves of ordinary relationships. The need for self-organization is catered for in that no resident staff are present to direct the clients, although a social worker may be on call for emergency problems in addition to the regular visits. Also, a committee member is available for such functions as payment of electricity bills and rent, the rent sometimes being underwritten by voluntary organizations who also redecorate and furnish when necessary.

While for the majority of residents the group home becomes their permanent abode, some may acquire sufficient independence to resume life in the community as a result of a spontaneous improvement of the illness, a useful response to the therapeutic ethos of the home itself, or the improvement of unsatisfactory social circumstances through rehousing, re-employment, or reunion of broken relationships. On the other hand relapse too may occur while the client is in the home, necessitating readmission to hospital, where treatment may often restore him to a state that allows him to return once again to the home. Whether residents remain permanently in the home or return eventually to life in the full community, the group home's overall aim is to supply a link in the chain of rehabilitation that leads patients away from the relatively restricted environment of the mental hospital or psychiatric hostel.

Skill in the initial selection of residents, and care with any subsequent additions, are of great importance. These functions are commonly carried out by a committee. The social worker and medical personnel supply the professional data about the proposed residents, and general discussion is then undertaken to achieve the most suitable balance of illnesses, temperaments and intelligence. In respect of each of these attributes there may be a wide scatter amongst individuals within any one home. And the homes themselves also vary in the criteria they adopt and the life-style they favour.

Assessment includes evaluation of the client's basic attributes, attempts to predict the form of any relapse in relation to possible antisocial conduct, such as violence or severely alcoholic behaviour, and the development of any less dramatic conditions that might lead to prolonged opting out of group relationships. Schizophrenic inertia is an outstanding example of the latter.

Within the established common pattern that clients must be able to use the social relationships provided, the concept of group homes is still an experimental and growing area, with room for changes and adaptations as experience accumulates. But it is already firmly established that they embrace a broad spectrum, ranging from those group homes in the community which house ex-mental hospital patients to those designed for clients with the milder psychiatric problems that have never necessitated hospital admissions or even day hospital attendances.

THE PSYCHIATRIC NURSE IN THE COMMUNITY

Among the most important of the developments in the second half of the present century for the management of psychotic illness within the community has been the birth of psychiatric nursing care conducted outside mental hospitals by specially selected nurses who are mental hospital trained and of senior standing and experience.

The system involves the provision of these nurses as an after-care service to schizophrenic people living at home, often alone, many of whom would otherwise need to remain in hospital permanently. By now it is a pattern of management, highly organized in some areas, through which these psychotic people are frequently enabled to live within their families, often contentedly and even with an ability to function successfully as the mother bringing up the children or the father maintaining the role of family bread-winner.

It is unnecessary to re-enunciate the basic attitudes on which community care rests. Naturally they apply as much to the nursing care service as to any other form of professional work on behalf of psychotic people in the community. But whereas the efforts of those working in the social services departments are primarily concerned with the alleviation of social problems or the resolution of inter-personal difficulties arising from factors that are often of a comparatively non-medical character, by contrast the work of those engaged in community psychiatric nursing is predominantly related to their medically-based background in the mental hospital. The community nurse's work is concerned essentially with the clinical manifestations of psychiatric illnesses, with their management in the community—usually by giving injections every two or three weeks and ensuring that any associated tablets are taken as prescribed—and with observation of the patient's progress and notification of it to the doctor in the event of need.

RELATIONSHIP WITH THE SOCIAL WORKER

The drawing of this broad distinction between the role of the social worker and that of the community psychiatric nurse also highlights the essentially complementary nature of these two branches of service. Although she is one of the central pivots on which the clinical welfare of the discharged patient turns, the community nurse herself also stands to gain a great deal of valuable insight into many types of problem whose solution in the main lies outside her own sphere but within that of the social worker. Social workers, on the other hand, can learn from the nurse much that is of value to them about the impact of these illnesses on their clients.

There are many different combinations of schizophrenic symptoms. The clearer and the more specific the information about the individual's illness that is passed by the nurse to the social worker, the better the social worker will understand the problems generated in her particular client. And the more closely integrated the joint understanding about the psychological reactions within the family achieved by the nurse and the social worker, the greater will be the individual contributions to be made by each.

One of the effects of intensive experience with psychotic patients, such as that acquired by the community nursing sister, is that it promotes the ability to translate a knowledge of the general into the particular—to relate more expertly and effectively the concepts of general theory to the details of particular cases. The nurse's liaison functions with the social worker therefore lie to a large extent in communicating to her any useful knowledge that she may have acquired about those symptoms in the particular individual that are most likely to occur in the event of his relapse. Since the social worker's knowledge of schizophrenia in the abstract is no substitute for a more specific familiarity with the clinical tendencies of the given individual, it follows that any system of working that procures cooperation—rather than leaving unchanged the comparative isolation of functioning so often found among people of different professional backgrounds—must be a force for benefit to the client.

The value of the social worker's liaison with the community nurse can be exemplified by the case of a recently widowed woman discharged from hospital partially disabled by schizophrenia, with children dependent on her for domestic and sometimes financial support and already known to the social worker before her illness—this social worker perhaps having been successful in assisting her with the claiming of social benefits and the organization of services for help in the home. As a result of lack of insight into her illness such a patient may begin to express to the social worker a developing reluctance to continue to attend the outpatient clinic for the maintenance injection treatment prescribed for her as a long-term measure when in hospital. Moreover she may become equally prevented by the illness from continuing to cooperate with the social worker over obtaining the financial help necessitated by her bereavement.

This reluctance for cooperation may have arisen as a result of an insidious, and perhaps unrecognized, spontaneous exacerbation of the psychotic progress, which required a prompt review of the situation in the light of a possible need to increase the dose or frequency of the injections as an urgent measure to avert further deterioration. Alternatively, at that particular point the reluctance to continue to cooperate may not have signified true relapse into illness, but merely a distaste for the inconvenience of travelling or an ordinary human hankering after self-sufficiency. But the very fact of discontinuing one or two injections often in itself leads to a recrudescence of the illness, and this recrudescence then brings its own loss of initiative or renewed upsurge of paranoid turbulence, either of which states will further deprive the patient of his already diminishing capacity to cooperate. When once this vicious circle has come into operation it usually continues, and more often than not gathers increasing force.

This concatenation of events is a fairly common precursor of avoidable readmission. But if the social worker already has a close and perhaps longstanding relationship with a wavering client, she may succeed in persuading him to continue or resume his treatment before further relapse erodes the possibility of his cooperating with anyone at all—or at least she may succeed in obtaining his agreement for her to pass the necessary information about his feelings of reluctance to the community nurse. The nurse may then be put in a position to use her additional influence in persuading him to accept treatment or to agree to an appointment for psychiatric review, where still further attempts may be made by the psychiatrist. Without these cumulative stages of persuasion, initiated by the social worker, the slow but insidious deterioration may progress to an end-point of blatant unmanageability requiring readmission to hospital where treatment may not by then be as quickly, or indeed as qualitatively, effective as would have been possible at an earlier stage.

The majority of psychotic people discharged from hospital in need of routine injections are observed by the community nurse in outpatient clinics when attending for their injections, either at a general or mental hospital. But one of her other main functions—that of visiting the patient's home—will sometimes be of greater advantage than the assessments she makes on an outpatient basis. These home visits, during which again she can both give the injections and observe the clinical progress, provide her with a ready-made opportunity of evaluating at close quarters the nature and influence of the home circumstances. Practical difficulties requiring specific measures for the information of the social worker, such as the need for assistance with finance or guidance about re-employment, together with many of the inter-personal problems in need of psychological help, may be seen far more clearly within the natural and everyday context of the home setting. But whether the nursing sister deals with the patient at an out-patient department or within the home, her predominant function is to administer the drugs prescribed for the control of the psychotic process, observe their effects on the patient's mental state, and assess the severity of any phsyical side-effects that may ensue.

EARLY INVOLVEMENT

How in terms of her daily routine does she carry out these functions? When once the patient has been launched back into the community she tries to see him at regular intervals, using her knowledge of the manifestations and treatment of schizo-phrenia already described. But her starting point, always in theory and as frequently as possible in practice, should be made at an earlier stage—within the mental hospital or in the psychiatric ward of the general hospital. It is very desirable for her to have had her first contact with her patient while he was ill in hospital, and to have discussed his illness and his home and occupational problems with the hospital staff.

The patient on the point of discharge is often apprehensive and uncertain about the arrangements to which he should conform after returning home if he is to maintain his improve-ment. He and his relatives will need to be informed in reassur-ing detail about the regime of management that will lie ahead when the direct support of the hospital has been severed or heavily reduced. For a patient to have the opportunity of making the acquaintance while still in hospital of the nursing sister by whom much of his treatment will be supervised after his discharge is therefore an important aspect, which should be included within the system whenever practicable.

If he is destined to require readmission at a later date, he will then be in a position to realize that the community nurse is herself part of the hospital team. And in the meanwhile he may be enabled to draw a sense of security from the knowledge that in the event of readmission she will once again act as a link with his familiar circumstances, even perhaps ensuring his reacceptance into his family circle after any subsequent admissions—sometimes a matter of disturbing doubt to him otherwise. The prospect that her continued understanding and supportive relationship may again be available to him during the difficult periods of early readjustment after any future discharges—and that these services may also lead to a prompt recognition and removal of any discomforts arising from changes in the dose of his medication over the course of time —can all combine to encourage him to leave hospital at the crucial stage when his vacillation might otherwise result in retreat from discharge; which might then lead to an over-dependence on hospital protection and occasionally even to ultimate institutionalization.

Another advantage in dual involvement in both the patient's hospital period and his follow-up management is the opportunity it can afford for comparative assessments along the course of his progress. Having seen the patient during the final stage of his illness in hospital, rather than merely meeting him for the first time when he may perhaps be largely free from symptoms after his discharge, the community nurse will be forearmed with a correspondingly clearer knowledge for detection of any changes that may herald a second attack—or, as they are termed in medical nomenclature, the prodromal manifestations. But whatever the previous circumstances the community nurse, because of her highly specialized clinical expertise, is in an exceptionally good position for recognizing the need for, and taking the necessary action to obtain, an earlier referral for any resumption of professional help that might otherwise be adopted too belatedly.

The value of early referral so that the patient's clinical condition can receive attention in its incipient stages carries two main advantages. Firstly, prompt action may entirely bypass the need for hospital admission—which might otherwise be eventually required later with great urgency because of an attack of acute schizophrenic excitability or a suicidal episode —with its dislocation of the family pattern, production of separation anxieties, and embarrassment caused to the client's children amongst their friends. Secondly, it may forestall a relapse into the type of subacute psychotic state which continues to smoulder for a prolonged or indefinite period at home at a level of intensity that does not quite reach one appropriate for hospital admission, but nevertheless renders the patient withdrawn, odd, emotionally cold, unreasonable, and prone to macabre delusional statement or hallucinatory experience. The crippling effects or this situation too on young children need no emphasis, nor the potential value to them that arises from successful efforts to forestall a parent's relapse into chronicity within the community.

THE SOCIAL WORKER'S SUPPORT

However skilful the clinical management in the community carried out for a psychotic patient by the general practitioner, psychiatrist or community nurse, there are many cases in which the community social worker's participation can be invaluable. The knowledge of the main psychiatric illnesses and their treatment outlined earlier is very important for the social worker. But it is not enough merely to know the course of the patient's illness. For long-term support it is important in addition to be able to predict as far as possible the constant or intermittent reactions of the various members of the family. This part of her assessment will call for a theoretical knowledge of the sort of defence mechanisms discussed in chapter 8. Practical experience will be required to enable her to perceive their occurrence and to understand their influence on the interplay of emotions arising between the particular patient and the members of the family concerned.

At the beginning she will need to discover whether the patient has a mental illness in need of formal psychiatric treatment, or whether alternatively his psychological management and that of his family can safely be allowed to rest exclusively in the sphere of casework. And it should never be forgotten that even if her client's condition is one in whose treatment she herself may have little primary part to play, such as perhaps an attack of mania necessitating a period of treatment in hospital, casework may still be needed with the family to help them to understand and adjust to the illness.

We are now in a position to take somewhat more detailed stock of the social worker's function of helping a family containing a schizophrenic patient discharged from hospital. Having armed herself with a knowledge of the likely course of the illness—let us suppose that it carries a probable future of continuously smouldering disablement possibly punctuated by recurrent exacerbations, or perhaps phases of temporary improvement—and having thought clearly about the significance of any social factors that may need remedy or which, as spurious 'causes' with little true bearing on the clinical essence of the illness, do not in fact justify any steps to change them, she should then turn her attention to the detailed practical planning to be carried out for the family's long-term future.

Practical support for the family

For the general planning she proceeds on the basis of two categories of function. She assesses the family's practical difficulties; and she assesses their psychological attributes, needs and the accessibility of its members to psychological support. To give a simple example of the former, if the history is one from which it is to be anticipated that the patient will play records during the night, then social factors such as the size of the house and the area in which it is situated—isolated or populated, tolerant or critical—will clearly be significant. The presence or absence of children and the particular stages and features of their emotional development in relation to the patient's symptoms—these being factors liable to indicate the importance or otherwise of periods of removal of the children from home to day nurseries or to relatives, or to holiday homes during the school holidays—are amongst those that come into this category. The social worker may have a vital role in recognizing the value of the whole range of diversionary social measures and supportive facilities for the client, taking an active part in persuading the relatives about the importance of these needs and implementing them when they have been discussed.

Decisions relating to many practical services to the family will rest on this combination of knowledge of available facilities and an understanding of the nature of the illness and its anticipated course. If the patient is a disabled man, the social worker may usefully try to discover whether he is likely at any time to become well enough to return to work; and if so she may usefully attempt to ascertain the general level of any earning capacity that can be reasonably anticipated.

Effective cooperation with the disablement resettlement officer may hinge on these efforts; and to obtain the best results from this source of expertise, enquiries about the potential value of vocational testing may be worth putting to those responsible for the overall psychiatric assessment. If it is a woman who is afflicted, the amount of initiative she will retain for her domestic functions, both material and psychological, and how far her domestic decisions will be reliable, are matters that may also need elucidation if possible, followed by careful thought and practical planning in the light of both short-term and long-term considerations.

Psychological support for the family

Whatever the concrete steps for the client's material welfare that occupy the social worker's energies, the need for attention to his psychological problems and those of the family must remain continuously in the forefront of her awareness.

Commonly this task demands prolonged and sustained effort. In the face of continuing distress or dissatisfaction in the relatives, the social worker may need to maintain a steadfast determination to resist any demoralizing effects on herself which these reactions can produce. To succeed in clarifying a complex situation, fitting the initially obscure elements of a perplexing predicament into a meaningful whole, may bring the satisfaction of a conundrum well solved. Moreover, to find any efforts at persuading reluctant relatives being crowned with success—for example in relation to their retaining or relinquishing a psychotic patient in accordance with the best interests of all concerned—can also bring a justifiable sense of purpose and achievement in the work. Equally, to secure on behalf of a stricken family any necessary financial advantages, or the services of one or more of the other caring professions, thus perhaps safeguarding the development of children or ensuring an improved adjustment in elderly relatives, may afford deep satisfaction.

By contrast with these satisfactions, attempts at long-term supportive work of a psychological kind may sometimes appear discouragingly slow or even entirely fruitless. Nevertheless in spite of its seeming lack of concrete results this service frequently ranks as highly in importance and ultimate effectiveness as any which a social worker provides; and it is all the more worthwhile because of the very difficulties it continuously presents and the great importance of maintaining a level of family cohesion—albeit one sometimes far below the ideal—rather than allowing mounting anxiety and discouragement to lead to either a subtle or an open breakdown of the family as a coping unit.

It is vitally important from the outset for the family to feel unreservedly supported. There is a particular stage at which this assurance needs to be conveyed with special initiative, namely during the phase when the patient's discharge from hospital is found to be approaching. A panic reaction amongst the relatives, involving the fear that they will now be permanently 'landed' with the patient and, at times, including the fear of physical violence, may evoke in them a vista of unending burdens and lead them to reject the patient even to the point of unwittingly overstating his symptoms, very occasionally almost deliberately provoking his relapse in an anxious attempt to ensure his removal again from the home. Once embarked on, these attitudes of mind have a tendency to become self-consolidating. And they may develop to proportions that are either totally resistant to efforts at reversal or can only be dispelled with great difficulty. Moreover although the patient may not be rejected on his return from hospital, he may well sense anxieties and undergo a further reaction of symptom-formation that can give apparent credibility to some of the more disturbing and even bizarre fantasies already held by the relatives.

These are situations in which early prevention by realistic explanations is better than attempts at cure. In this important work of forestalling potential family rejection, the social worker may find herself placed in an invidious position between the hospital and the family. Anxious relatives looking for directions into which to channel their turbulent emotions, which may understandably possess a frustrated need for concrete action, are sometimes prone to resent the hospital for discharging the patient 'only half cured', their anxieties impelling them to regard this act as indicative of indifference, incompetence or negligence on the part of the hospital.

If the social worker then visits the hospital and sees, for example, some form of undesirable incident, such as one patient causing distress to another, she may become perplexed and alarmed about the role of her own involvement. Indeed if she walks on to a ward and is unable to see the ward sister she may overreact and spoil a relationship that would otherwise prove very helpful to everyone concerned. But these occasional reactions will be less prone to occur if she realizes more clearly that the hospital staff themselves have strong regrets about all the limitations—feelings that are essentially comparable with her own. She will then appreciate that here is an area that gives practical illustration to the adage that half-truths unrecognized as such can readily mislead. However well meant and sympathetic her collusion with the family's incorrect reactions, it will seldom lead to any real improvement in the situation.

How then should she present to the relatives, in the light of her understanding derived from the data outlined, a useful and reliable explanation of the role of the hospital? Firstly, while not neglecting to convey that their reactions are understandable and indeed commendable in the context of their determination that the needs of the family as a whole should be served, she can indicate that they spring from lack of experience of the nature of chronic schizophrenic illness, whose effects are often regarded as incomparably more devastating than is nowadays frequently the case.

The vestigial influence of ancient folklore lies close to the surface in many relatives. Unjustified fears of sexual assault, of violent behaviour, or even of macabre and bizarre murders will sometimes remain unexpressed outwardly and indeed only loosely formulated internally. They may well constitute an unspoken state of distress that will escape the social worker's notice if it occurs in individuals who in other respects are calm, intelligent and sophisticated. When fears of this sort are deeply ingrained it is hardly surprising that they give rise to unfortunate suspicions that the patient's discharge from hospital has arisen from a callous indifference.

By first removing some of this widespread ignorance and fantasy surrounding chronic psychotic illness, the social worker can often succeed in eliminating the destructive misunderstandings that have existed about the hospital's role. She can then proceed to supplement these efforts by drawing attention to a particular facet of mental illness. It is an aspect that has sometimes been appreciated in general terms. But for its importance to be fully grasped it often needs to be emphasized specifically. This problem is the grave propensity to become 'institutionalized' that affects many patients in hospital.

'Institutional neurosis' is a very real entity. It can erode self-confidence and even increase the existing disability to a point that renders discharge from hospital impossible. For these reasons good hospitals are reluctant in the interests of their patients to retain them longer than necessary. In stressing this point to relatives, the social worker can make clear to them that what may perhaps have seemed a premature discharge from hospital may in fact have been far preferable to the psychological side-effects that could have resulted from more prolonged admission. A clearer knowledge of these considerations by relatives can soften their anxieties when they have previously assumed that their own difficulties were bypassed by the hospital. They should be helped to realize that the staff understands and sympathizes with their feelings, and that if it transpires that well-founded anxieties exist the hospital is usually able to consider reasonable steps for 'compromise', such as prolonged leave-periods before final discharge or perhaps the delaying of discharge while the social circumstances are receiving any further attention that may be thought desirable and practicable. Furthermore, in suitable cases all possible efforts will be made to readmit the patient promptly at times of crisis, if indicated, or if unmanageable deterioration appears about to occur.

Having helped with any such criticisms or misunderstandings about the role of the hospital—though they are the exception rather than the rule—the social worker may need to remove other areas of ignorance. Families of schizophrenic patients discharged home from hospital may find themselves ignorant of the effects of the illness partly because, like many families of mentally subnormal people also, they were too overwhelmed when the information was presented to them to grasp it clearly. And even if they succeeded in doing so, they frequently consider, correctly, that insufficient ongoing advice is available.

Much of this advice can be supplied if a community social worker is available. In the first place, families may have failed to realize that the condition is widely believed amongst clinical psychiatrists to be essentially a physical illness, in spite of the present lack of understanding of the physical details, and that when maintenance medication is required the situation is broadly analogous to the need for insulin by diabetic people— whose disabilities, as in schizophrenia, require chemical measures to combat the physical factors that lie behind the symptoms. Similarly, even in the group of schizophrenic people left with residual defects for which maintenance treatment is of no benefit and therefore is not prescribed, the responsibility is equally to be laid at the door of an unfortunate physical development. Through this realization, which can be understandingly conveyed by a good social worker, all concerned may be spared both self-accusation and the blaming of others.

One means by which ignorance can sometimes be removed is through free communication with families who themselves have, or have had, a schizophrenic relative. Apart from their psychologically supportive value these families will often have had experience from which considerable practical advantages can be drawn. Such intra-family communications should not of course be forced, but they may be usefully encouraged.

Certain symptoms are particularly apt to lead to unnecessary difficulties if misunderstood. Amongst the most important are the physical inertia, the poor concentration, the solitary behaviour, the indifference to relationships which may have its effects both on members of the family and also on the family's friends and neighbours, and the diminished sexual interests.

Each may usefully be considered in turn. Mental inertia can lead the sufferer to abrogate so much responsibility, which then devolves on other members of the family, that with the passage of time their initial sympathy and understanding may become gradually replaced by resentment and eventual loss of insight into the still pathological nature of his mental inactivity. What is at first seen in its true light may ultimately become regarded as an exploitation—a contrived technique of using the illness for opting out. The social worker may help to prevent this fallacious change of belief.

The schizophrenic client's diminished concentration can also be a source of misunderstanding, usually because although recognized as a symptom its degree is often not fully appreciated by the family. It may in fact be such a strain on him as to be almost exhausting, and he may retire to bed in consequence. Abortive attempts to sustain concentration may have been made by a client with laborious though invisible efforts; but when their lack of success results in behaviour unpalatable to the relative—for instance walking away aimlessly when sharing the companionship of reading or watching a simple television programme whose threads he cannot in fact retain—then the relative may feel aggrieved and perhaps inclined to react by retaliatory withdrawal.

The physical inertia is sometimes equally misunderstood. In its extreme it may take the form of remaining in bed throughout the day rather than attending to the lightest of tasks clearly within his physical strength. This situation too can easily be misconstrued as wilful exploitation of his psychiatric history. In actuality the lack of drive arises from the effect of the illness on motivation, the powers of motivation being more impaired than are some of the processes of thinking. This motivational loss, however, is equally pathological and can be even more crippling.

Ill-understood indifference to relationships may not only be hurtful within the family but embarrassing amongst neighbours. It may lead to loss of friendly communication between individuals and even between families. Suitable enlightenment can prevent estrangement within the family. And frank explanations to friends and other families that his offhand manner is due to a blunting of his emotions by the illness can remove more widespread reactions of offence. The afflicted family may require some encouragement to approach other families for purposes of explanation, and occasionally may need to be assisted by the social worker's direct action on their behalf. However, considerable restraint is clearly required in pressing this suggestion in the face of a family's reluctance. The social worker's role is primarily to enlighten the family and open up possibilities of readier discussion rather than take executive action.

Distress about a schizophrenic person's decline of sexual interest is sometimes expressed by the marital partner. Once again a component of misunderstanding may be present. It may not have been fully realized that loss of sexual inclination may not only form part of the emotional and physical deficits of the illness itself. It can also be a side-effect of medication. When the illness is seen to have improved in general while a corresponding return of sexual interest has failed to materialize, the marital partner may wrongly conclude that personal loss of affection has occurred.

These considerations apply to particular symptoms. But sometimes it may be necessary for the social worker to give help of a sort that relates to the basic psychodynamics within the family rather than to misunderstandings of the symptoms themselves. This aspect requires more circumspection.

Overprotectiveness, with its limitations on the return of the patient's self-confidence and capacities, can easily arise through a misplaced solicitude by the relative, which takes the form of a kind of unhealthy collusion with him over the features of the illness. Such relatives are apt to catch too readily on to the diagnostic label. In other cases, particularly when emotional deprivations exist in other areas of a relative's life, over-possessiveness may develop and bring its own undermining effects. Where significant feelings of hostility were already present, attitudes of denigration may become adopted, reducing the patient's confidence in his ability to distinguish reality from unreality. The normality of even those areas of his thought processes which previously were unaffected may then be at risk of erosion.

It sometimes happens that the presence of a schizophrenic person in a family causes or catalyses a split between the families of the two partners, the patient's relatives blaming the partner or vice versa. In these circumstances an explanation to the relevant people about this seemingly physical nature of the illness may go far towards reversing the hostility, providing all concerned with an area for common sympathy.

Naturally the children also can experience disturbing emotions. These children may find themselves caught in a whirlpool of guilt, a sense of almost clinical responsibility which it is beyond their emotional or intellectual development to meet, and reactions of resentment towards a schizophrenic parent's appearance of sulkiness or the embarrassment he causes in relation to their peer group. Like the adults, they too may stand in desperate need of talking through their feelings. On occasions, therefore, the social worker may usefully ask her schizophrenic clients if they would like her to talk to their children who refuse to approach them or do so in a disturbing manner. It should always be remembered that it is the schizophrenic person, and not merely the family, who is the client; that he himself should be consulted; and that he, like the other relatives, stands to benefit from the family help as a whole. But it will sometimes be found that these children's defence mechanisms, or their imitative responses giving rise to secondary problems, even point to the need for attendance at a child guidance clinic to restore and bolster their waning security.

Finally, while alleviating guilt by emphasizing the essentially physical nature of the illness, the social worker should keep in mind that social stresses themselves may cause relapse. The social interactions involved in going to a party, for example, may constitute an intolerable stress to some clients; or struggling with unsuitable work may militate heavily against recovery. Steps are commonly required to reduce general social stresses as well as those which can arise from family misunderstandings.

THE DAY HOSPITAL

A psychiatric day hospital offers an opportunity to treat a wide range of patients within the community in a manner which is unique. Sometimes it is sited away from the main hospital, carrying the advantages of being in the community; in other instances it forms part of the complex of a general hospital. As far as possible day hospitals are placed in situations accessible by public transport and within easy reach of a town or shopping areas.

A day hospital may be used in various ways. It can act as a bridge between in-patient care and discharge home, the patient first attending during the day for a week or two while continuing to sleep at the hospital and perhaps going home for weekends. In this way he can come to know his fellow patients, the staff and the day hospital routine in readiness for his discharge. Secondly, it is used as a means of continuing treatment for the discharged patient while he is living at home, thus helping to avert readmission and the deleterious effects of removal from family life. This pattern of support is particularly helpful for mothers of families, though other patients too are often enabled to carry on with their jobs if they can take the time away from work to attend the day hospital for regular sessions, sometimes only for one day per week.

A third group of patients also appears in a day hospital, namely those whose general practitioners consider them to be in need of some form of communal psychiatric help but who are not ill enough for admission. These are often patients who before the advent of day hospitals would only have been seen at out-patient clinics, or possibly treated solely by the general practitioner.

The overall aims of a day hospital are to help preserve the identity and individuality of the patients and enable them to return with as full an independence as possible to their normal everyday living. These functions embody various forms of psychological treatment, sometimes in conjunction with physical treatments by drugs or E.C.T., and an assessment of the effects.

A relatively informal atmosphere is aimed at. But a well-balanced and realistic programme is essential. The activities comprise projective techniques, projects, pottery, art, music, drama (chapter 7), 'socials', informal outings, gardening, quizzes, records, table games, relaxation exercises, dressmaking, cooking, shopping and group therapy, that can vary from analytically orientated groups to supportive meetings and simple discussion groups. Some patients attend only for the group sessions.

Groups may include mothers' groups (most mothers needing psychiatric treatment have difficulty in coping with their children), young people's groups, and so on. Marital therapy for family problems may also be carried out there. Often the ideal criterion for group membership is not merely an ability to verbalize, but some ability or potential ability to comprehend, and sometimes also to verbalize, the feelings experienced in relationships. A suitable balance of participants needs to be achieved. Details of the various forms of activity provided, and the conditions treated, will not be entered into here. But of the many conditions helped in day hospitals agoraphobia is worth special mention since it is a condition in which a previously intractable resistance may be particularly open to treatment within this setting. Both group therapy and behaviour therapy, which in a comparatively crude form constitutes graduating periods outside the hospital, e.g. walking to the corner, then to the shops, then to catch the bus, may be of great help with this condition if suitably persisted in. To progress to the local shops, and thence into the town, into bigger shops and even into supermarkets—with the patient accompanied in the initial stages by the therapist—may eventually lead even to complete independence after the 'weaning away' period.

All the patients are encouraged to look outwards from a day hospital. An important step back to a full and satisfying life in the community may sometimes be achieved through the medium of voluntary work, arranged by the voluntary services liaison officer, through the social services department, or through joint efforts between these two fields. A group of patients may undertake projects for the local community, such as gardening, decorating, visiting, or shopping for people unable to manage for themselves. The voluntary services liaison officer may also help the day hospital by arranging visits by speakers on various topics which stimulate new interests and the finding of new hobbies and relationships.

Essentially a day hospital functions through a multi-disciplinary approach, with medical, nursing, psychologist, occupational therapy and social worker staff all participating in the care of the patients. All staff members have their own specific contributions to make, both by training and individual personalities. A patient may sometimes relate best to, and thus gain most from, even the most junior members of the team.

THE DAY CENTRE

Whereas ideally the day hospital should provide diagnostic and treatment facilities comparable with many of those in the mental hospital, by contrast the day centre supplies a simple supportive role, with much less medical and related forms of supervision than exist within the hospitals. Indeed, in some day centres no medical involvement is considered necessary.

Some are designed to provide long-term care in a sheltered environment for patients who are unemployable; others supply short-term care, bridging the gap either between mental hospital and full return to the community (with or without support in the latter from various paramedical professions) or between the day hospital and the community. While attendance at a day centre may reflect the need for a relatively long stay or even help for a chronic disability, in some circumstances it may represent progress in that no medical cover is required.

Although it often has little or no medical cover the day centre's function is nevertheless a positive one, designed to provide a social atmosphere, occupation, and work therapy. The various working activities contain comparatively conventional and straightforward concepts of the need for social relationships, providing work facilities generating ordinary bonhomie for those in whom isolation would otherwise be gravely deleterious.

But valuable elements of more tangibly practical utility also enter into the system—for instance kitchen activities contained in an 'activities of daily living unit' such as cooking, together with the most basic activities of dressing and looking after toilet needs, may all be included. However, the day centre's concern with the broad socializing objective, rather than the deeper and specialized treatments, constitutes the essential difference in ethos and aim between the day centre and the hospitals, whether day or residential.

The numbers attending range from fifteen to a hundred, and the types of client vary from the physically handicapped and mentally subnormal to those with a history of mental illnesses which have left them incapable of self-support. The occupational therapy carried out with these patients is of a supervisory rather than executive nature, since even though the socialization and work have their therapeutic value it is the support and shelter offered by the centre which constitutes its main *raison d'être*. And while the occupational therapist's overseeing of the patients' daily working patterns may be a pivot of the day centre, the detailed daily implementation of much of the activities is carried out by technicians skilled in special work such as carpentry, paid 'helpers' and voluntary workers.

DOMICILIARY OCCUPATIONAL THERAPY

Occupational therapy (chapter 7) for those living in the community may be carried out on a purely domiciliary basis, in a day hospital, or a day centre. But in each of these situations its psychiatric function relates both to diagnosis and treatment. The activities prescribed for patients in the community will vary according to whether or not they remain entirely at home. If they attend a day hospital or day centre they will be involved there with any of the activities already mentioned under these headings; if they work entirely at home they may be given activities such as cooking, sewing, or light assembly work made available within the home by the occupational therapist.

Nevertheless the role of the occupational therapist with the client who is living at home or in a hostel is, like that in the hospitals, wider in its scope than simply providing him with activities to be carried out. The bulk of her work is in fact concerned with assessment and follow-up. Her contribution to this diagnostic process rests not only on her direct assessment of the client's presentation in the home setting, but also on her enquiries about a whole spectrum of factors from other sources. These enquiries may need to elucidate the client's home relationships, his successes or failures in his job, the extent of his social activities in mixing with individuals or within clubs, or his functional level in his hostel. The sources from which with the client's permission the information may be sought include members of the family, home helps, hostel wardens, doctors, hospital staff, social workers, community nurses, psychologists and disablement resettlement officers.

Psychological, physical and social elements all require to be considered specifically in their significance to the home context. Clients' everyday behaviour in relation to family and work, as well as their capacities for functions such as cooking, housework, shopping and personal care, have an important bearing on the occupational regime to be decided on.

Thus the attitudes of one partner to another, as observed in the home setting, may throw useful light on the mental state. The current level of intensity of a paranoid illness for example or the nature of a psychoneurosis, as revealed by observed marital reactions, may point to the presence or absence of clinical progress; and these revelations can provide data for the occupational therapist which may very usefully enhance her contribution to group therapy at the day hospital as well as individual activities. Similarly, a home in a state of material disarray may point directly to the existence of depressive retardation, schizophrenic apathy, etc., which might otherwise be less clearly appreciated. In addition to formal medical measures, practical action for obtaining a home help or other steps to reduce the burdens of household tasks, may be undertaken on this basis.

In some respects domiciliary work assists with different aspects of the clients' problems from those concerned in the occupational therapy carried out in a hospital. In hospital the framework of rehabilitation is more tangible; the other disciplines are more easily available for contribution to assessment, and psychological features and personal relationships can be reviewed more closely and constantly. The hospital system is more economical of the occupational therapist's time, but the home may provide a more realistic setting. Patients in hospital may too readily dissociate themselves from their problems and perhaps become over-reliant on others. In their home environments these inclinations may occur less readily. A potentiality for self-awareness and adaptation may be seen, and participation in ordinary life more effectively and meaningfully encouraged.

The occupational therapist's first visit to the home can be usefully accompanied by a social worker. The social worker may already be known to the client, and a smoother introduction may be accomplished on this basis. Also a more valuable joint assessment can be facilitated.

In the domiciliary setting the occupational therapist's preventive role is particularly important. She is sometimes the first professional worker to note any impending relapse, when her involvement can be very helpful for notifying the family doctor, the psychiatrist, the nurses involved in the Moditen clinic, or the social worker. The social worker may be alerted to increase or alter her casework techniques. The particular steps taken by the occupational therapist will naturally be determined by the nature of the illness and the circumstances. Arrangements for day hospital or day centre attendances, without the less desirable alternative of hospital admission, may result from a report on the situation presented by the occupational therapist after she has obtained the client's personal consent to provide it.

THE INDUSTRIAL UNIT IN THE COMMUNITY AND THE HOSPITAL
FOR THE MENTALLY SUBNORMAL

Industrial units in mental hospitals have been referred to in chapter 7; those in the community are broadly comparable. But in general the industrial unit in the community allows for greater flexibility of selection than does its counterpart in the mental hospital, because as a community resource it draws from a wider range of psychological states and problems.

Different geographical areas have somewhat different methods of allocating the physically handicapped, the mentally handicapped and those disabled through mental illness to the various forms of day centre or industrial unit that may be available. Differences in allocation are determined by the availability of the facilities in the locality and the criteria for the clients. The latter can be endlessly variable. The attributes of the individual himself, in addition to the particular policy appropriate for his diagnostic category, are weighed in the decision. Mixtures of physical and mental abnormalities are commonly to be found in these units.

Day centres and industrial units have an important part to play in the management of children leaving schools for the educationally subnormal. In their last few weeks at school such children may spend some of their time in attending an industrial unit—either a unit situated within a day centre or one that exists as an entity on its own. After leaving school mentally subnormal people may attend on a basis of living in the community while going to the centre or unit daily— possibly with periodic admissions to relief beds so that the relatives' burdens can be eased.

Alternatively, continuous life in a residential institution may be needed. Over the years there has been an increasing tendency towards using the small type of hostel or local community residential home rather than the larger institutions of the type which in a previous era were termed mental deficiency colonies. Nowadays these former colonies are hospitals for the mentally subnormal; and in spite of the move towards the smaller establishments they still have much to offer those in need of their special form of help.

The fundamental philosophy of the hospitals for the mentally subnormal rests on the concept that every attempt should be made to help mentally handicapped individuals towards life in the community. And while these efforts are being made, the hospitals provide the handicapped person with shelter. For those who suffer from multiple handicaps or who for other reasons are incapable of existence outside the hospitals, long-term shelter is provided. Subnormality hospitals also aim to provide suitable individuals with short-term or day care, carrying out various forms of training which may include operant conditioning (chapter 6). The system of day care may be very helpful to those individuals who are not acceptable to industrial units. In some of these cases the aim will be to assist them in returning to the community when they have been rendered suitable for industrial units by the work done by the hospital in eradicating, or at least reducing to acceptable proportions, any behaviour problems that had deprived them of this opportunity.

These hospitals form part of the services available for children, though those requiring the hospital's long-term shelter may continue to receive it on reaching adult life. Nevertheless, an educationally subnormal child leaving a school for educationally subnormal children may well come to regard the small hostel or institution as a more individual home, its very smallness making this reaction more natural. It should of course be relatively near the family home, so that social contacts and family connections can be closely maintained, and as near as possible to the day centre or industrial unit for daily attendance.

THE PSYCHOGERIATRIC UNIT

A resource whose functions should be well understood by the community social worker is the psychogeriatric unit, to which is attached the psychogeriatric community nurse.

These units may be sited either within a general or a mental hospital. Although they vary from area to area they are primarily designed to supply support to families who contain an elderly and mentally infirm relative, fulfilling much of this function by temporarily accepting the elderly person into the hospital unit on a residential basis, often as a desperately needed measure, for periods of several weeks' duration and at intervals that range from once fortnightly to six monthly or yearly depending on the severity of the problem. Usually however they also contain day facilities, so that old people can travel daily to receive the various forms of help, often with great relief to their families, even though the old person continues to sleep at home.

The community psychogeriatric nurse who deals with the mental health of the elderly is, like the Moditen clinic nursing sister for schizophrenic patients, first trained in a mental hospital; but later she works predominantly in the community. Her activities should become thoroughly familiar to the social workers in her area, since here again a close cooperation between the two disciplines is required.

THE COMMUNITY PSYCHOGERIATRIC NURSE

Fundamentally the role of the community psychogeriatric nurse is threefold; firstly, to look at the possible indications for inpatient admission to the unit and to participate in further assessment of this need if on discussion with the family doctor it seems required; secondly, to consider similarly any need for day facilities; and thirdly, to supply relatives with explanations about the patient's condition and provide them with practical advice and psychological support.

ADMISSION TO THE UNIT

We should therefore look briefly at each of these functions. The social worker's role in relation to admissions will necessitate a clear understanding of the system adopted by the particular psychogeriatric units in her area. Usually the assessment will involve such factors as the extent of an elderly person's tendencies to wander into danger, to follow relatives to a point that becomes impracticable or realistically intolerable, to develop severely faulty eating habits or unmanageable incontinence, to interfere with the grandchildren's homework repeatedly or seriously to distort their emotional development. The criteria for hospital admission, and assessment of its optimal frequency, must thus take account of the various attributes of the family members, such as their vulnerability or accessibility to psychological support and the possibility of alternative systems of suitable support becoming available within the home. However, when a thorough evaluation has revealed an inevitable need for temporary admission, the relatives must be left in no doubt from the outset that it will operate as only a temporary measure and that the old person will be returned to their care.

Often it must be emphasized to them that its temporary nature does not negate its value. Resilience is a real commodity among relatives, but its existence is often beyond their own powers of recognition when they are feeling desperately anxious and emotionally moribund as a result of continuous strain. But in spite of their initial pressures for permanent admission, which are usually administratively unrealistic, the necessary resilience will often declare itself when they have regained some of their equilibrium as a result of the relief they experience through even temporary admission.

In the interests of the community these temporary beds must be made available to the largest possible number of those in need. This aim is achieved by a system of frequent turnover for the patients from the general community, rather than permanent immobilization of a bed by any individual from a particular family. In addition, in relation to the clinical interests of the individual patient himself, permanent removal can bring severe disadvantages. These disadvantages may need to be pointed out to relatives. For example, when he is at home an old person may receive care from one or two people who know him as an individual. In hospital he becomes one of a number; and the care he receives there is inevitably less closely geared to his individual needs and will necessarily be carried out by a number of different people. But in general elderly people do not appear to become further confused by recurrent moves from home to hospital, provided that each admission is into the same unit and into similar circumstances on each occasion.

Sometimes it is found that a patient's intake of medication has fallen seriously out of balance due to failure to take it as prescribed. Deterioration may therefore have taken place, with an unnecessary lack of control of the tension that would otherwise prove manageable. There may have been a lapse into an untreated but reversible depression, which then falsifies the diagnostic picture; or a large assortment of medication may have been hoarded and the current intake become hopelessly obscured. Admission for observation, stabilization of medication, and more thorough steps to ensure the subsequent supervision of this aspect of management may be an urgent though temporary need.

Another indication for a brief period of admission may be the need to clarify the diagnosis even before medication has been instituted. Schizophrenic preoccupation or depressive psychomotor retardation for example may each produce in the elderly a picture closely resembling dementia, needing experienced evaluation. At times a degree of underlying dementia may indeed be present and may become manifest when the symptoms of accompanying conditions have been reduced or abolished in hospital. But even if present, the element of dementia may prove markedly less severe than the initial appearance of the compound of symptoms suggested—and steps for control within the community, previously thought entirely impracticable, may now be undertaken more rationally and effectively.

Sometimes however it is sadly evident that the family's reactions to the stresses imposed by an elderly client are destined to become so unmodifiable by any supportive efforts, and the elderly person's needs destined to be so seriously neglected in the home environment, that other placements are on balance to be preferred. Their practicability should then be fully explored.

In those cases where the prediction can be confidently made that for an elderly person in mild dementia the balance of advantage will eventually lie in the need for permanent removal from the family environment, a welfare home can be considered. As a rule these homes are designed to cope with comparatively well preserved people. Again, however, the individual criteria of the particular welfare home will be amongst the most important determinants. And its criteria, ethos and reputation should all be assessed in relation to the needs and attributes of the particular client and the particular family.

ATTENDANCES ON A DAILY BASIS

For those situations in which help other than hospital admission will suffice, but where the client is nevertheless in need
of diversionary activities and the family needs some relief,
attendances at the hospital unit merely on a daily basis may
be very useful. The client may be living alone, or amongst
relatives unable to supervise him because of their own emotional strain or physical frailty, and may be unable to guard
himself from ordinary dangers or demented to a point that
endangers others—underfeeding, turning on gas taps, indifferent to fire, and wandering without the ability to return home
or avoid the hazards of traffic or falling. On occasions this
assistance, although non-residential, may therefore be of life
saving importance.

The features of psychotic illnesses also, such as paranoid
psychoses involving insufferable interference with neighbours
or their children, can sometimes be assessed and dealt with
quite simply on the basis of day attendances. And with the less
dramatic but very significant disability of the increasing apathy
of dementia (chapter 13)—equally deserving of attention
even though not associated with antisocial behaviour—these
attendances at the unit may serve to stimulate healthy interests,
preserve self-esteem, halt the blunting of awareness and furnish
facilities for constant supervision of medication.

In all these circumstances this system of daily attendance is
likely to be beneficial for the clients themselves. The group
activities at the unit—music and bingo, occupational therapy,
and the facilities for nursing attention to hygiene—may all
play effective parts. On the other hand, social factors in the
environment may limit the value for the relatives. Attending
from 9 a.m. to 4 p.m. can usefully lighten the load on a
daughter or daughter-in-law who is otherwise in continuously
tiring contact with the client. Yet the son or son-in-law out
at work during the day, or the children at school until tea
time, return to find their own circumstances seemingly un-
catered for. Irrational and perhaps unspoken resentment can
follow.

These situations again highlight the principle, basic to all social work, that problems and reactions of individuals must be viewed within the total relationship system of the family. And not only must the individual members be viewed within the family, but factors relating to wider spheres of involvement must be looked at along a forward-looking time-scale. Hence if a client is later to receive day care, any admissions thereafter should be made whenever possible into the ward in the same unit as that in which the daily attendances are to be provided, to spare him the potentially confusing efforts involved in adapting to new circumstances. The circumstances of both the medium-term management and also the eventual outcome should therefore be kept in mind when the arrangements for day care are first being planned.

EXPLANATIONS TO RELATIVES

The third major function of the community psychogeriatric nurse—that of providing explanations to relatives about the client's condition and supplying psychological support—is often the most demanding.

There are no hard and fast procedures. Visits may vary from once weekly to once a month. A natural first step in these explanations can be to point out that the brain cells are in a state of mild deterioration, that a further degree of deterioration is unfortunately to be anticipated, but that its course may be slow and its effects fluctuating and pleasingly responsive to a system of shared caring.

This concept of shared caring should be emphasized strongly and enlarged on clearly. Responsibility is neither totally removed from, nor totally left with, the burdened relatives. The participants involved in the sharing process with the relatives may include the community psychogeriatric nurse, the hospital staff, the health visitor, the district nurse and the social worker.

A simple explanation of the symptoms and the effects of the illness is often important. Its features are widely known. But when they insidiously insert themselves into a family unaccustomed to psychiatric ways of thought, the recognition of the clinical essence is liable to become submerged beneath reactions of anxiety, frustration and resentment. Not only should reminders be given about the tendencies, incorrigible in the more severe cases, of the elderly to repeat themselves interminably, to dwell on the past with tedious inconsequentiality, and to fail to grasp facts so simple and ordinary that these failures can easily be construed as a wilful indifference to the interests of the other members of the family. There may in addition be an unmistakable egocentricity which closely resembles, but in fact is different from, the selfish motivations which in earlier life could portray a more deep-seated lack of affection. As an abstract concept it is commonly realized that the crotchety and selfish old person is a psychological victim of his years; within the family he is liable to be wrongly regarded as a voluntary renegade from ordinary social conformity. This point too should be particularly emphasized.

Warnings of these developments as unhappy and impersonal possibilities should be presented clearly but in a manner designed to avoid arousing alarm. On a more active level, however, there are a number of practical measures to be adopted. Old people in this state should remain as closely as possible within the family group, involved in its relationships, participating in its activities as far as reasonable, and regularly carrying out any congenial simple tasks to which they are accustomed, such as dusting and laying the table.

These activities may help them maintain their dignity and preserve a sense of usefulness. An inadvertent neglect of this need may result in a further lowering of the level of functioning from one which was still adequate to a state of deterioration which it may soon become impossible to reverse. Confusion, restlessness, aimless wandering to a stage of unmanageability, and increasing withdrawal through lack of interests, followed by incontinence, can all supervene. Isolation in a bedroom for instance may rapidly produce these effects.

The advent of incontinence does not in itself betoken mishandling. But it may become associated with urinary infection which adds both toxic and emotional elements, accentuating the confusion and perhaps then exceeding the relatives' capacity to cope. A number of other disturbances too may be forestalled by timely comment. It should be explained that it is very common for relatives to feel guilty about their ordinary resentments and practical shortcomings; that their embarrassment in relation to friends is a normal reaction; that their social lives may become restricted, both because of this embarrass-ment when friends visit in the presence of an incoherent person and also because of the impossibility of leaving the old person alone, that marital difficulties can thus become grafted on to the practical problems unless the risk is recognized and sensibly discussed; and that relatives' failures to realize fully the high incidence of these situations in the community as a whole often produce an unjustified sense of isolation which is at variance with everyday experience of those familiar with these problems.

Drugs are sometimes required. Tension may need assuaging or a psychotic condition may coexist requiring treatment in its own right and recognition of the relative significance both of its own symptoms and of any side-effects produced by the drugs given for its control. From these facts it will be appreci-ated that a complex network of features may require disen-tanglement. If the social worker has reason to believe that this is the case she should mention her impression to the psychogeriatric nurse, who will seek medical opinion when necessary.

Health visitors attached to the practices of family doctors are sometimes the first workers involved, since it is to the health visitor that the doctor is often most likely to turn for immediate assistance. District nurses and health visitors, with their valuable backgrounds of hospital experience, may under-standably set high store on action of a concrete type. Immediate attendance at a psychogeriatric unit may commend itself as the most practical and therefore the most desirable measure. After full diagnostic assessment, however, home management sup-ported solely by the advisory work already discussed will often be found feasible and sufficient. This form of management should never be readily discounted or bypassed, particularly if the advantage of nursing facilities is also at the disposal of the family.

In a few areas in England the psychogeriatric nurses in the community are also attached to family doctors' practices. This link-up may enable them to attend any practice meetings held with the health visitor, district nurse, social worker and occupational therapist, when they can advise these other workers on the most likely progress of mental symptoms, and all can discuss such matters as the apportionment of roles.

Though implying a dichotomy that is often largely imponderable, very broadly it is the ratio of medical to social factors that will determine whether the visits will mainly be from one of the nursing personnel or the social worker. However, even if the problems are predominantly medical it will still be desirable for the social worker to be involved to some degree if only because in the eventual need for transfer to a welfare home, rather than to a hospital bed, it is a social worker who will be called on to attempt the necessary arrangements. If she is conversant with the particular problem through longstanding familiarity with the family situation, her understanding will be more meaningful and her recommendations correspondingly more convincing.

Some physical illnesses: the social worker's role

SOME GENERAL CONSIDERATIONS

In this chapter we shall be considering a few of the physical illnesses that can produce mental changes and consequent social difficulties liable to bring the social worker into medical situations.

Health visitors may have had experience of these conditions. But for a social worker to concern herself with physical illnesses might seem an irrelevant excursion into foreign waters—or even a dangerous travesty of her basic function, since the diagnosis of physical illness often poses perplexing and complex problems to the doctor himself. Moreover techniques of nursing care require specialized training and experience that lie outside anything encompassed within the background of the social worker. A little knowledge is a dangerous thing, and meddling in amateur medicine is clearly a pursuit that should often be discouraged rather than fostered.

Yet, since physical illnesses are part of the human scene, to recognize this fact with suitable restraint but judicious and helpful interest need not constitute meddlesome interference. From a social worker this recognition may prove to be of service both to the patient and to the medical profession. Obviously, dissemination of medical knowledge does not necessarily lead to scaremongering or hypochondriasis. It may result in early detection of illness and the securing of appropriate help. The successful spreading of medical information by the public health authorities and mass media is an established activity testifying to the value of sound health education.

The role of the social worker brings her into daily contact with clients who have run into difficulties of many types and

origins. Poverty, unemployment, practical problems consequent on bereavement, or any of a whole host of social misfortunes may result in her involvement. Sometimes these social
difficulties may themselves have led to mental symptoms;
sometimes on the contrary a mental illness, recognized or unrecognized, has caused a failure in the social sphere or the
development of physical symptoms; sometimes no serious
problems in the social sphere exist intrinsically, but the client
has unintentionally placed undue emphasis on social difficulties in order to obtain help in the unburdening of emotional
problems through the simultaneous opportunity thus afforded
for their discussion; and, finally, physical illnesses may give
rise to mental changes.

It is the last group that will provide the main content of the
rest of this chapter. Many physical illnesses can result in
psychological effects. The very fact of feeling unwell, from
whatever physical cause, clearly embodies changes in the mental outlook; conditions as common and various as a cold in
the head, a chest infection, a gastric upset, or an attack of tooth-
ache can all produce their mental accompaniments. Our concern will be with those physical states that are known to lead,
when severe enough, to mental changes as a direct and sometimes inevitable consequence through physical involvement of
the brain in some way.

The physical illnesses falling into this category are numerous, ranging from maladies that are fairly clear-cut and easily
recognizable to, for example, states of subtle biochemical
change. We shall merely select a small number of the better-
known examples to serve as illustrations of this principle and
to alert the social worker to the importance of recognizing
them.

UNDERNOURISHMENT

In the category of general diseases, possibly the condition of
most immediate interest to the social worker is malnutrition.
The nature of her work is liable to bring her into contact with
people in whom poverty, ignorance or geographical isolation

have resulted to a greater or lesser extent in malnourishment. Other reasons for inadequate feeding include physical frailty, the mental enfeeblement of dementia (chapter 13) or the reluctance to eat that can occur in psychiatric conditions such as anorexia nervosa, schizophrenic inertia, depressive loss of interest in food or paranoid illnesses containing the belief that food has been poisoned. Loss of ability to embark on shopping expeditions, due for instance to severe agoraphobia, may be another important reason among the psychiatrically afflicted. Further causes can lie in dental factors such as pain on mastication, ill-fitting dentures or an inability to look after them or use them correctly.

Clients may also be encountered who are overweight but nevertheless malnourished as a result of a poorly balanced intake of nutrients with a resulting storage of more than is required, while the consequent obesity not only brings its own processes of physical degeneration but also deflects attention away from the underlying lack of various elements essential for sound health. Excessive weight, with its physical dangers, may occur in psychoneurotic clients who overeat for solace. But the 'tea and biscuits syndrome' may spring from the fact that the simplicity of preparing such meals renders them the most readily available to those whose mental infirmity, however it arose and whatever its nature, precludes their engaging in the more elaborate procedures of thought and action necessary for balanced intake. Meat, fish, and vegetables, for example, are less likely to be eaten by such clients.

The social workers should therefore be alert to all these possibilities amongst patients discharged from mental hospitals, who live alone or under circumstances that provide only limited dietary supervision. On occasions minor signs of specific nutrient deficiencies may coexist with the obesity—such as unhealing sores due to vitamin C deficiency, cracks around the sides of the mouth resulting from lack of vitamin B, or the dryness of the skin associated with poor intake of vitamin A.

Severe syndromes of dietary deficiency, either alone or in association with the obesity of selective feeding, are uncommon in this country. Nevertheless blatant obesity requires medical assessment in its own right; and while the excessive weight may be due to the drugs necessary to control a schizophrenic illness, it may also be a reflection of a dietary imbalance that calls for a review of feeding habits and remedy of faulty patterns of selection and preparation.

Although malnutrition may be revealed by obesity of this sort, its most directly recognizable feature is of course loss of weight, commonly associated with mental lassitude and physical weakness. Again signs of specific dietary deficiencies may or may not be present. In any case their clear recognition lies outside the scope of the social worker.

This loss of weight may well prove on examination to have been the direct expression of a primary dietary insufficiency—and a shrewd guess about the likelihood of underfeeding can often be made from the known attributes of the client's mental state and his social circumstances. But many possibilities may need to be excluded by medical examination before the dietary aspect can be confidently regarded as the sole or even the most significant causal factor. Diseases causing malabsorption from the alimentary canal, for example, or conditions such as cancer or tuberculosis may lie behind the weight loss.

The first function of a social worker meeting these situations will therefore be to arrange for the client to be referred for medical opinion, and not merely to encourage better feeding habits. If dietetic alterations are then found to be indicated the doctor will advise on the procedures to be followed, if necessary recommending the involvement of a responsible relative, the dietician or a health visitor. The social worker should be conversant with current administrative systems for cooperation, since the steps to encourage her clients to take a sound mixed diet will often require her collaboration, at least in the first instance, with someone having specialized knowledge of dietetics. The machinery for securing this collaboration may vary. An important step, however, will be to involve the patient's own doctor.

The social worker's contribution may be twofold; firstly, to explain to her dietician colleague the psychiatric client's intellectual, emotional and financial limitations so that they can be given the necessary weight when planning the most expedient system of advice and support; secondly, to provide follow-up supervision so as to ensure that these recommendations are being carried out.

Each case needs to be dealt with on its own merits. In many instances the client's mental faculties will be well enough preserved for full reliance to be placed on his ability to carry out recommendations. At the other end of the scale, the intellectual grasp or emotional drive may be so lacking that recourse to exclusively 'convenience foods' containing essential nutrients, such as Complan, may be required.

The initial construction of a diet and any later modifications embody a number of important principles. The most basic is that it must contain adequate protein, minerals and vitamins. Fat in the diet need not be specifically catered for, since it occurs in association with protein in such foods as meat, eggs, cheese and milk. Thus it may well be more important to reduce fatty foods than to focus on the need for their intake.

Any knowledge the social worker acquires about the food sources of the various nutrients can be helpful; but it is important to avoid involvement in areas beyond her experience. If she has reason to suspect that a psychiatric client's diet is unsatisfactory, verification and help from those with the necessary training in this field are likely to be required.

A few general principles, however, can be usefully remembered. Young people need more food than the elderly, a person engaged in sedentary employment should receive less than an active physical worker, and the ill and the old may thrive better on a diet of 'little and often' than on three daily meals each of which is of overtaxing quantity. And when bolting food and eating irregular meals are known to be contributing to a patient's ill-health and are open to rectification, the social worker may play a very valuable part in the restoration of his physical health and the consequent preservation of his mental well-being if she can help to rearrange the pattern of his life into one in which these adverse influences become modified or eliminated.

DISEASES OF THE NERVOUS SYSTEM

These conditions are often extremely complicated, since in implicating the brain and the central nervous system they affect the most intensely intricate and elaborate of all the systems of the body. The social worker merely needs, and without medical training could only hope to acquire, the most general and rudimentary knowledge about them. Yet it will be important knowledge, for those conditions which afflict brain functioning are amongst the most distressing of the chronic illnesses which patients and their families are called upon to contend with, and for which the social worker's assistance may be required.

To consider organic diseases of the nervous system in relation to the social worker's involvement, the best approach will probably be to discuss examples under two overlapping categories: first, those in which an early diagnosis is essential; secondly, those in which the outstanding requirement is for help in the management of long-term problems. The examples we shall consider from the first category are epilepsy and tumours growing inside the skull: from the second, the speech impairment known as aphasia.

EPILEPSY

Epilepsy is a condition that may be defined as a paroxysmal disorder of cerebral function that is short-lived and recurs from time to time. It is sometimes thought of as a purely physical condition consisting of 'fits' or 'faints'; but while the assumption that it is primarily and basically a physical illness is correct it inevitably brings about—being a disorder of cerebral function—a temporary disorganization of thinking and feeling. Although it is not a mental illness, and commonly involves little if any abnormality of personality, it cannot be thought about in isolation from the psyche.

Before embarking on any discussion of its causes and manifestations, reference may be usefully made to some of the dangers associated with failure to recognize it. Four will be mentioned. In the first place, the illness may have begun as a result of the development within the skull of a condition such as a tumour or a dilation of a blood vessel, whose pressure on the brain substance has fired off the epileptic condition. This underlying causal pathology can be of a potentially lethal nature, and in need of immediate remedy in its own right. In these circumstances the warning symptom of epilepsy may well prove a blessing in disguise.

Secondly, these attacks, of whatever origin, are associated with loss or alteration of normal consciousness. Therefore they need to be brought under control as quickly as possible, to avert the risk of injury or death due to falling, and to stave off other calamities that could occur from sudden loss or clouding of awareness in situations such as swimming or driving.

Thirdly, though by no means invariably, a state of irritability may precede or follow the attacks; and this unfortunate state may lead the helpless sufferer to behave in a floridly antisocial way or with an unkindness that is entirely out of character with his usual feelings and strongly at variance with his outlook when in a state of normal placidity. This state of irritability may lead him to inflict emotional trauma on his nearest and dearest so deeply cutting that forgiving and forgetting may prove an impossible task for them, however much they may wish to achieve it.

Amongst the patient's relatives, young children and insecure or unsophisticated adults are particularly liable to develop unfortunate reactions on this basis; and family patterns of mutual misunderstanding and sometimes reciprocal recriminations may proceed to ingrain themselves and become virtually ineradicable. The possibility that such disturbances will develop in the family is itself a strong reason to attempt early amelioration of the illness provoking them. And if epileptic attacks of irritability happen to be very severe, they may even give rise to outbursts of physical violence that subsequently become a source of bitter regret to the perpetrator as well as perhaps serious injury to the unfortunate victim.

Fourthly, in the sphere of gainful employment any intermittent disturbances of concentration produced by the illness may be misinterpreted as incompetence or as indicative of an

improvident indifference towards work; whereas intrinsically
the patient may be of solid worth, distressed by his failure to
sustain the standard of attention to his work to which he
genuinely aspires. The man whose job is at risk, or the child
under unjustified accusation of laziness on this basis, are two
examples of this principle in operation. To acquire the knowledge necessary to initiate action to remove the sources of these
misunderstandings in their incipient stages is clearly worth any
effort the social worker may make for the purpose.

What, then, are the features of epilepsy about which she
should become especially aware? She needs a working knowledge but not any profound understanding of the illness.
Indeed in going too deeply into the details of this subtle condition she might become too preoccupied with it and lose the
inestimable advantage of the ability to exercise ordinary
common sense with confidence and balance.

Two forms of epilepsy are commonly described—grand
mal, or convulsive attacks; and petit mal, or minor epilepsy.

Grand mal

That grand mal epileptic fits involve falling to the ground,
followed by violent movements of the limbs, blueness of the
lips, and sometimes frothing at the mouth will already be
known to the social worker. These facts are also widely known
to the general public. Naturally therefore the decision that
medical aid should be obtained when a person has been found
to develop features of this sort will often have been taken
without any direct reference to the views of a social worker.
But even in these circumstances any knowledge she possesses
about the illness may prove highly relevant. As an informed
participant brought in by the various secondary social problems to which the illness—or its hysterical imitations—have
given rise, she may find herself in a position to help in the
gathering of data that will be of considerable use. She may be
able to help the client to find suitable accommodation and
employment and, if she happens to have witnessed his attacks
or is able to interview anyone who was present, she may be

able to pass on to the doctor information that will assist his diagnosis.

The facts to be ascertained in particular are those that will assist in distinguishing between an attack of epilepsy and a different illness—hysteria—which though not of an epileptic nature may nevertheless, especially in its convulsive forms, mimic the epileptic condition sometimes fairly convincingly. This hysterical mimicry, however, is only represented with a degree of realism or a lack of it that are determined by the patient's knowledge of the illness, his skill in theatrical performance, and the strength of his motivation to perform. In addition, if the state is in fact hysteria, the onlooker's own powers of perspicacity and qualities of imperturbability will play important parts in minimizing the level of violence and the duration of any hysterical episode.

It is therefore important that the social worker should preserve her own equanimity and capacity for detailed and detached observation. She may be helped to do so by remembering that the severity of the patient's illness, and any dangers it involves, are by no means commensurate with the height of the melodrama presented. If she herself shows signs of becoming disturbed by the violence of the eruption, which can easily occur unless she is aware of these facts, an hysterical incident is likely to become all the more prolonged and all the more cripplingly repetitious.

The main distinguishing features are that in hysterical attacks the onset tends to be more gradual than in epilepsy, the patient sometimes screams almost continuously, injuries as a result of falling are minor or more often non-existent, the attacks do not occur during sleep though sleep may be feigned, they are staged in the presence or potential presence of an audience, and often the hands remain continuously clenched. The tongue is not bitten, incontinence of urine does not occur and the incident may be prolonged.

The epileptic attack, on the other hand, often starts with a weird-sounding cry, which though horrifying does not signify pain and is in fact merely due to the mechanical factor of the passage of air through the narrowed opening in the throat. The arms are slightly bent, and the legs and back are extended and rigid. A striking feature is the blueness of the face, alarming to witness but merely due to a temporary cessation of the movements of breathing.

The stage of violent movements of the limbs begins about half a minute after the sudden fall and comprises strong jerking movements of the arms, legs and head muscles which cease after about a minute and give place to a relaxed state of unconsciousness which may last up to as much as half an hour. Frequently the patient then passes into a deep sleep.

It may happen that relatives are reluctant to bring these occurrences to the notice of a doctor, fearing loss of employment or grave illness of which they prefer to remain in ignorance. There may be an associated sense of shame, since even in these medically-enlightened days this illness has not entirely lost the impediment of unjustified stigma by which it was formerly surrounded. Total reluctance for medical aid in this form of epilepsy is in fact unusual; but when present it will call for the social worker to exert her influence for persuasion, explaining that treatment is indispensable if the patient is to lead the fullest and safest life possible.

More often the main element in her role will be to act as a reliable intermediary in the process of bringing to the attention of the doctor as clear and detailed a description as she can possibly obtain. The doctor will then be concerned to establish, at least provisionally, the differential diagnosis between these two conditions. His success in doing so will rest heavily on the description given him, with special reference to the points of comparative data already mentioned.

Petit mal

Another form of this illness, petit mal, can be highly significant in psychiatric situations. And unfortunately, being less blatantly pathological, it is more likely to escape detection. For both these important reasons the social worker should acquire some familiarity with its manifestations also.

Petit mal is a condition whose symptoms sometimes resemble so closely the attributes of normal fluctuations of manner and behaviour that their underlying significance is liable to escape the attention of the average person. And even amongst those who are aware of the possibilities contained in these 'turns', the situation often poses considerable difficulty of elucidation. The old adage that 'all children with measles have spots, but not all children with spots have measles' is nowhere more applicable, and productive of anxious perplexity, than in the evaluation of this moderately common clinical state.

The difficulty in diagnosing petit mal arises because the condition consists of brief attacks of 'dreaminess', which unless closely observed may appear quite unremarkable.

Owing to the wide diversity in the degree and content of these attacks, there exists a correspondingly wide scope for ambiguity of interpretation. Much may be lurking in the guise of little. But equally an over-ponderous lavishing of attention on the commonplace may itself promote in the patient a multiplication of symptoms bringing their own problems of diagnosis and disability. One of the most important prerequisites for reliable evaluation is, of course, close experience of the illness. Nurses accustomed to these patients often become skilled at noting changes of state, and acquire a useful astuteness in distinguishing between the trivial and the radical.

A brief analogy from another sphere may illustrate the principle that underlies the difficulties encountered in the diagnosis. It will readily be appreciated that the problem of shortness of breath—to take a symptom with many possible origins—is one that can cause considerable diagnostic difficulty. Such disparate factors as diseases of the heart muscle, pressure on the heart from tumours or fluid or even from a distended stomach, obstructions to the airway, diseases of the lungs, diseases of the blood, excessive weight, smoking, allergic reactions, and purely or predominantly emotional factors may all account for this symptom. Some are grave; some are minor.

The causes of 'dreaminess' are comparably protean. Its possible origins range over a wide spectrum; and hence its significance may be very difficult to deduce. 'Dreaminess' is so common, both as a trait of personality and as a reaction to stress, that to view every person who displays it as being a possible sufferer from petit mal would be to condemn a high percentage of the normal population, and an even higher percentage of those who are psychiatrically disturbed, to a clinical suspicion that would not only be unjustifiable but would be manifestly undesirable.

It is important therefore that the social worker has in mind as reliable a picture as possible of the clinical evidence that may point to petit mal.

The essential feature consists of a brief period of loss of awareness that may last for as much as a minute but often for only a few seconds. Naturally the shorter its duration the greater the likelihood of its being overlooked. Failure to answer a question, a short break in the flow of conversation, or a fixed stare or absent-minded gaze may be the only indications to be seen.

From this description it will now be appreciated even more fully that indisputable evidence may be difficult to obtain. Each of these features can be quite unremarkable in isolation, and unfortunately even in the aggregate they may constitute an equally nebulous entity. However, when the social worker suspects that the condition is present she should try to render the picture more concrete by focusing on two specific aspects.

One is to attempt to ascertain whether or not a true loss of consciousness occurs. It must be remembered that as part of its very essence the condition involves a dissolution of awareness; but since the patient seldom falls, the absence of physical collapse is immaterial in the diagnosis. It is this presence or absence of true suspension of consciousness during the attacks that forms the crucial fact to be established. Although if the attack lasts, let us say, for three quarters of a minute, the verification will be easier than if its duration is only for a second or two, the latter, despite its short duration, is of equal importance in proclaiming the illness.

Although brevity of symptoms can give no grounds for complacency in diagnosis, understandably relatives may cling to this aspect when seeking for factors to alleviate their underlying fears. The briefness of the attack, therefore, must not be allowed to deflect attention away from diagnostic essentials.

The vital question is whether the patient was for any length of time, however short, genuinely 'out', even on his feet.

The second of the two more tangible features needing consideration is the patient's colour during the attack. Characteristically, although by no means invariably, the face turns pale; and when this change of colour takes place it constitutes strong corroborative evidence. It is not wholly indicative, since episodes of pallor may occur as a feature of simple fainting tendencies, for instance, or as physical correlates of anxiety attacks. Nevertheless it adds likelihood to a diagnosis already suspected on other grounds. Hence attacks of pallor should always be confirmed or excluded by enquiry from a reliable observer, and when present should never be allowed to pass unmentioned to the doctor. The closest of observation may be required, since at times this change may be only momentary.

Either of these attacks—grand mal or petit mal—may be preceded by a phenomenon known as the epileptic aura; and each may be followed by one that is termed post-epileptic automatism. These phenomena are important both as diagnostic indices and also because they can carry important social effects. The social worker should therefore be aware of their characteristics also.

An aura is a brief phase of changed mental experience, sometimes accompanied by objective manifestations. Indeed on occasions its own manifestations may be more prominent than the unconsciousness it foreshadows. It may last for only a second or two, and takes place immediately before the loss of awareness. Although a frequent precursor, it does not occur invariably. As a convenient aide memoire and guide to how the social worker can best make use of her knowledge of its characteristics in detecting its presence, she can think of the aura in two ways. Firstly, there are those features which she or another witness to the attack may notice as observers—the objective component. Secondly, she must be familiar with the subjective type of sensations which the patient himself may experience but which do not reveal themselves to her own direct observation.

The subjective features can only be communicated by the patient himself. Therefore, while taking care to avoid eliciting from the patient any statements based merely on his suggestibility or fantasy, she should ask him at least in general terms about their occurrence, if none is spontaneously mentioned. The objective manifestations, on the other hand, must usually be sought from a witness to the seizure. They may consist for example of the twitching of a limb, or perhaps only a muscle, prior to the onset of the attack. Occasionally the sufferer may run in circles or rush forward for no obvious reason.

The subjective features, which the patient may experience clearly but only be able to convey inadequately through the spoken word, may consist of the strangest of physical and mental changes. Many of these feelings that defy clear description by the patient may involve attacks of numbness, noises in the head, flashing lights and strange sensations of movement quite foreign to his everyday life and currently dominating his consciousness, their sudden pervasiveness grossly fragmenting his mental processes and heralding the loss of consciousness. Bizarre thoughts, weird but indeterminate emotional states, and even hallucinatory experiences may overtake him on the instant.

These sudden mental changes may also contain marked anxiety; but the nature of its origin is a matter of speculation. Since epilepsy is essentially of physical origin this distress must in the final analysis have arisen from physical factors. But how much in any given case it is an integral part of the primary state, or arises from the secondary physical changes that sometimes occur such as an alarmingly excessive consciousness of the beating of the heart, is a moot point. Of even more speculative significance is the strange part that may be played in anxiety production by the strange mental happenings themselves. Sensations of changes in body-size, for example, are not unknown in epileptic seizures, and perhaps have some resemblance to those described in fiction such as *Gulliver's Travels* and *Alice in Wonderland*. At all events they can reasonably be regarded as likely to generate states of anxiety-laden perplexity in any patient having experiences so grossly out of accord with normal existence and with the laws governing everyday human experience. On the other hand states of ecstasy are also recorded.

These subjective experiences are sometimes regarded as part of the central epileptic attack rather than its aura. But such considerations are only of academic interest in relation to the social worker's function. The essential point is that she should suspect their possible epileptic nature when they occur.

It may be recalled that another phase of abnormality liable to be associated with an epileptic seizure is the state termed post-epileptic automatism. Sometimes this state is in its own way of even greater significance than the features preceding it since it may lead to behaviour of an antisocial type, possibly resulting in court proceedings. The fact that this behaviour is automatic must be recognized to prevent both its recurrence and any miscarriage of justice.

For post-epileptic automatism to be seen, or at least inferred, as arising from epileptic activity a knowledge of its potential content is required. Without this knowledge its significance can pass unrecognized. Furthermore, a limiting factor in its recognition is that an attack of petit mal preceding the automatism may have been so trivial as to have escaped notice. Here again it cannot be too strongly emphasized that the degree of the disturbance caused by the automatism may bear no obvious relationship to that of the brevity and seeming insignificance of the loss of awareness that preceded it. Hence acts of irresponsibility, such as undressing at inappropriate times and in inappropriate places, or criminal acts such as senselessly violent behaviour, may be regarded as culpable when in fact they are essentially mechanical in their origin and nature.

Temporal lobe epilepsy

The reason for the apparently spontaneous nature of epileptic episodes lies in their invisible origin in sudden changes of the physiological rhythms of the brain which then manifest themselves in corresponding changes which include alterations in the psychiatric state. In the condition known as temporal lobe epilepsy the patient becomes engulfed in a tidal wave of his own emotions, which erupts suddenly from this basis and sweeps him into an intense but temporary state of emotional helplessness that is the psychiatric correlate of the physiological upheaval. It can easily be overlooked, however, since collapse and convulsions do not occur. The condition has already been referred to in chapter 4 and mention will only be made here of the fact that these episodes are sometimes accompanied by weird sensations and aimless muscular movements, which although on the ordinary level are nonsensical nevertheless possess their own rationale in terms of the corresponding area of the brain whose functions are in disarray. Sometimes there are also mental changes, which include unrealistic feelings that a new situation is familiar or a familiar situation new.

Hallucinations of any of the senses may arise, and also sudden attacks of depression and fear which, having regard to their origin, can be reasonably thought of in the classic layman's phrase of 'fits of depression or anxiety', even though the convulsions of epilepsy are not involved. The most striking and disruptive feature, however, may be attacks of senseless and even violent rage which can bring the sufferer into severe conflict with his family or the community. Between the attacks, though yet again not invariably, abnormality in the personality may exist, and lead to predicaments for which the social worker's assistance is requested.

Difficulties abound when attempts are made to decide as to whether or not unprovoked outbursts are in fact sufficiently suggestive of temporal lobe epilepsy to warrant special diagnostic procedures. She can only attempt to achieve such a degree of balance in assessing the position as can be brought to bear from a basis of informed common sense combined with a general awareness of the potential existence of the condition, and when in doubt recommend medical opinion.

Clearly, from the frequency of gratuitous irritability amongst highly strung children, the rapidity of the normal ebb and flow of childhood emotions, and the fact that it frequently transpires in many cases that there was an apparently meaningful provocation to the outburst, it follows that it is not always easy to disentangle the contributory factors, or to categorize them into causes and effects. In addition to the difficulty of recognizing whether the episode is spontaneous or reactive, the interpretation of the significance of its actual contents may prove perplexing. Even when there is some impairment of memory concerning the episode or the surrounding circumstances, the situation is still open to doubt. Clouding of memory may have an organic origin; for instance, head injuries can lead to loss of recall of the circumstances preceding or following the injury, or electric convulsive therapy can produce the transient and insignificant amnesia sometimes associated with its use. But amnesia may also occur as a manifestation of hysteria, as was discussed in chapter 9; and in these circumstances it may vary from slight aberrations of memory, arising from minor degrees of selective inattention, to the gross examples of psychoneurotic loss of recall that take the form of wide-ranging memory blocks for long periods of life.

The degree and duration of the explosiveness can be comparably unenlightening. Extreme temporary violence is a characteristic of the adult aggressive psychopath, whose immaturity of personality, low tolerance to frustration, and uncontrollable though rapidly passing explosions have much in common with the tantrums usual in young children. Assessment can thus be very difficult; and since the possibility of malfunction of the temporal lobes can clearly provide endless opportunities for the riding of epileptic hobby-horses, the balanced expertise of those with experience and the necessary skill in this field is often required.

Treatment

Once a diagnosis of this condition has been justifiably made the treatment of all forms of epilepsy will require highly expert assessment. Both medical and surgical methods may need consideration. With medical methods a reduction may be achieved in the frequency of the attacks. Unfortunately, however, owing to the fact that the attacks themselves tend to relieve the patient of his tension, the mental state in general may, at least in theory, on occasions be worsened by the very freedom from attacks brought about by the use of the drugs.

Nevertheless medication should not be neglected if prescribed. On the surgical side the reader may remember that certain areas of the brain are more sensitive to oxygen lack than others, the temporal lobes being particularly vulnerable. When temporal lobe epilepsy has resulted from damage to this area, various forms of surgical treatment may prove helpful; but not every patient with this condition is suitable for surgical treatment, and complex investigations and weighing of many factors are essential in every instance.

Help through the social worker

Recognition of the features of epilepsy is only one part of the social worker's contribution. She has other services to render both to the individual with whom she is directly concerned and to the general community, amongst whom she may be able to exert some much-needed influence towards a clearer understanding and removal of prejudice.

The remarks made here about the social worker's role in the management of these afflictions are not primarily addressed to those working in neurological units or special centres. Social workers in these establishments accumulate rich and concentrated experience; and they will in any case have more direct and detailed access to the type of knowledge they require. Even to these centrally placed workers, however, insoluble problems arising from public prejudice and lack of formal provisions will inevitably be encountered.

To those social workers whose work does not primarily revolve around this group of clients, the frustrations and uncertainties are accentuated by their comparative inexperience and lack of relevant contacts. For this majority group of social workers, guidance may be obtained from a variety of organizations, statutory and voluntary. A good starting point for these enquiries may be the British Epilepsy Association, a voluntary body that came into existence in 1950.

The particular clinical features of the individual client will naturally form the basis on which the social worker will plan her help. The symptoms need not be reiterated. A broad point, however, must be underlined in relation to management. One of the reasons why this condition is held in such stigma even today is that it is widely regarded as comprising a single set pattern of symptoms which characterizes all cases.

This belief is erroneous. The symptoms and their effects in fact occur in an infinite variety of severity and frequency. Many sufferers experience only trivial inconvenience, with many months or years of complete freedom from attacks, in spite of the fact that the nature of the condition's pathology is to be classified as having a chronic tendency to relapse. To equate these mild cases, which constitute a high proportion of people suffering from the condition, with those whose severity has given rise to the dramatic and sometimes chilling image possessed by the public as a whole is as destructive as it is fallacious. Furthermore, many of the landladies and employers who refuse permanent or holiday accommodation as soon as they suspect that a diagnosis of epilepsy exists are no doubt far from being inhumane or unduly anxious in general.

In assisting the victims of this malady to obtain and maintain the gainful employment and opportunities for social relaxation that are an essential condition for mental health, the social worker should therefore assess each case not in terms of a stereotyped misapprehension but on its own merits, seeking the necessary data from all the relevant sources open to her.

It is to be hoped, then, that this error of stereotyped assumption made without regard to the individual facts is one into which no social worker will fall. For she is one of the key persons within the community who has the opportunity to put it into reverse. Until this reversal is achieved, the vicious circle of guilt, anxiety and resentment produced in the sufferer by his sense of 'oddity', and the apparent confirmation to him of his oddity in the eyes of the community that results from those very reactions in him which his own feelings about himself engender, is one that easily continues under its own momentum. And such problems as the rejection over accommodation and employment which are thereby created will diminish any benefits—all too inadequate in the past—which official efforts may offer in attempts to mitigate these problems.

Not unexpectedly there is a high unemployment rate

amongst these sufferers. There can also be a high refusal rate
when living accommodation is applied for. The social worker's
ability to present a balanced account of the details and import
of the illness may therefore do much to make or mar the
epileptic person's prospects of achieving acceptance in each of
these spheres.

It is the attacks of grand mal, rather than petit mal, that
lead to the most revulsion and dread amongst landladies and
employers. When faced with the task of enlightening an understandably reluctant layman, therefore, it is valuable for the
social worker to have acquired some skill in combining her
warning of the dangers with an effective form of reassurance.
The witnessing of a grand mal attack may be horrifying at first
sight. Nevertheless it may become progressively less so with
each incident observed. Moreover a prior knowledge of its
details may protect the layman from the full impact of the
anxiety that arises when an attack occurs unexpectedly. Panic
among bystanders in the presence of loss of consciousness
from any cause is a common reaction. But unless the patient
sustains an injury from falling, the most serious physical effect
to be anticipated in an adequately safeguarded epileptic person
is usually little more than the possibility of a bitten tongue.

Regular medication may be required. But it can be explained
that protection against open fires, heights, or any of the other
hazards whose avoidance is dictated by ordinary common
sense, is the only other preventive measure needed—except for
a calm acceptance of the unaesthetic nature of the cry (not due
to pain), the harmless violence of the muscular movements,
the blueness, the frothing at the mouth, the incontinence, the
temporary confusion and the need for sleep. These features are
repellent partly because they present unaccustomed sights.
Knowledge of the necessary procedures can dilute this reaction.
The only first aid required is loosening of the clothing and
insertion of a mouth gag if possible. Further medical aid is not
a routine requirement. Each case will need assessment and
description on its own merits. If for example there is a history
of antisocial conduct following an attack it should be mentioned. But on the whole this occurrence is a clinical rarity and
need not be stressed if the history in this respect is clear.

If therefore a suitably sympathetic, calm, confident and in-formative account of the patient's disability is presented to landladies, to personnel concerned in receiving applications for convalescent or holiday placements, to employers, staffs of industrial units and vocational training schemes, sheltered workshops, Remploy factories or day centres leading to shel-tered employment, then the social worker's epileptic client may be accepted instead of turned down, and spared the demoralizing experience of repeated rejections that can arise from a mistaken but well-meant overconcern by those on whom his material welfare and self-respect will heavily depend.

The three main areas of service, therefore, in which the social worker may help her epileptic clients are guidance in applying for work and accommodation, explanations when necessary to the people involved in selection, and general supervision and psychological support for those clients unable to obtain em-ployment or plagued with the anxiety and self-consciousness which the uncertainties attached to this condition can so easily bring.

BRAIN TUMOUR

The discussion of epilepsy leads logically to another condition in which the machinery of the nervous system is implicated, namely cerebral tumour, or, as it is known in everyday terms, tumour of the brain.

Earlier in this chapter reference was made to the fact that epileptic manifestations may sometimes arise as a result of pressure on certain areas of the brain exerted by a tumour or dilation of a blood vessel, and it was mentioned that the development of epileptic features in these circumstances can be a blessing in disguise. However, many other organic conditions interfering with the normality of brain tissue may produce epileptic responses. Damage to the brain substance by syphilis, processes of degeneration, small clots in the blood vessels associated with high blood pressure and disease of the walls of the arteries, violent injury to the brain, and pressure from fractured bone can each result in mental changes and con-vulsions. Loss of proper oxygen supply due to certain types of heart disease or asphyxia may induce similar results. Poisoning from liver or kidney failure will at times lead to convulsive attacks. Invasion by viruses may involve the brain and therefore be followed by convulsions and alterations of awareness.

The reasons for describing to the social worker the clinical picture caused by a cerebral tumour is that sooner or later a tumour will produce gross impairment of mental ability; and the resulting failure by the patient in the management of his affairs, which may even include loss of employment, can lead to anxious calls for help in the solution of these particular difficulties. But in reality the primary need will be for her to initiate urgent medical help.

On what grounds may the social worker suspect that the reason for a client's failing mental processes is a tumour growing within the skull? The manifestations fall into two groups. In the first are the features determined by the particular position of the tumour, which are known as its focal manifestations; in the second are those features that develop from the general increase in pressure produced within the skull. Neither group of manifestations will contain the features of every cerebral tumour.

The character of the focal features and the significance they may portray as to the site of the tumour are not subjects on which the social worker can usefully dwell at length. All that need be said is that because a tumour is a gradually expanding entity inevitably any focal manifestations will be progressive. Therefore any gradually increasing weakness or incoordination in one or more limbs, any unsteadiness in walking, any squint, double vision, or drooping of an eyelid or indeed weaknesses of any of the muscles of the face, any flashes of light, strange sensations such as numbness, tingling or pins and needles must necessarily be regarded with serious suspicion when they take place in conjunction with the mental incompetence whose effects have led to the social worker becoming involved. They may be of totally different import, but they should be assumed guilty until proved innocent.

It need hardly be added that if a tumour involves areas of the brain in which mental processes are not primarily concerned, any of these manifestations may occur without mental enfeeblement or psychological peculiarities accompanying them—at least in their earlier stages.

This first group, then, contains localizing features by means of which it may prove possible to identify the site of a particular growth. The second set of features comprises those general manifestations that are induced by the overall development of increased pressure within the skull. Features of both groups may coexist, and the various manifestations from each may present themselves in numerous permutations and combinations. Moreover a number of pointers to increased pressure within the skull will, when it is severe enough, arise irrespective of the locality of the tumour and the particular focal manifestations it may have generated.

With the general pressure inside the cranium increased above a certain level of tension, therefore, come the tell-tale features of this development, namely headaches, vomiting and deterioration in the eyesight. Depending on the nature of the tumour there are variations in its speed of growth. But all will produce these general effects in the fullness of time if the patient survives to this stage and is left untreated. Intervention must be effected before the victim becomes overtaken by disaster that proves irretrievable.

A few points are necessary in amplification of the headaches, vomiting and visual deterioration. Once established the headaches tend to be continuous; often they are relatively mild in the first instance, but they are prone to undergo variations in their intensity according to circumstances. For example, a headache caused by a cerebral tumour is frequently at its worst after a prolonged period of lying down. Hence in the early mornings they may impinge on the patient's awareness with a particularly unpleasant intrusiveness. And any other factors significantly increasing the pressure within the skull, such as stooping, coughing or physical exertion, may similarly fire off an intensification of the discomfort, perhaps transmuting a dull ache into a paroxysm of frank and distressing pain. These exacerbating factors tend to be common to all headaches that have a physical element—migraine, for instance. Nevertheless, headaches in which these attributes exist from the outset, or which take the place of others that previously lacked such features, should undoubtedly sound a warning note. They constitute a situation that must receive immediate attention if tragedies are to be avoided.

The vomiting is usually a comparatively late development. Even its total absence, therefore, is no valid argument against the existence of a tumour. When present this symptom, like the headache, is apt to occur on waking; in addition it has a tendency to take place during the night. With regard to disturbances of vision, some of the ocular changes may embody focal symptoms of localizing value—as when they have their origins in pressures exerted by the tumour against those nerve tracts directly concerned with vision or with innervation of eye muscles. In the latter case squints and loss of control of individual eye movements may develop. But other visual disturbances may derive entirely from the increase in the general pressure within the cranium.

The doctor, knowing the appearance of the normal retina, which is the 'photographic screen' behind the eye, may detect the relevant changes on examining it by means of a light from an ophthalmoscope shone through the pupil of the eye. Engorgement of blood vessels, small haemorrhages that have occurred as a result of their rupture, blurring of the edges of the retinal disc due to the stasis of the lymph fluid whose movement has been obstructed, and various other signs in the retina will all signify to the experienced examiner that a rise of intracranial pressure, ominous in its portent, has developed.

The point to be remembered is that although in its gross degrees this state in the retina gives rise to visual impairment and ultimately to blindness, in its earlier stages there may be no alteration of visual capacity that can be noted by the patient himself or by ordinary observers. Here again, therefore, as was the case with the symptom of vomiting, the governing principle must be that the absence of any obvious changes in this respect should not remove suspicion of cerebral tumour if it has already been reasonably raised on other grounds. A misleading sense of security, perhaps calamitous in its outcome, could be the bitter sequel to this faulty process of diagnostic elimination.

The investigation of these cases after they have come under medical care is beyond the scope of the present discussion. A few tests, such as X-ray of the skull and electroencephalo-graphy, may be conducted on an outpatient basis; but investigations in hospital will be required if any doubt about the diagnosis remains. The outlook too is a matter on which the social worker cannot comment. Some tumours are highly malignant and prove fatal within a year of the development of symptoms; some may carry an expectation of a number of years of life; some are slow-growing and satisfactorily susceptible to surgical treatment.

There is little further than can usefully be said to the social worker about the diagnosis of this condition except to re-emphasize the principle that any progressive loss of alertness, the development of an increasing and unaccountable apathy, or on occasions the development of an uncharacteristic faceti-ous jocularity associated with failing mental faculties, should all be viewed with suspicion as possible indications of cerebral tumour. And if they are accompanied by any of the focal manifestations previously mentioned the need for immediate assessment must assume priority over any other aspect of management, such as the social or psychological help which the situation as a whole may require.

ORGANIC SPEECH IMPAIRMENT

Some fundamental aspects

In the pathological states of the central nervous system so far dealt with, namely epilepsy and cerebral tumour, the main stress has been placed on the possible part to be played by the social worker in assisting in their detection with the immediate object of securing medical treatment followed by any supportive help then required. Before leaving the nervous system we should focus in greater depth on the organic speech impairment termed aphasia, or in its lesser degrees dysphasia. These terms do not refer to the slurring of speech due to the mechanical factor of loss of power of speech muscles, a condition known as dysarthria.

In this group of conditions (aphasia and dysphasia), a diagnosis should lead not only to formal professional treatment, but also to a better long-term understanding of the patient's social difficulties and a consequent improvement in the quality of approach offered him by those on whom his immediate comfort will depend. The set of concepts relating to these particular states may seem rather more elaborate than those previously considered; but the practical value of understanding them clearly in order to provide some of the much-needed help for these patients will certainly repay any effort made.

Many of the situations looked at in this book are ultimately studies in isolation. In general it is those states of psychological isolation stemming primarily from the psyche that are receiving attention. But isolation from one's fellows may spring from many sources, physical as well as psychogenic. And the states of intellectual and emotional isolation that follow from organic impairment of the function of speech are among the most important of the mental changes originating from physical damage.

This form of verbal isolation has as its basis the dead and dying state, and the subsequent disappearance, of those cells of the brain responsible for the expression and comprehension of concepts through the medium of words. Damage to the intelligence as a whole, though commonly coexisting to some extent, is not in itself the essence of the disability. The crucial loss is specifically in relation to the brain machinery for verbal activity. The impairment of this special faculty of verbal understanding, which is vital for the two-way communication necessary for personal relationships, as well as for clear abstract thinking and the elaboration of sentiments on all but the simplest level, brings psychological isolation.

The anatomical basis

In general, damage to the left side of the brain is apt to affect verbal skills, whereas damage to certain parts of the right side affects more heavily the intellectual processes involved in mechanical manipulation and the perceiving of relationships in the visual field. In other words, specific mental functions are impaired in accordance with the particular areas of the brain involved.

It may therefore be helpful to consider this phenomenon of anatomical localization in relation to the impairment of speech. In right-handed people the centres controlling the organization of speech and language are almost invariably situated on the left side of the brain, which is termed the dominant hemisphere. At the present point it must be emphasized that it is the organization of language and not the mechanical production of speech which lies in these centres. The control of the muscular activity subserving the mechanical functions of speech—such as the innervation of the muscles of the mouth and tongue—is governed by a different set of centres and tracts within the brain, which are situated in areas other than those we are considering.

It is axiomatic that unhealthy emotional as well as physical factors can militate against the healthy capacity for normal communication, sometimes inhibiting communication and sometimes, on the contrary, reducing the level of inhibition. In the latter case the person will be verbally uncontrolled, garrulous and perhaps tactless.

The effects of these emotional factors may be obvious, as in states of severe verbal inhibition in which the patient's power of expression is grossly diminished. In other cases the emotional inhibition may simply lead to a somewhat reduced level of verbal competence that falls, perhaps chronically, below the person's intrinsic ability. The degrees of disinhibition too may sometimes be only slight, as in the earliest stages of hypomania. But whether unhealthy emotional factors, major or minor, are present or absent is irrelevant to the essential principle that the intellectual processes involved in the production and comprehension of words—written as well as spoken—lie basically within this special speech area of the brain and the associated pathways that enter it and emerge from it.

The brain is composed of several parts. The outer surface is called the cerebral cortex and comprises two hemispheres situated on the left and right.

Speech and language disturbances occur as a result of damage to the dominant (usually left) cerebral hemisphere. The areas are usually termed Brocas' area and Wernicke's area, which are confined to the outer surface of the brain. The practical corollary is that speech disturbances of the type which we shall be looking at shortly can only result from damage to this outer layer and the underlying tissue in its immediate vicinity. Damage to the deeper areas of the brain, even when producing severe symptoms, will not be accompanied by the sort of disorders of verbal functioning we are considering, unless at the same time a relevant area of the cortex is also harmed. In other words, organic brain disease does not necessarily produce loss of verbal ability leading to social difficulties.

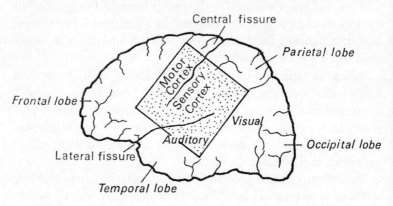

The second matter to which we should give some attention, since it is concerned so fundamentally in the chain of events lying between the damage to the machine and the consequent manifestations of its malfunctioning, including social disabilities, is the question of the pathways by which these speech centres are connected with other areas of the brain.

There are three main sets of nerve pathways that enter the speech area. Each comes from its own area of the brain, the normal function of which will naturally be the factor determining the nature of the symptoms produced when it is diseased. One set arrives from the area in which are situated the visual centres; another comes from that containing the auditory centres; the third emanates from the region concerned with sensations arising from the movements of articulation. However, not only do the speech centres receive pathways into them. They themselves also supply outgoing pathways, one of which passes to an area in which vocal speech is activated, while the other goes to the area similarly concerned with written speech.

It is understandable that the nature and significance of these mechanisms may not always be comprehended easily by those unaccustomed to thinking in these terms; but at least the reader will have usefully grasped the following two points. Firstly, conditions that cause damage to the functions of the speech centres do not necessarily lead to a degree of mental enfeeblement in other directions commensurate with these more specific defects. This fact has a practical significance that will be returned to later. Secondly, in the light of the reference made to 'visual centres', 'auditory centres' and 'sensations associated with movements of articulation', it will be appreciated that a form of 'blindness', 'deafness' and 'disorder of articulation' will follow respectively from damage to the area relating to them.

The vital point, however, is that the 'blindness', 'deafness' or 'disordered articulation' carry a specific quality which takes them out of the categories of disability which we normally understand when we use these words. The patient is not blind, deaf or paralyzed in the ordinary sense.

What, then, is the sense in which we are in fact using these terms? They are also described as auditory and visual agnosia and verbal dyspraxia. The essence underlying all these terms, however, is that the patient has an inability to interpret the sensory stimuli which are conveyed to the brain. All these points represent logical stepping-stones to an understanding of symptoms. As has been seen, the disabilities are directly attributable to the anatomical factors described. We are therefore now in a position to look at the symptoms themselves in some detail on a basis of clearer deductive reasoning.

It will be recalled that the overall term for these symptoms of verbal impairment arising from cortical damage is 'aphasia'. The state is subdivided into two types known as motor aphasia and sensory aphasia, also known as expressive and receptive—and more recently as input/output—disturbances. Symptoms from each type will commonly be found in any individual patient, because of the rich interconnections of nerve fibres within the brain; but in any given case those of one type will predominate. For this reason, and for clarity of understanding, it will be helpful for us to consider the features of each type separately.

In motor or expressive aphasia the essential disability is a loss of power to express ideas in words, both in speaking and writing, although the muscular capacity to make the necessary movements is unimpaired. Since the general intelligence is also often relatively unaffected, the unfortunate sufferer knows what it is that he wishes to say. But whilst he can formulate the vague conception of the material he wishes to convey, and has the power in his lips and fingers with which to speak and write, he is nevertheless unable to utilize these capacities because of the specific cerebral deficits to which he has fallen victim. A chain is only as strong as its weakest link, and on this basis he finds himself deprived and unable to communicate.

Given this knowledge, it is not difficult to imagine the distressing sense of impotence within which he must feel imprisoned, foreign to all his previous experiences and itself incapable of being conveyed to those people who, were they only aware of his true predicament, would respond with informed sympathy and with more efficient and effective methods of approach based on clinical enlightenment. Such, unfortunately, is often not the case. Isolated, incapable of refuting errors of judgement made by those who regard him as a 'mindless vegetable', and frustrated by his powerlessness to convey his own needs or to relieve the distress of onlookers, he will often stand in desperate need of reasoned help.

One of the most striking features of motor aphasia is the great diminution in the number of words available for use. And with this drastic and disabling cut in his fund of words may also come a diminished power of fluency in the use of even those words he still retains. The result is that his speech may be reduced and his sentences may bear more resemblance to those used in telegrams than to the speech of normal usage. Stammering may also arise for the first time in his life, and the tendency to reiterate a word or phrase, known as perseveration, also forms a highly characteristic feature.

At times it is possible to elicit a more subtle manifestation, termed nominal aphasia. As the name implies, here the patient has lost his ability to name objects. An interesting and diagnostically significant point, however, is that he has retained his ability to demonstrate by his actions the use of the object whose name he cannot express. Moreover, contrary to what one might assume, he is able to describe its use in words also. Thirdly, he often retains the names of many other objects.

If a patient with nominal aphasia is shown a key, for example, he may be unable to name it when asked. But he may well answer 'for putting into locks', and make a turning movement of his hand to express its function. Asked if it is a cup, he indicates his recognition of the falsity of the suggestion, shaking his head. But if the word 'key' is then spoken or written he nods to express his confirmation that the name is correct.

Motor aphasia, however, is usually not confined to impairment of the spoken word. Often a cluster of similar difficulties, proportional in degree, exists in relation to the words that the sufferer attempts to write. The presence of this disability, named agraphia, will provide useful confirmation. If motor aphasia is suspected, therefore, his writing should be inspected if possible, not only for evidence of the general paucity of his words and the telegraphic nature of his sentences, which as we have seen characterize the speech of aphasia, but also for the presence of perseveration of written words too. In written material, as well as in that which is spoken, the same word or phrase may be continuously reiterated.

The other type of aphasia, sensory aphasia, is also known as receptive aphasia. As can be deduced from the term, this condition means that the patient cannot receive words; or, put in another way, just as he cannot communicate with the onlooker verbally neither can the onlooker communicate verbally with him. When we were discussing the anatomical basis of these difficulties, we noted that when the pathways between the speech centres and the visual and auditory centres are interrupted, blindness and deafness in the ordinary sense do not result. What does result, it may be remembered, is 'word blindness' (the technical term for which is dyslexia—a condition which, as is well known, may also occur as a congenital anomaly) and 'word deafness'. The patient can see and hear the words but he cannot recognize them. They mean little or nothing to him. Visually, printed words are meaningless shapes; auditorily, spoken words may be as of an unknown foreign language.

Out of the 'word deafness' there also arises a condition called 'jargon aphasia'. Jargon aphasia arises from unmonitored speech. It is associated with the fact that in addition to his reduced ability to understand the words of other people, the patient is to a greater or lesser extent unable to understand his own words. They too are relatively meaningless to him, and correspondingly meaningless sounds therefore emerge in his own speech. In effect there is thus embodied within the sensory aphasia a disorder of the executive mechanism of his speech also. Hence the comprehensibility of his own speech will be impaired for others. In marked cases the observer may even find this jargon aphasia indistinguishable from the 'gibberish' of extreme psychotic dilapidation. And the sufferer is unaware of his own mistakes; but this form of speech abnormality is not an index of psychosis. The reader may now understand more clearly the seeming paradox of the statement made a few pages ago that 'disordered articulation' occurs in spite of the fact that there is no paralysis of the muscles of articulation.

Finally, each of these conditions may have bound up with it a cause that produces additional symptoms of its own in the total picture. These symptoms will again have sprung from whatever anatomical areas of the brain that have been additionally involved. Thus the disease state sometimes extends deeper than the cortex, encroaching on to the area containing pathways whose interruption leads to a true blindness in the right half of the visual field. Similarly, if the condition producing the aphasia occurs in the major artery supplying blood to the portion of the brain that contains not only the speech area but also the areas innervating the movement of limbs, then a right-sided paralysis of the arm will coexist (although the affected artery is in the left side of the brain, the limbs of the right side are implicated because the anatomical pathways cross to the other side on their course below this region). Later in the chapter we shall see how these anatomical factors relate ultimately to the practical aspects of the social worker's involvement.

Helping the client

So much for the nature of the machinery, and the effects that logically result from damage to it. We have arrived at the point, therefore, at which we can consider the management of these afflictions in relation to the role of the social worker in more meaningful terms than would have been possible on a purely empirical basis.

The social worker will find that any technical knowledge acquired from the previous discussion will not be wasted if it is accompanied by an interest and opportunity to serve this group of patients. Anatomical knowledge facilitates logical understanding; objective understanding helps towards reasoned sympathy; and enlightened sympathy that springs from both mind and heart helps towards a capacity for the type of rapport which is essential for the patient if he is to be rescued from the darkness of his isolation.

Her rapport, then, will lie at the centre of the patient's needs. As to the practical techniques related to the scientific aspects, while she cannot emulate much of the expertise of the speech therapist, nevertheless any simple skills she seeks to learn from the therapist about the art of communicating with the aphasic patient will be of great value.

She will soon find that this art will not only be exercised within the limitations imposed on the patient by his intellectual loss. In addition, changes in his emotional state, known as emotional lability, often accompany the intellectual deficit. This state has also been described as emotional incontinence. By these two terms is meant that episodes of sudden changes from smiles to tears, or vice versa, may take place with pathological readiness.

This phenomenon of emotional lability is one of the manifestations that may occur in brain damage in general, and is not confined to states of aphasia. But it is frequently found in aphasics, where in one sense it is a blessing in disguise, since the patient is spared the unhappiness of a continuous state of anger from his frustrations. On another level, however, it is a grave handicap, in that his lack of capacity for sustained receptiveness renders the task of firmly implanting new skills correspondingly more difficult.

One cannot clearly delineate those areas of therapeutic activity in which the social worker should involve herself from those that will lie outside her potential for service, if only because no two cases of brain damage are alike. But one point is clear. In this field mere book learning is inadequate. She can only be of help if she discusses the particular case with the speech therapist. The speech therapist may then try to advise her on any functions that may fall within her range of competence.

Nevertheless there are a number of therapeutic principles that can quickly be understood from preliminary studies, in addition to the more detailed techniques of procedure which she may then acquire through personal discussion and demonstration with the speech therapist. Within these more general principles of management by which she can equip herself in advance, a cardinal point is the need for the knowledge required to help the patient to feel at ease. Although reduced in certain directions, his general comprehension is often quite well intact, and insult should not be added to injury by approaching him with a patronizing though well intentioned manner appropriate to a young child. The social worker's own speech should therefore be natural, and her manner sympathetic but free from any traces of the maudlin sentimentality to which his genuinely poignant state can easily lead.

For several reasons her own articulation should be clear and also slow. For example, any sense of hurry must be scrupulously avoided because the patient needs time to search for words and alternative phrases. Another reason why she should speak slowly is that with so many words reduced to meaningless noises he will need to fill in the gaps by intelligent guesswork akin to that required in translating a foreign language. And when aphasia is severe, as may occur after a major stroke, there is often a superadded loss of ordinary intelligence. His predicament therefore demands slowness, tolerance and great patience.

But it is also important for the social worker to realize that slowness alone is not enough. Repetition may be an equally important need, so that the patient will have enough time to consolidate his learning without being forced to decode a new message before he has adequately grasped the first. Repetitions and waiting periods must be alternated before fresh material is presented. In addition, his intense though transient reactions to frustration will need to be allowed to subside, without prolongation by the flustering effect of any impatience shown by others.

The techniques adopted by the speech therapist which can also help the social worker in her own attempts to communicate cannot be spelled out as easily as the general principles already described. But there is one further point that can usefully be stated. Any help required must be instituted at an early stage. In other words, specialized professional advice should be sought quickly.

Experience has shown that a marked tendency to improve may occur spontaneously during the first few months, but that subsequently it is only by relearning that further advances can be made. Accordingly it is extremely important that the patient's natural potential for improvement during this initial stage should not be impaired by emotional factors. Learning blocks can easily result from discouragement. Unless they are overcome promptly—which to a large extent means preventing their becoming ingrained through an inadvertent accentuation of a sense of failure—the point of no-return for spontaneous recovery may be passed. It is necessary from the outset to ascertain from the speech therapist the skills that have been least impaired, and to know whether there is any method by which they can be successfully made use of—both for the value of the skills themselves and as a medium of encouragement.

Early on in her assessment the speech therapist will be likely to try to determine what the patient has retained, perhaps by noting his capacity to recognize common words, understand simple phrases, repeat digits, write, spell, copy or recognize the value of coins. Having done this she may then try to formulate a scheme for rebuilding on this foundation, using any automatic speech powers that are still found relatively intact.

Her methods of rebuilding cannot be gone into here, apart from noting that her object will often be to start with the patient's best functions—gestures, for example—and try to associate simple verbal skills with them. Any capacity for pointing, copying, tracing, or for recognizing concepts in pictorial form, may be exploited therapeutically; and skilled techniques may be applied for helping him to circumvent his difficulties by the use of substitute words, to memorize, and to sort out objects with common properties by means of which he can regain his power to classify. Many other techniques will be known to the speech therapist. The greater the social worker's knowledge of fundamentals the more intelligible they will become to her.

The social worker will now have achieved a certain understanding spanning the gap between theory and practice. This gap can be closed further by referring back to three symptoms to which attention was drawn earlier in the chapter. It may be remembered that when we were considering the physical substrata of aphasia we saw the anatomical reasons why many patients with severe aphasia suffer at the same time from paralysis of one side, blindness of one half of the visual field, and personality changes. The practical corollary to this constellation of symptoms will be obvious. A team approach is indicated. The doctor, the speech therapist, the physiotherapist, the occupational therapist and the social worker will each have a special part to play. But none can serve the patient with full advantage, or even without incurring the risk of unwittingly exacerbating his difficulties rather than easing his problems, unless all relate their work to that of each of their colleagues.

This discussion of aphasia began with the concept that establishing a diagnosis should result in a better understanding of the patient's difficulties and a consequent improvement in the quality of approach offered him by relatives and others.

With a little effort of imagination the social worker will now be able to picture to herself the sort of frustrations with which the patient is constantly flooded. He is able to hear his relatives clearly, but is unable to understand the meaningless noise level which their attempts to communicate with him produce; he broadly understands the need to pay bills but is unable to read their content or sign a cheque; his attempts to speak produce an incomprehensible language of whose meaningless nature he is unaware since he cannot interpret his own verbal sounds—while his relatives fail to respond to the sense which he thinks he is making; he cannot ask verbally for objects of practical need or comfort, such as bread and butter, and must often rely on gestures that may not lend themselves to presentation with sufficient finesse to convey the necessary detail; he may wish to know the time, appreciating the need to do so, but cannot read the clock. In any case his efforts at communication are shortlived owing to the transient quality of even such capacity for concentration as his misfortune may have left him; and reciprocal irritation and shortness of manner may be evoked amongst those on whom he must rely for his emotional as well as his practical support.

And, as will be appreciated from the anatomical factors described earlier, if the damage to the cortex affects other centres in the brain he may look at the environment and see only one half of the field of vision, or perhaps try to raise his right arm only to find that it remains an immobile weight. However frantic his efforts to overcome the unfamiliar obstacles and strange experiences, failure is the common end-point.

These are a few of the disasters that can betide anyone unfortunate enough to suffer the fairly common calamity of a stroke. But causes other than apoplectic seizures may lie behind aphasic difficulties. First, as a passing occurrence aphasia may even accompany migraine or epileptic attacks. Secondly, as a permanent state its causes may include any of those discussed under the heading of dementia. Thirdly, as a feature indicating the need for urgent medical investigation it may form part of the picture produced by a cerebral tumour, abscess or removable clot of blood following a sometimes seemingly trivial head injury sustained often a short time previously or perhaps within the preceding few weeks.

The development of aphasia will therefore necessitate a medical opinion. The subsequent requirements will be dictated by the diagnostic findings. But whatever its underlying cause, when the condition is protracted the patient will need not only the special expertise of a speech therapist deeply versed in the relevant techniques of communication, but also as knowledge-able a type of befriending as possible from other workers with the time and readiness to supply the basic warmth of a caring and suitably informed relationship. And from his relatives in particular he will need the patience derived from an adequately detailed understanding of the difficulties from which he suffers but which he is unable to convey. From them, more than from anyone, he will need the acceptance arising from a recognition of the essentially impersonal nature of the tendency to tire quickly, the querulousness, moody behaviour and shallow domineering that are liable to accompany damage to the brain.

If the social worker can help relatives towards an intelligent appreciation of all these facts, and support them in their efforts to act on it, their relief will often be directly expressed; and that of the patient, while not conveyed through the medium of verbal expression, may prove discernible through his dimin-ished irritability and improved appearance of contentment. Though necessarily fluctuating because of the nature of his mental damage these features will nevertheless testify, if only inarticulately and intermittently, to the value of the humane attitude, buttressed by the element of technical understanding, which he is receiving in his misfortune.

DEMENTIA

An important mental disability which is the direct result of physical deterioration in the brain is the condition termed dementia. Correctly used it denotes a permanent, organically-acquired deterioration of the intellect which is usually accom-panied by emotional changes. And, unfortunately, by the very nature of its pathology true dementia cannot improve beyond the limits imposed by the destructive process in the cerebral cortex. Loosely-used phrases such as 'demented with fear', though popularly accepted, are a travesty of its clinical meaning.

A frequent cause of dementia is a state of senility, with its well known features of loss of memory for recent events often accompanied by an increased vividness of recollection of earlier experiences, and a tendency to fill in memory gaps with false recollections. Loss of ability to grasp new situations, proceeding to general apathy and confusion and sometimes punctuated by lucid phases, is not unusual in senile states. A diminishing range of interests, an increasing rigidity of attitude, resistance to change, and slowing of thought processes with faltering and repetitive speech are other common findings. Loss of depth of feeling, with an associated irritability, restlessness (particularly at night) and lack of inhibition, are also characteristic. It need hardly be emphasized, however, that while minor mental disabilities are moderately common in advanced old age, they are still often accompanied by an appreciable capacity for adaptation, though in the unfortunate events of sudden change of surroundings, infection, or major trauma such as fracture or surgical operation, an intensification of senile features may occur and may be followed by residual defects.

It is important that senile dementia be distinguished from dementia due to other causes, and in particular from those conditions, such as syphilitic brain deterioration, which may be susceptible to halting by treatment.

In dementia produced by arterial change, which may occur at an earlier stage of life, the distinctive features are a tendency for the personality to remain more intact and for confusional episodes to be more short-lived and in more striking contrast to the general mental state. In alcoholic dementia the patient's own statement about his alcoholic consumption, often plausibly presented, is best accepted with some reservation. However, the plethoric facial appearance and a combination of charm in company and morose irritability at home may suggest the condition. In some cases there may be a history of delirium tremens. In syphilitic brain damage—the possibility of which should obviously not be raised—the classic extravagant delusions of grandeur are uncommon; but boastfulness, impaired powers of judgement, a dogmatic attitude and irritable egocentricity are more characteristic. Physical examination may reveal the diagnosis. In epileptic illness, dementia may supervene after years of frequent fits. However, the condition should not be confused with the symptomatic epilepsy of an intracranial tumour accompanied by mental deterioration.

Other conditions causing dementia will not be discussed here. However, it is important that some non-dementing conditions which may superficially resemble it, such as depressive retardation, schizophrenic apathy, and in severe cases preoccupation with obsessive ruminations, are not wrongly regarded as dementia itself.

DISORDERS OF THE THYROID GLAND

Three other physical conditions particularly likely to produce psychiatric problems involving the social worker are known as thyrotoxicosis, myxoedema, and cretinism. Each of these conditions is produced by an alteration in the action of the thyroid gland in the neck. In myxoedema and cretinism the secretion produced by this gland is diminished; in thyrotoxicosis the gland is overactive.

Thyrotoxicosis

Thyrotoxicosis is a condition which always produces—and sometimes appears to be produced by—emotional disturbance. Its mental changes are mainly those of severe tension, of which irritability and restlessness are apt to be the most marked features. The sufferer over-reacts with intense anxiety to stimuli which before the onset of the condition would have produced no such response. The rapid mood changes, bouts of tears, and the restlessness which often carries over into severe insomnia, may easily lead to the belief that the condition is 'purely psychological', the social worker being called in to help either with the problems which the client's behaviour creates, or, in those cases in which the onset was preceded by obvious stresses, with these supposedly primary causes in the environment. Unless she is familiar with the clinical features of the illness she may, like the relatives, oversubscribe to assisting with the social aspects of situations whose significance, though the source of her own involvement, is not the essence of the condition.

Great difficulty may be experienced in distinguishing this condition from a state of 'pure' anxiety, and sometimes a period of hospital observation is required. Nevertheless, certain points may alert the social worker to its possible existence. Palpitations, a moist skin and a dislike of warm weather, an increased appetite which is actually associated with loss of weight—though occasionally there is weight increase—and attacks of diarrhoea may all point to thyrotoxicosis. In some cases, but by no means all, the eyes may protrude in a characteristic manner. A very important feature is that the illness not only renders the patient a burden to himself and others; if left untreated it will be likely to prove lethal through its effects on the heart. If for no other reason, therefore, its detection is essential. When it can be reasonably suspected, steps to obtain medical opinion must be the social worker's first concern.

Myxoedema

In myxoedema the bodily processes are slowed rather than speeded up. On the whole it is a condition of middle or later life, usually developing spontaneously but sometimes arising in a person with long-standing thyrotoxicosis, possibly as an exhaustion state of the gland. Broadly its features are opposite to those of thyrotoxicosis, and hence it is usually those problems produced by sluggish thinking and behaviour that lead to the social and family difficulties. Apart from general apathy there is a gain in weight, a dry coarseness of the skin, undue sensitivity to cold weather, poor appetite and constipation, all in striking contrast to the features of thyroid overactivity. Also the hair often falls out, this feature characteristically including the eyebrows. Fortunately it can respond satisfactorily to simple treatment with tablets which supply the missing chemical to the body. Its possibility should always be kept in mind.

Cretinism

Another example of thyroid inadequacy is found in the condition termed cretinism. If an insufficiency of the normal thyroid hormone exists in infancy, the result is a failure of brain development that may be gravely incapacitating mentally and grossly stunting physically. Only by treatment with a suitable preparation at a very early stage of life—preferably well within the first few months and certainly at the earliest possible moment after the diagnosis—may any worthwhile benefit be obtained. Happily the condition is rare; but it should be suspected in an infant whose mental apathy is accompanied by a rough dry skin, limbs that are short in relation to the general body size, eyes that are puffy, and a skull that may seem unusually long. Timely treatment may at least assist in physical development, and if instituted in very early life may forestall the arrest of development of intelligence which is otherwise inseparable from the condition.

PHENYLKETONURIA

A further condition comprising a type of mental subnormality in which medical treatment in infancy is of vital importance is the condition known as phenylketonuria. This state is also very rare. But its capacity to respond to treatment, the possibility of early detection by special tests, and the gravity of the subnormality to which the untreated condition gives rise necessitate routine testing of every child during early infancy. Essentially it is caused by an inborn failure of a chemical termed phenylalanine to be converted to another chemical substance. The result is an accumulation of phenylalanine, and chemical abnormalities which render normal development of the brain impossible. When found to be present, however, it may be treated by special diet preparations, low in phenylalanine, designed to produce the chemical environment necessary for the well-being of the brain.

To safeguard against the illness escaping detection, tests should be carried out routinely on every newborn infant. In some areas of the country these tests are carried out on the child's blood a few days after birth; in others a urine test is conducted after about two weeks. Normally the blood tests are supervised by the midwife, and the urine tests by the health visitor.

The routine for these purposes is laid down by official policy, and the procedures involve no significant discomfort to the baby. In the urine test a small piece of special 'chromatography' paper is placed against the baby's napkin. The mother herself may carry out this little task, having had certain details of the procedure explained by the health visitor. If, however, it is felt that the mother cannot be relied on to do so, the health visitor undertakes the function on her behalf. It is therefore rare for any hitch to occur in the arrangements. Obviously, however, this possibility cannot be entirely excluded. If for example a mother, particularly when mentally unwell or un-intelligent, moves to another area it may occasionally happen that the need for testing becomes lost sight of. A social worker involved in these circumstances should if necessary immediately inform her health visitor colleague in the relevant area, so that the position can be verified and any necessary action taken. In spite of the rarity of the condition, even one case overlooked will constitute a grave tragedy.

Conclusion

The system of presenting disguised case histories has not been adopted in this book. The most instructive, vivid and memorable cases for the social worker to study are those she encounters in her daily work. And the most effective method of grasping the psychological concepts discussed will be for her to think about them in relation to these cases known to her where their relevance can be reasonably suspected.

This experience of repeatedly observing the reactions of the clients within their families, together with gradually increasing skill in applying knowledge of psychological theory to both the assessment of the factors prompting these reactions and the consequences to which the reactions may lead, will then reveal case after case in which the principles touched on in this book will be seen at first hand to lie behind the problems for which the help has been sought.

In the final analysis the most basic means of acquiring professional understanding will be through case discussions among suitably experienced colleagues. Given this opportunity it will often be comparatively easy to make correct assessments. But to maintain imperturbability and to sustain a sense of purpose in the face of disappointments, and at times ingratitude, are ends which at least initially may be more difficult to achieve.

In dealing with psychologically disturbed clients, workers are apt to have personal aversions. Some have difficulty in coping with attitudes of aggressiveness; some are repelled by dishonesty; some by slovenliness, some by lack of social grace, and so on. It is therefore helpful for every social worker to be as aware as possible of those particular attributes which she herself inwardly finds the hardest to accept and the most difficult to adjust to. To the extent that she possesses this self-understanding of her own attributes and their likely influence on her assessments and management of the particular situations with which she is constantly confronted, her value to her clients will be correspondingly enhanced. But unless she also detaches herself successfully from serious prejudices of this sort, there will remain many occasions when all theoretical and practical knowledge will count for little.

Similarly an attitude of reasoned balance will be necessary in relation to the more general considerations about which from time to time her professional role must inevitably impose the need to form a personal opinion. Every bandwagon destined for only passing significance has its over-ardent champions, and every passing phase its avant-garde. Sound understanding, capable of evaluating periodic claims likely to prove of merely transient topicality, and an ability to distinguish between enthusiastic assertions and reasoned arguments while giving each the value of its proper weight, are necessary qualities of outlook which tend to come with the passage of years. Seeking to understand developing frontiers, and cultivating powers of discrimination coupled with an equal readiness to participate in the new and worthwhile, are clearly aspects of social work which have their own general importance as well as a direct bearing on the individual families with which the social worker will be personally involved.

PROFESSIONAL COMMUNICATION

The need for as much communication as possible between professional workers has been repeatedly stressed throughout this book. It will therefore be fitting to end with some brief comments about the relevance of this principle to the relationship between the two main groups of professional readers to whom it is addressed. Frequently the practical and psychological functions of the social worker and the health visitor closely overlap; in such cases any lack of communication is apt to be to the detriment of everyone.

The health visitor, for example, may sometimes gain considerable advantage from advice from the social worker in connection with problems over housing, social security, suitable lodgings and foster homes, the difficulties of single homeless people, and so on. Moreover the experience gained by social workers among families in the intermediate age range may be of considerable help to health visitors involved in assisting with the psychodynamics occurring in this phase of life, since in general health visitors carry a decreasing responsibility for families as the children grow older.

The health visitor, on the other hand, possesses invaluable experience of family problems relating to young children in their crucial formative years, or the problems of the elderly, which is more detailed than that of the social worker. Another special contribution that may be available from the health visitor derives from her rich experience of the problems of pregnancy. In addition to the psychodynamics arising within the family, an understanding of the social circumstances that commonly surround the antenatal period can be very useful to a social worker.

Neighbours, for instance, may exert a profound effect on the sensitivities of a pregnant woman. Pregnancy can seldom be a private matter; and the emotional attitudes of those around, possibly involving criticisms, gloomy prognostications, or maudlin or spurious sympathy, can all undermine the confidence of the young or immature. And although these attitudes are comparatively uncommon, an environment of friendly outlook being more usual, unfortunately in modern life a suitably supportive environment is too often unavailable.

Not only is the pregnant woman apt to remain at work until an advanced stage of her pregnancy. After the birth she frequently finds that her neighours are working away from home throughout the day. Moreover the pregnancy may be clouded by vague anticipations of coping alone with infantile convulsions or other fancied emergency situations, with no help available from the empty houses of the neighbourhood. Unexpressed fears of loneliness may be increased by the added stress of change of home accommodation. The need to move to a larger house to accommodate the child can bring the dual stress of loss of existing friends coupled with the loss of mobility by means of which new friendships could be acquired.

In these and other environmentally-determined circumstances, some degree of reactive depression during the pregnancy and its puerperal period is understandable. A social worker may therefore gain valuable information by approaching an experienced health visitor for discussion of problems suspected of falling into this category.

Another reason a social worker may sometimes need to approach the health visitor is for family information of a retrospective kind. Even when a health visitor no longer has any contact with a particular family—though often contact is in fact maintained over many years—she will still sometimes have a memory or record of important details relating to earlier stages at which, for example, marital or child/parent difficulties may have taken root. This data may then throw a great deal of significant retrospective light on the current situation, unavailable to the social worker by her own unaided enquiries from members of the family whose memories of this early phase may well have gradually receded under the weight of the very problems to which these original problems later gave rise.

Confidentiality is of course a principle which both professions observe. Nevertheless to introduce into an uncertain situation a health visitor whose earlier experiences with the family may be of help in the present predicament, providing essential data about the family members' problems, though with relevant regard to their feelings, is a form of cooperation that can sometimes lead to advantages to clients and their children which cannot be conferred by any other means.

As we have seen, both disciplines have their own fields of emphasis and each performs certain aspects of work that cannot be carried out by the other. But both also share much psychological work that is essentially similar. It was for this reason that in the introduction to this book the statements were made that 'for convenience of presentation the term "social worker" rather than "social worker and health visitor" is used throughout. However, it should be constantly remembered that all remarks are addressed equally to health visitors.' Any separation of the basic psychological functions of these two groups of workers, made either by a writer in presenting to readers the relevant principles of psychiatry or by the participants themselves in their practice of much of their daily work, would be an artificial division, significantly lessening the value of each of these fields of activity both to the community and to the two related professions themselves.

Selected Bibliography

The following short list of publications relates to the most important of the topics dealt with in this book. It is intended to provide guidance for those concerned to increase their psychiatric knowledge but is designed to be short enough to avoid perplexing choices of alternatives or time-wasting duplication of too much information.

The present time is an important era of experimentation in the fields of psychiatric concepts and resources, and a search of the literature has revealed a comparative dearth of single publications summarizing in suitable form the overall psychiatric scene for social workers and health visitors, though official reports supplying various statistical trends, perhaps with recommendations arising out of them, are likely to remain a prominent pattern of the future.

For illuminating accounts of developing services, reliance must sometimes be placed on articles or books describing particular establishments or projects. Such data is apt to carry the restrictions of the individuality of the particular institution or project described. Nevertheless publications of this nature are sometimes well worth consulting for their own interest, for any practical applications of their details and for their references to other works. A few have therefore been included.

Books

BALBERNIE, R.   *Residential work with children.* Oxford: Pergamon Press, 1960

BARKER, P.   *Basic child psychiatry.* St Alban's: Staples Press, 1971

BARTON, R.   *Institutional neurosis.* 3rd Edn. Bristol: Wright, 1976

CROW, L. D. and CROW, A. *Adolescent development and adjustment.* New York: McGraw-Hill, 1956

CUNNINGHAM, P. J. (Ed.) *Nursery nursing.* London: Faber & Faber, 1974

DAX, E. CUNNINGHAM *Experimental studies in psychiatric art.* London: Faber & Faber, 1953

DE MARE, P. B. and KREEGER, L. C. *Introduction to group treatments in psychiatry.* London: Butterworth, 1974

D.H.S.S. *Non-accidental injury to children.* London: H.M.S.O., 1976

EDEN, D. S. *Mental handicap: an introduction.* London: Unwin Educational Books, 1976

FREUD, A. *Ego and the mechanisms of defence.* London: Hogarth Press, 1941

GORE, E. *Child psychiatry observed.* Oxford: Pergamon Press, 1976

HAYS, P. *New horizons in psychiatry.* Harmondsworth: Pelican Books, 1964

JAMES, R. *Understanding medicine.* Harmondsworth: Pelican Books, 1970

JOLLY, H. *Book of child care.* London: Allen & Unwin, 1975

KAHN, J. H. and NURSTEN, J. P. *Unwillingly to school.* 2nd Edn. Oxford: Pergamon Press, 1968

MACDONALD, C. *Occupational therapy in rehabilitation.* 4th Edn. London: Baillière, Tindall, 1976

POST, F. *Clinical psychiatry of late life.* Oxford: Pergamon Press, 1965

PRIESTLEY, M. *Music therapy in action.* London: Constable, 1975

ROGERS, B. N. and STEVENSON, J. *A new portrait of social work.* London: Heinemann, 1973

SHEILDS, R. W. *A cure for delinquents.* 2nd Edn. London: Heinemann Educational Books, 1971

SIMPSON, Sir John Roughton, *The Mental Health Act 1959.* London: H.M.S.O.

SKYNNER, A. C. R. *One flesh, separate persons: principles of family and marital psychotherapy.* London: Constable, 1976

STORR, A. *The integrity of the personality.* Harmondsworth: Pelican Books, 1960

TIZARD, J. *Mental retardation: concepts of education and research.* London: Butterworth, 1974

TUSTIN, F.   *Autism and childhood psychosis.*   London: Hogarth Press, 1974

VAN RIPER, C.   *Speech correction.* 5th Edn. London: Constable, 1972

VARAH, Chad,   *The Samaritans in the '70s.* 3rd revised Ed. London: Constable, 1977

VARMA, V. P. (Ed.)   *Psychotherapy today.*   London: Constable, 1974

WEBB, L.   *Children with special needs in the infant school.* Gerrards Cross: Colin Smythe, 1967

WEST, D. J.   *Young offender.* Harmondsworth: Penguin, 1970

WING, L.   *Autistic children: a guide for parents.* London: Constable, 1971

Articles

BENTOVIM, A. and LANSDOWN, R.   Day hospitals and centres for disturbed children in the London area. B.M.J. 1973. 1. p. 536ff.

BOXALL, M.   The nurture group in the primary school. *Therapeutic Education.* 1976. 4(2). pp. 13–17

CALLIAS et al.   Use of behaviour modification techniques in a community service for mentally handicapped children. Proc. Roy. Soc. Med. 1973. 66. pp. 50ff.

CAPSTICK, N.   Group homes. Proc. Roy. Soc. Med. 1973. 66. pp. 1229ff.

CASPARI, I.   What is educational therapy? *Therapeutic education.* 1976. 4(2). pp. 19–25

FOTTRELL, E. M.   A ten years' review of the functioning of a psychiatric day hospital. Br. J. Psychiatry. 1973. 123. pp. 715–7

GATH, A.   Emotional needs in a new family. Nursing Mirror. 1977. 144. pp. 52ff.

MCCARTHY, D. et al.   Children in hospital with mothers. Lancet. 1962. 1. pp. 603–8

MORRICE, J. K. W.   A day hospital's function in a mental health service. Br. J. Psychiatry. 1973. 122. pp. 307–14

MORRIS, D.   The Doctor-Patient-Midwife relationship. *Midwife and Health Visitor.* 1972. 8. pp. 23ff.

STRONG, P. G. and SANDLAND, E. T.   Subnormality nursing in the community. *Nursing Times.* 1974. 70. pp. 354ff.

Index